"Thoroughly tested until proved perfect"

The Art of French Cuisine

1st Edition
Recipes translated and adapted from original family French recipes.

Copyright© Copyright Holders: K. L. Déaux and J. A. Reiner

All rights reserved. No part of this publication may be reproduced, stored in a retrieval system or transmitted in any form or by any means, electronic, mechanical, photocopied, recorded or otherwise without the express prior written permission of the publisher.

Published by:
UBT (EU) Ltd, Exchange Place, Poseidon Way, Warwick CV34 6BY

Authors: K. L. Déaux, J. A. Reiner
Photographer: K. L. Déaux
Translated by: J. A. Reiner
Editor: P. J. Reiner

Art of French Cuisine

L'Art de la Cuisine Française

Volume 1

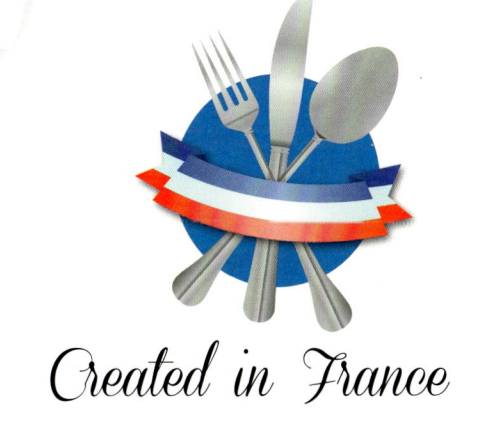

Created in France

Preface

> Le 10 novembre 2010, le repas gastronomique des français était inscrit au patrimoine culturel immatériel de l'humanité, le repas reserve le cercle familial et amical et plus généralement les liens sociaux "the art of french Cuisine" est là pour célébrer le repas non seulement français mais aussi le fait de partager ces bons moments de convivialité dans tous les pays du monde. Dans cet ouvrage magnifique de plus ouvert à tous avec la langue international qu'est l'anglais, vous découvrirez des recettes simples de tradition, ludiques et faciles à réaliser. À chaque page vous allez être surpris par la qualité des photos qui donnent vraiment envie de réaliser ces recettes.
>
> Qui dit nutrition dit santé, vous trouverez des conseils pour cuisiner de façon plus équilibré avec des informations sur la valeur nutritionnelle des produits.
>
> the art of french Cuisine, c'est plus qu'un livre de cuisine, c'est avant tout l'engagement de passionnés, d'une équipe qui savent donner de leur temps, de leur générosité pour aider les personnes en difficultés. C'est un bel exemple pour nous tous, parce que l'achat de ce livre permettra de financer différentes actions sociales et humanitaires : recherche médical, l'aide après une catastrophe naturelle, sauvetage en mer, et bien sur un soutien appréciable à l'éducation et à l'enseignement
>
> c'est ça l'art de la cuisine,
> donner sans retour, une belle preuve d'amour.

Régis Marcon

> 10th November 2010, the French gastronomic meal was inscribed as the intangible cultural heritage of humanity, the meal that binds the circle of family and friends and, more generally, social links.
>
> The *Art of French Cuisine* is to celebrate not only French meals but is also to share those moments of conviviality in all countries of the world. In this beautiful book, more accessible to all being in the international language of English, you will discover recipes, simple by tradition, which are fun and easy to make. Each page will surprise you by the quality of the pictures which truly tempt you to make these recipes.
>
> Nutrition means health; you will find tips to cook in a more balanced way including information about the nutritional value of products.
>
> The *Art of French Cuisine* is more than a cookbook, it is, above all, a commitment of enthusiasts, a team who know how to give of their time and their generosity to help people in difficulties. It is a good example for us all, because the purchase of this book will fund various social and humanitarian actions: medical research, help after a natural disaster, sea rescues, and of course a substantial support to education and teaching.
>
> That's the art of cuisine,
> to give without return, a beautiful proof of love.

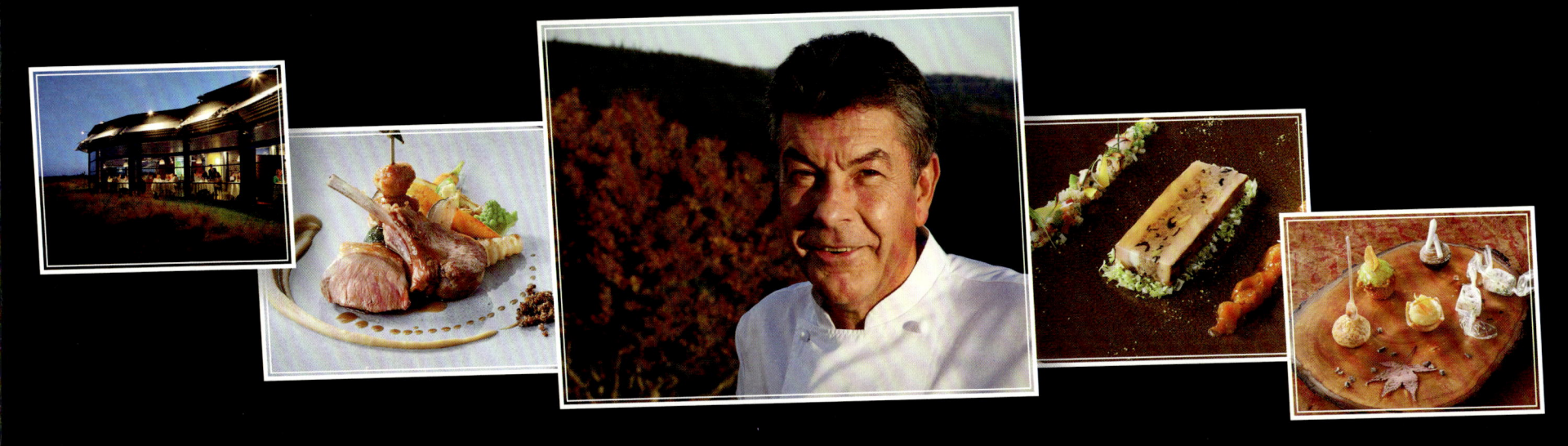

Régis Marcon

Having been a chef for more than 30 years, Régis Marcon was joined by his son, Jacques, in 2004 and opened a gastronomic, 3-star restaurant in the heights of *St-Bonnet-le-Froid*, between *Velay* and *Vivarais* in *Haute-Loire*.

They have no fixed menu—*à la carte*—as their recipes are the reflection of the surrounding nature and very important traditions of the Marcon family. Everything is guided by the four seasons and, although for them cuisine is innovative, they respect traditions, and great classics are not forgotten.

Régis won the *Bocuse d'Or* (1995), *Prix Brillat Savarin* (1992) and *Prix Taittinger* (1989).

"The Marcons' cuisine pays tribute to mother nature, as does the superb glazed building. Autumn is their favourite season, when they go out hunting for mushrooms in the thick undergrowth covered in a carpet of reddened leaves. Try the local reared meat, green lentils from *Le Puy*, regional cheese and hand-picked mushrooms."
MICHELIN guide inspectors.

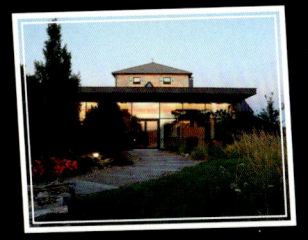

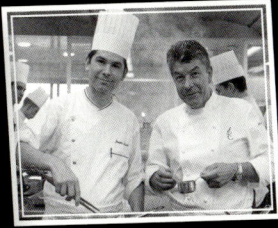

Hôtel Restaurant Régis et Jacques Marcon
Larsiallas
43290 SAINT-BONNET-LE FROID
www.regismarcon.fr

... terrine les œufs, le sucre, le sel ; battez donc... jusqu'à ce qu'il soit devenu... le mélange... Ajoutez la farine, mélangez... et coulant... le beurre et... à la ... puis ajoutez ... pendant 4 ou 5 minutes ... Vous obtiendrez une pâte ... Laissez-la reposer.

... mondées et entières de taille égale : 1 d... ... ... environ.

Manière de procéder

Choisissez un moule à manger... Beurrez le ... puis prenez gros comme un œ... de la "pâte support" et du bout des doigts étendez-en une épaisseur d'un demi-centim... surtout le fond.

Crème au caramel (cuisinier...)

Introduction

ART OF FRENCH CUISINE
... unveiled secrets and savours from France ...

Voilà ! A French cookery book with genuine classic French recipes translated from preserved family originals. But more than that...

For those who are familiar with French cuisine, this book is filled with nostalgic scenes and stunning photos; childhood memories of *grand-mère's* kitchen, filled with aromas, will return vividly to your mind; long-forgotten dishes can be tried again, but this time with guaranteed success, as every recipe has been trialled and adjusted until correct.

And for those who are not so familiar, it will open up a whole new repertoire of food and tastes. Basic, rudimentary ingredients can be made use of—which you may well appreciate cooking with in a day of frugality. Typical French cuisine can be explored through a fascinating and captivating collection of recipes with spectacular photographs that will teach you tips and secrets of how to master the art.

For hundreds of years, people all around the world have been seduced by the unique style and manner of French cooking, and not only that, but the way cuisine is interwoven into the very culture and character of this most intriguing and varied country. In fact, you could say France and cuisine are almost synonymous! This book, which has been created from memories, ideas and cooking experiences, will create—for those who haven't already got it—an interest and passion for French cuisine.

Where every dish has a history or a reason for its being, recipes can be tried, tasted and adapted—if necessary! The *Art of French Cuisine* is ideal for those starting out in their first steps of cookery—to make them into experts; or for those who have already some experience—to enhance their culinary skills.

In your own surroundings, discover different techniques, taste new, subtle flavours which have been carefully chosen and combined... as we unveil to you some of our secrets and savours from France.

Bon appétit!

Contents - Volume 1

P. 4   Preface
Préface

P. 76   Starters
Entrées

P. 260   Cheese
Le fromage

Contents - Volume 2

P. 4 — Preface / Préface

P. 6 — Introduction / Introduction

P. 10 — Details are important / L'importance des détails

P. 12 — Mastering the art of patisserie / Maîtriser l'art de la pâtisserie

P. 20 — Gateaux and patisseries / Gâteaux et pâtisseries

P. 54 — Desserts / Entremets

P. 102 — Tarts / Tartes

P. 128 — Breads and sweet pastries / Brioches et pâtes feuilletées

P. 132 — Mastering the art of bread making / Maîtriser l'art de la confection du pain

P. 160 — Biscuits and confectionery / Biscuits secs et confiseries

P. 180 — Jams / Confitures

P. 184 — Mastering the art of jam making / Maîtriser l'art de faire de la confiture

P. 196 — Drinks / Boissons

P. 212 — Basic recipes / Recettes de base

P. 214 — Tips for making successful pastry / Astuces pour réussir les pâtes à tartes

P. 224 — You are what you eat / Vous êtes le reflet de ce que vous mangez

P. 252 — Freezing recommendations / Les recommandations pour congeler

P. 262 — Gluten free / Sans gluten

P. 274 — Glossary / Glossaire

P. 280 — Conversion tables / Tables de conversion

P. 282 — Index / Index

Details are important...

All these recipes have been tried and tested and have proved to be successful and delicious! However, there are certain points to consider:

BEFORE STARTING

Before trying any of these recipes, we strongly recommend that you read through the glossary first so that you are familiar with the terms used, and also take time to follow the pages that are included to provide **tips for success.**

Always read a recipe through carefully, at least twice, before starting. We have taken great care to add anything we feel is important. *By following every recipe step by step, correctly and accurately, we can assure you of success.*

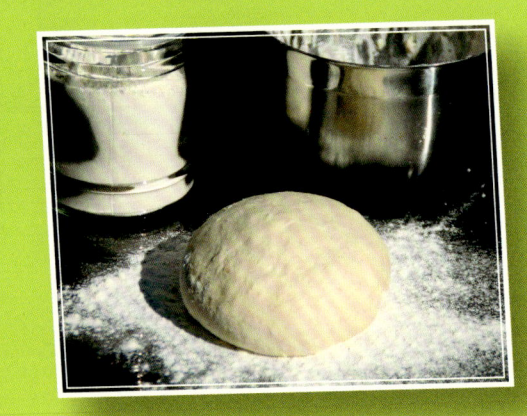

SERVING QUANTITIES

Most of the recipes included are recommended for a certain number of persons. This is only approximate, bearing in mind that in France a larger quantity of vegetables and salads are eaten and a smaller quantity of meat as compared to other countries.

COOKING AND OVEN TEMPERATURES

Cooking is a very important step in a recipe. We have given a cooking temperature and time but remember, fan assisted, electric and gas ovens all work differently and you will have to adjust the temperature and time accordingly for your oven. *Remember, you're the chef, and it's up to you to judge if something is cooked or not.* (This is especially important for cakes and patisseries.)

Unless otherwise indicated, the oven must be at the correct temperature before commencing cooking.

Important note: All recipes tested in this book have been cooked in fan assisted ovens.

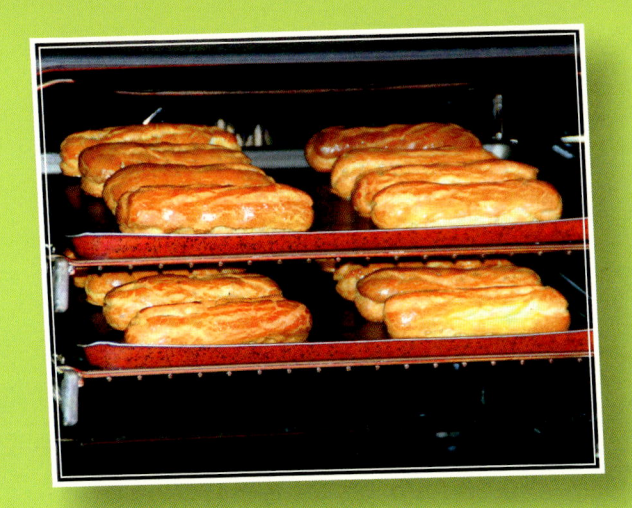

SECRETS OF SUCCESS LIE IN THE DETAILS

If after following all these instructions you are disappointed with the result, do not think that the recipe is a failure. Read through the instructions again to check that there is not a little detail that you have overlooked. **This little detail could have been the secret to success!**

French gastronomy

LIBERTÉ, ÉGALITÉ, FRATERNITÉ, and... GASTRONOMIE!

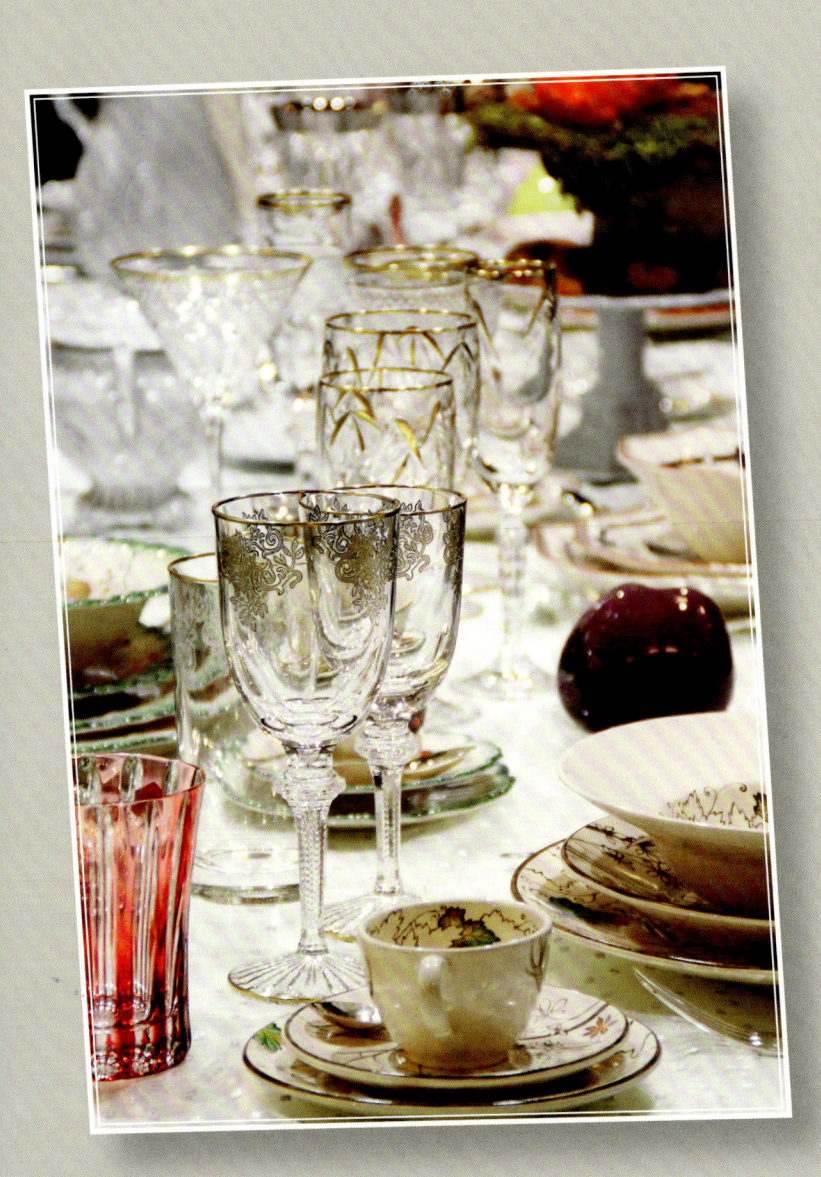

Yes, GASTRONOMIE! For the French are famous not only for their commitment to the great principles of democracy, but for their culinary excellence.

No country in the world compares with *La France* for her *Art de Vivre*—the special bond of French people with their food. No wonder UNESCO has listed the **Gastronomic Meal of the French** as intangible Cultural Heritage.

This includes, of course, great cuisine. But it also includes how even the simplest of meals can be prepared and presented with elegance and style. For a meal is not just about eating. It includes the little rituals—how wines are paired with food, how the table is dressed—that make a French repast such a uniquely enjoyable experience.

Did you know that French people spend an average of two hours a day sitting at table, eating? Three meals a day is at the heart of French eating habits. Every meal is a special time to share—experiences, sorrows and joys—with family and friends.

The heart of every good meal is good food! The finest ingredients prepared with care and presented with panache!

FRENCH GASTRONOMY, a centuries-old legacy

Origin

The history of French cuisine dates back to the Gauls, who, in pre-Roman times, developed a culture of eating and drinking well, and this has continued through the centuries.

It was during the reign (1643-1715) of Louis XIV (b. 1638) that French cuisine became great. Meals became a staged presentation organised by the head waiter and this type of French service reached its peak in the 18th century. Soon recognised internationally, it paved the way to structuring meals by starting with soups and starters, followed always by roasts, and finishing with desserts.

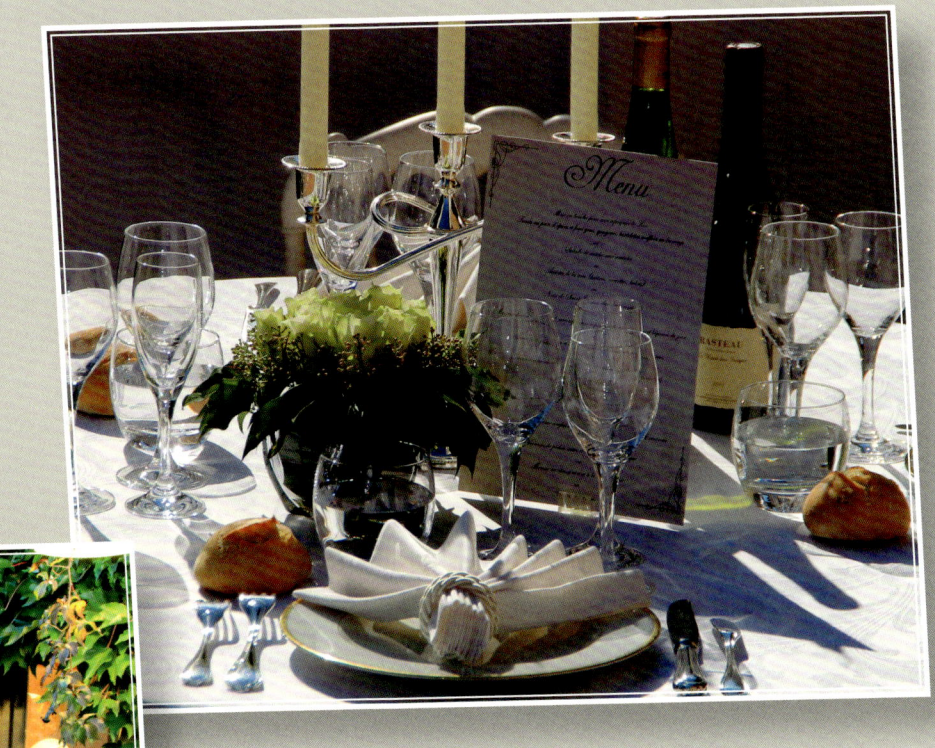

French gastronomy

Two styles of French cuisine—*haute cuisine* & *cuisine régionale*

That French cuisine has been appreciated and proclaimed for centuries is no doubt due to the richness and quality of the products used, but also, especially, to talent, innate taste and the technical ingenuity of chefs and *cordon bleus*.

Chefs wanted to prove that there were better and more refined ways of mingling or breaking down products to achieve absolute harmony between tastes. Encouraged by King Louis XIV, **haute cuisine** began in France and is still practised in top restaurants and hotels today. It is the elaborate, expensive style which requires the experience and talent of great chefs, rare products and ingenuity. Common ingredients are replaced by more expensive ones.

Cuisine régional is the more familiar, family style of cuisine, prepared in homes, cafés and *bistros* all over France. This style is relatively economical using local, fresh, raw ingredients of high quality, which, subtly mixed with herbs and seasonings, form the basis of the cooking. *Cuisine régional* can be subdivided into many types of cooking as each region has its particular cuisine just as much as it has its particular architecture, customs, accent, costumes, songs, folklore and furnishings.

Regional culinary traditions and recipes are mostly passed down orally from generation to generation, each family having its own particular method of preparing and mixing food.

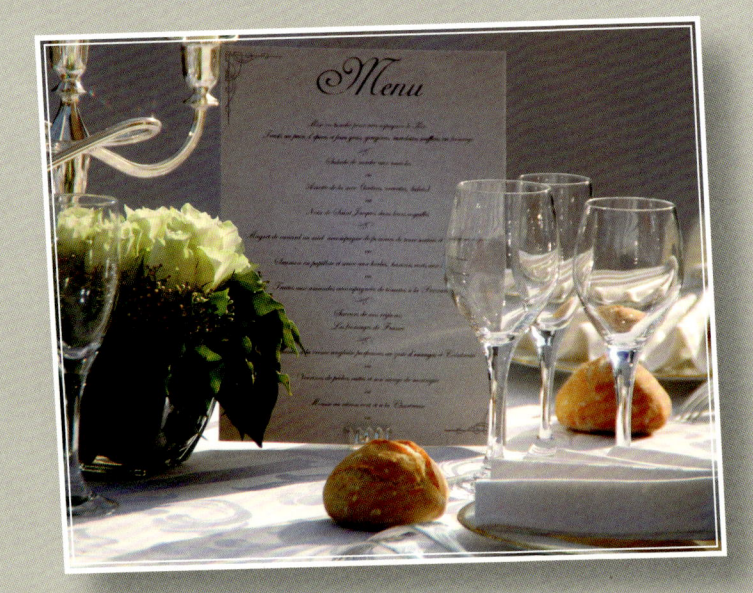

A gourmet meal, French-style

A French-style gourmet meal is a ceremonial procedure, with a succession of courses served in immutable tradition amidst continual conversation across the table.

It begins with an *aperitif* and ends with a *digestif*, with at least four courses in between, namely a starter, fish and/or meat, cheese and a dessert. Every course is not only accompanied by bread, but also by wines associated with each dish.

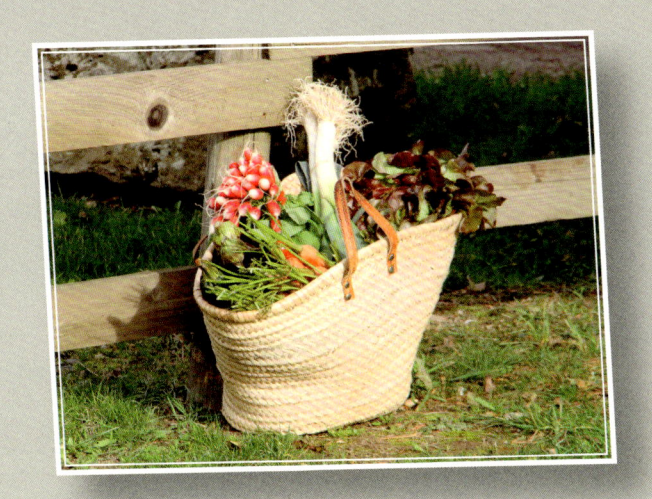

The choice of ingredients

A trip to the market is prerequisite before entertaining friends or family. The season, occasion and different taste preferences of those invited will determine the menu and dishes.

Markets, a French tradition

Markets are held in every town or village in France, once or several times a week, where local farmers can sell their own selection of fruits, vegetables, meat, fish or cheese. This tradition dates back to medieval times when they were very important for the distribution of food. Visiting a market is an opportunity to discover the local flavours and to be tempted by the fresh local products.

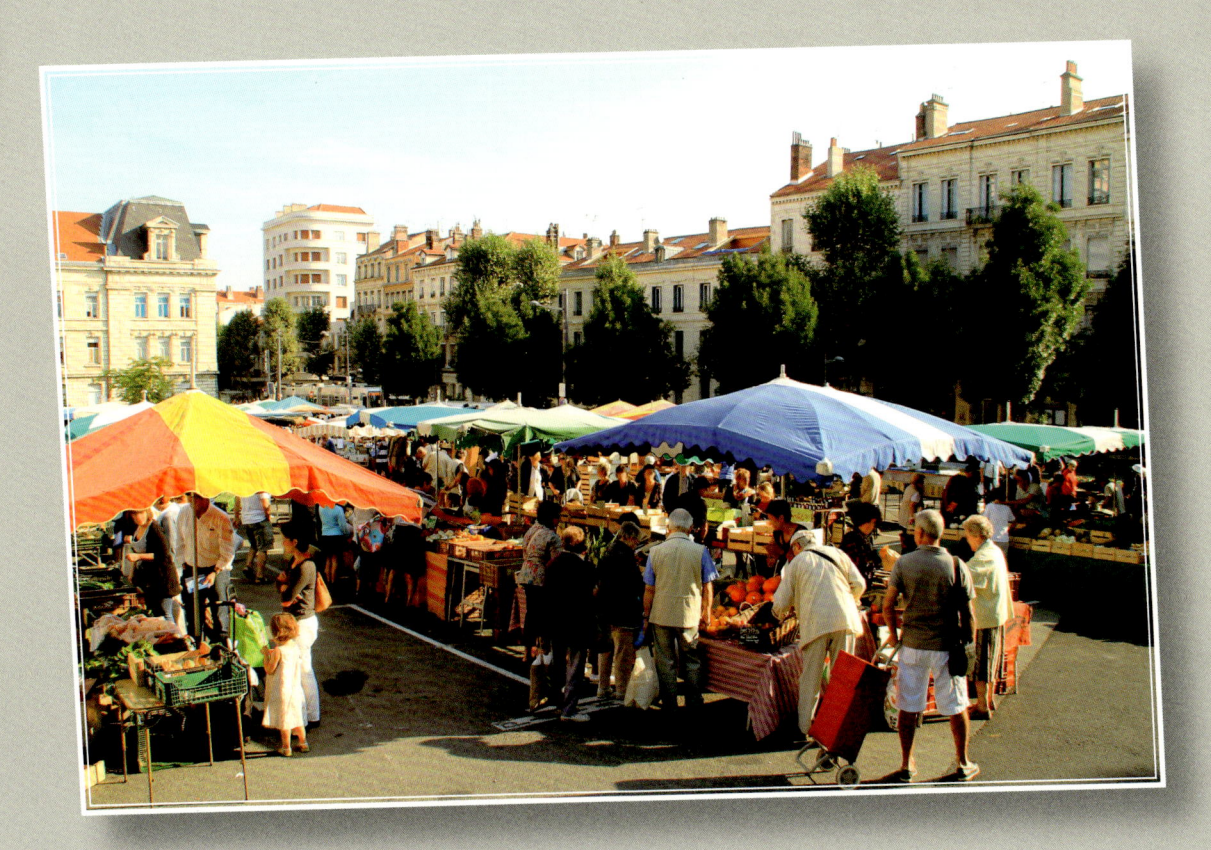

French gastronomy

Animated, colourful, warm, scented—the markets are teeming with shoppers armed with shopping baskets, from first thing in the morning, when the best choices of ultra-fresh products are available, until just before the stalls are dismantled, when the remaining produce is often bargained.

In the South, where the climate is hotter, markets are particularly rich in colour and smell; varied sun-soaked fruits and vegetables such as plump apricots, sweet cherries, bulging peaches, fresh green almonds, brilliant shiny peppers and dark purple aubergines; bunches of sweet-smelling herbs such as mint, lavender, rosemary and basil; fresh-caught fish from the surrounding Mediterranean; green and black olives drenched in oil. Bright-coloured parasols shade and protect the stalls from the blazing sun. It's a favourite place for the gourmet as well as the tourist!

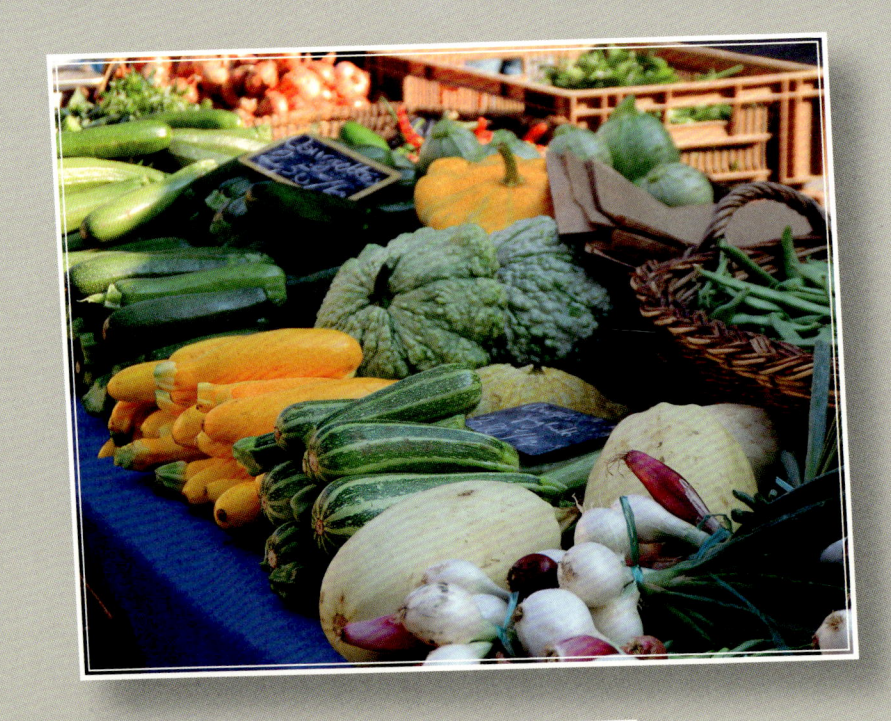

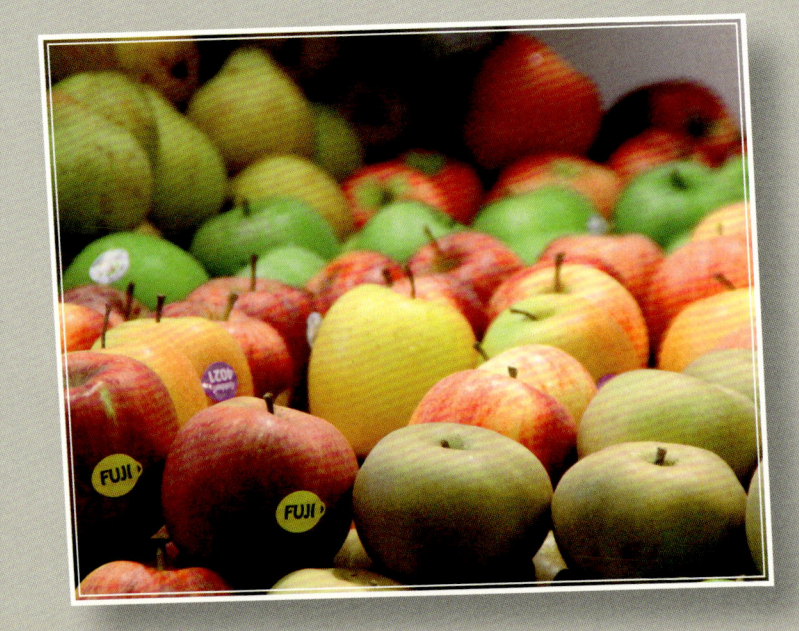

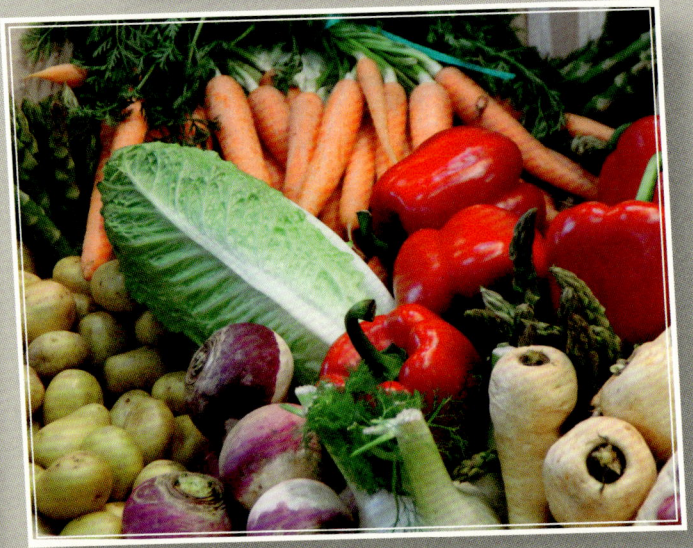

SPECIALITIES

France has such an extensive gastronomic heritage that a complete list of its specialities would be too long to provide. Just the more significant ones are therefore selected here.

Foie gras

One of the most prestigious dishes of French cuisine is *foie gras*, a prized French delicacy. It is a special, very expensive, type of *pâté* particularly popular for Christmas and other festivals when it is served on small slices of toast or bread, or fried and melted on meat.

It comes from the enlarged liver of a force-fed goose or duck, where the liver is enlarged up to ten times. (An average duck's liver normally weighs 50 g but, when enlarged, can be up 500-600 g.)

Goose *foie gras* is slightly richer and mellower than that of duck *foie gras* which has a hint of wine flavour. Today, over 85% of *foie gras* produced in France is made from duck rather than goose.

Goose or duck *confit* is traditionally made from the meat of birds that have been fattened for *foie gras*. Cooked long and slow in their fat, the meat is tender and matures to a delicious rich flavour.

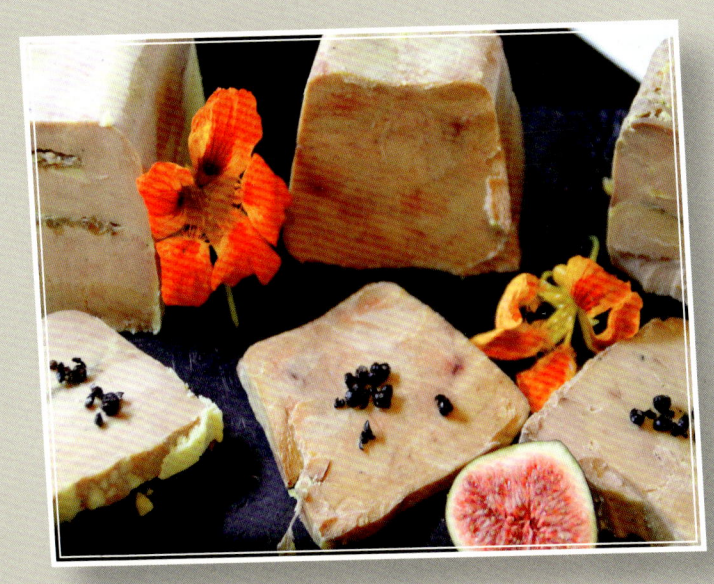

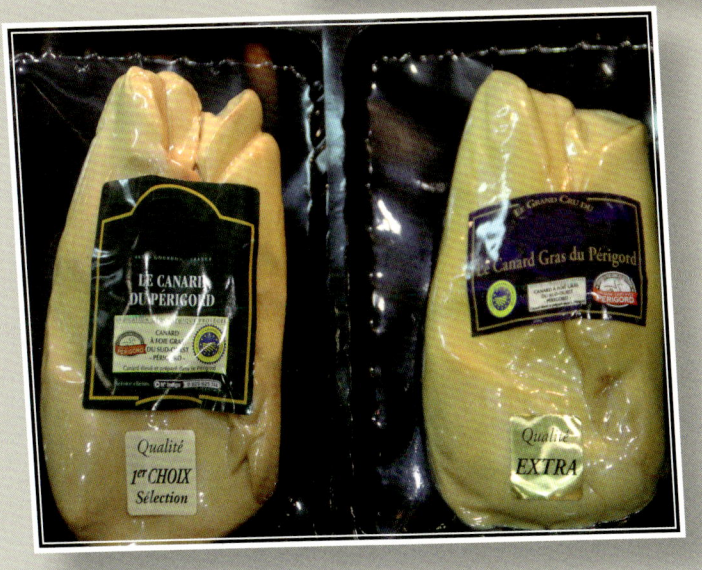

French gastronomy

Truffles

Very rare and expensive, but peculiar to certain regions, are the famous truffles, often known as 'black diamonds'. These are precious, unusual mushrooms which grow underground on the roots of certain trees, namely, oak, hazelnut, lime or beech, and are the crowning glory of *haute cuisine* where they are used to flavour sauces, and chicken and veal dishes. They can transform a simple omelette or scrambled egg into a fine dish.

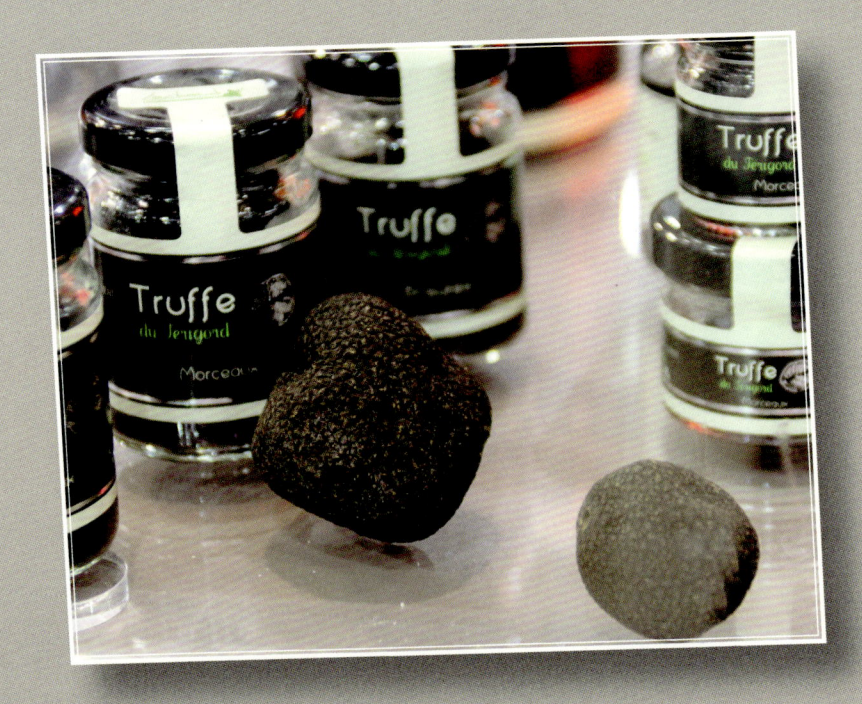

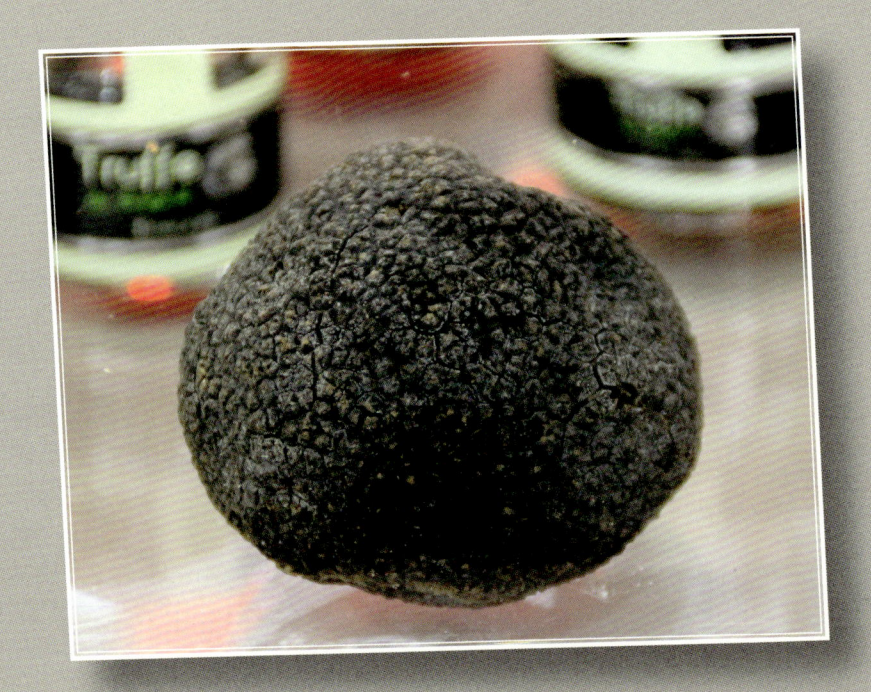

Truffles may take 5 to 8 years to develop before they are harvested using trained dogs or pigs to sniff them out and then finally gathering them by hand. Traditionally, pigs were always used, but, as they often ate them once they were discovered, dogs were found to be more reliable and are mostly used nowadays.

Truffles are fairly small (about the size of a walnut), although larger ones can be found. They have a very strong flavour—one small one produces enough flavour to pervade the whole dish.

Seafood

With 2700 km of coastline, it is hardly surprising that fish and shellfish are extensively used in French cooking with every region in France having its own style of preparation.

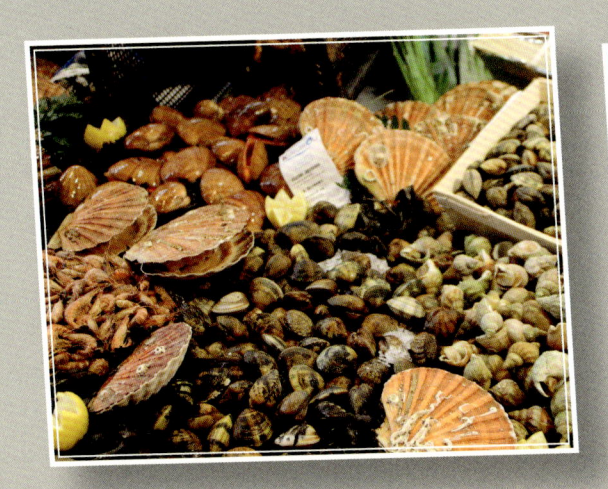

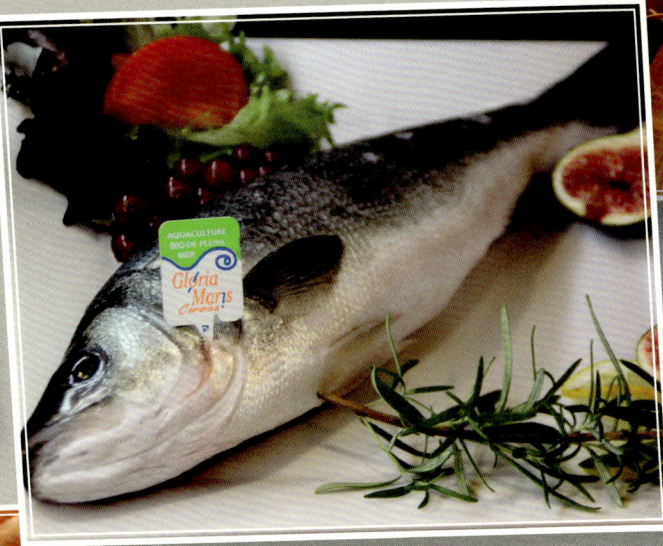

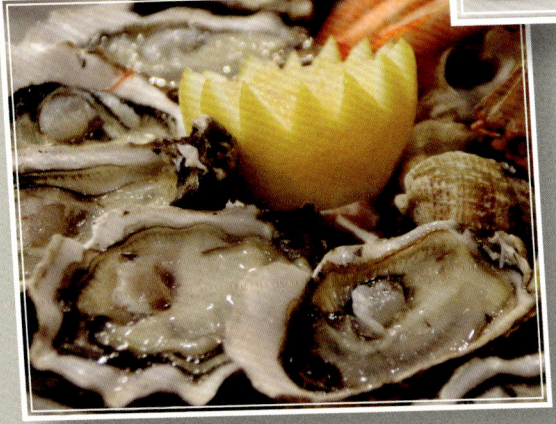

Oysters are a specialty in the Atlantic regions and are normally eaten raw with lemon and salted butter. These molluscs are very popular among the French and they often accompany *foie gras* at festivities.

French gastronomy

SNAILS AND FROGS

Snails and frogs are an integral part of French culture when it comes to gastronomy!

Snails

Although snails are consumed in various places all over the world, France is the most famous for this remarkable delicacy, and they are a popular festive dish, mostly consumed at Christmas. Although there are several snail farms in France, (about 200 throughout the country) there are not enough to supply the high demand for them, so many snails eaten in France are imported from other Eastern European countries.

Before killing them, they have to be purged from the undesirable contents of their digestive system by fasting or feeding them on a wholesome replacement such as flour during several days. They are then killed by plunging them into boiling water, removed from their shells and cooked (generally with garlic butter, chicken stock or wine). They are placed back in their shells with the garlic butter and sauce for serving.

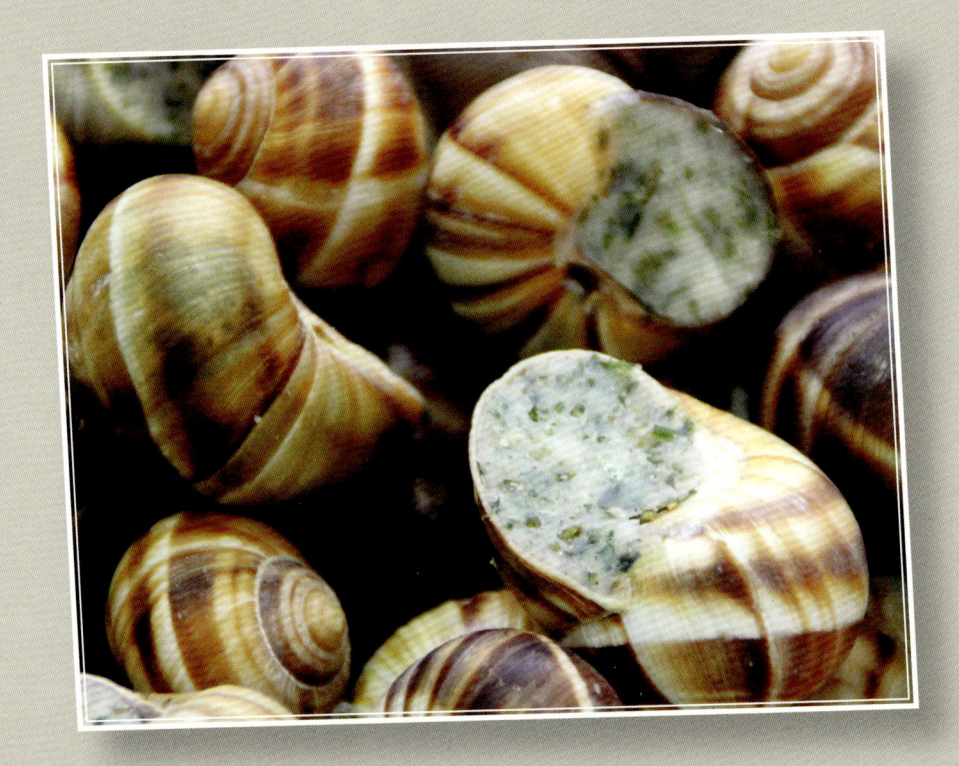

Frogs

Frogs' legs are eaten in other European countries as well as Quebec, the United States and the Caribbean, but somehow they have become emblematic of French cuisine. Farmed only for the consumption of the legs, they are cultivated in certain wet or marshy areas around France such as in the *Dombes*, *Vendée*, *Jura*, *Alsace*, *Auvergne*, *Bretagne* and *Bourgogne*.

Whether they are made into soups, omelettes, or stews; enhanced with cream and finely-chopped herbs; fried, sautéed with chopped parsley and garlic, or baked in a sauce... frogs' legs have found a place on the tables of great restaurants around France.

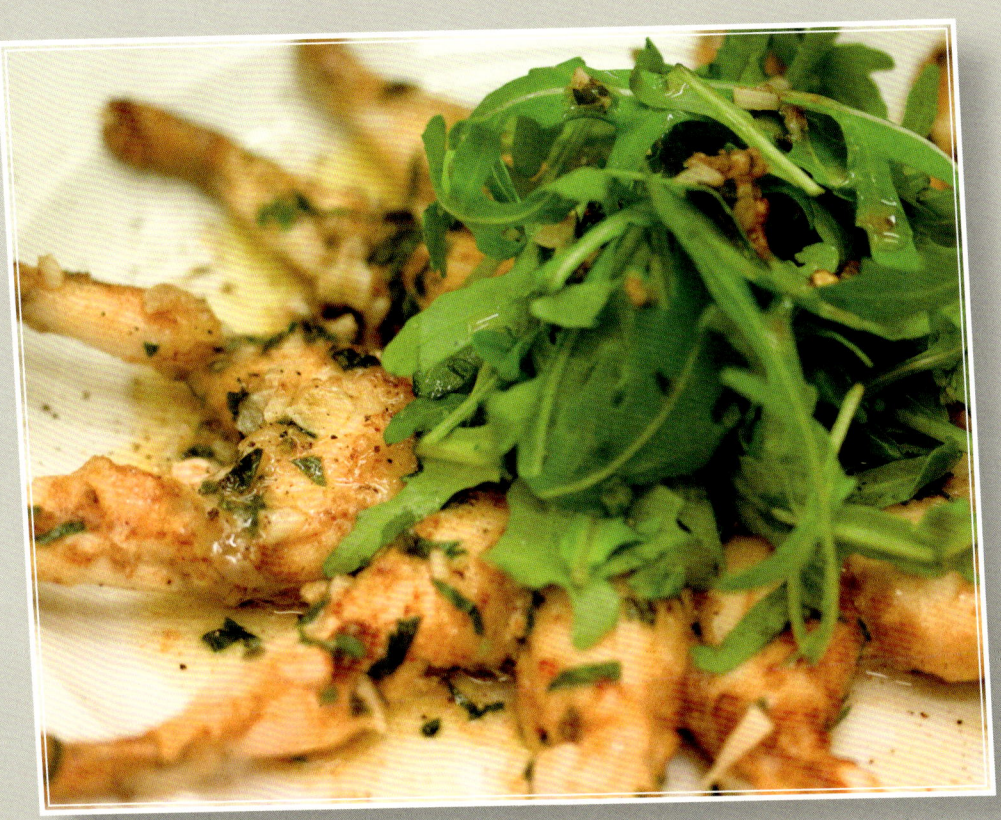

French gastronomy

Cheese

Probably the best known product associated with France is **cheese**. Charles de Gaulle (1890-1970), French president, military leader and statesman, once commented, "How can you govern a country which has more than two hundred and forty-six varieties of cheese?"

Far removed from packaged, supermarket produce, are the hand-made artisan cheeses produced from the milk of not only cows, but also sheep and goats. Cheese is traditionally served with red wine and crisp, fresh bread at the end of the main course, and before the dessert.

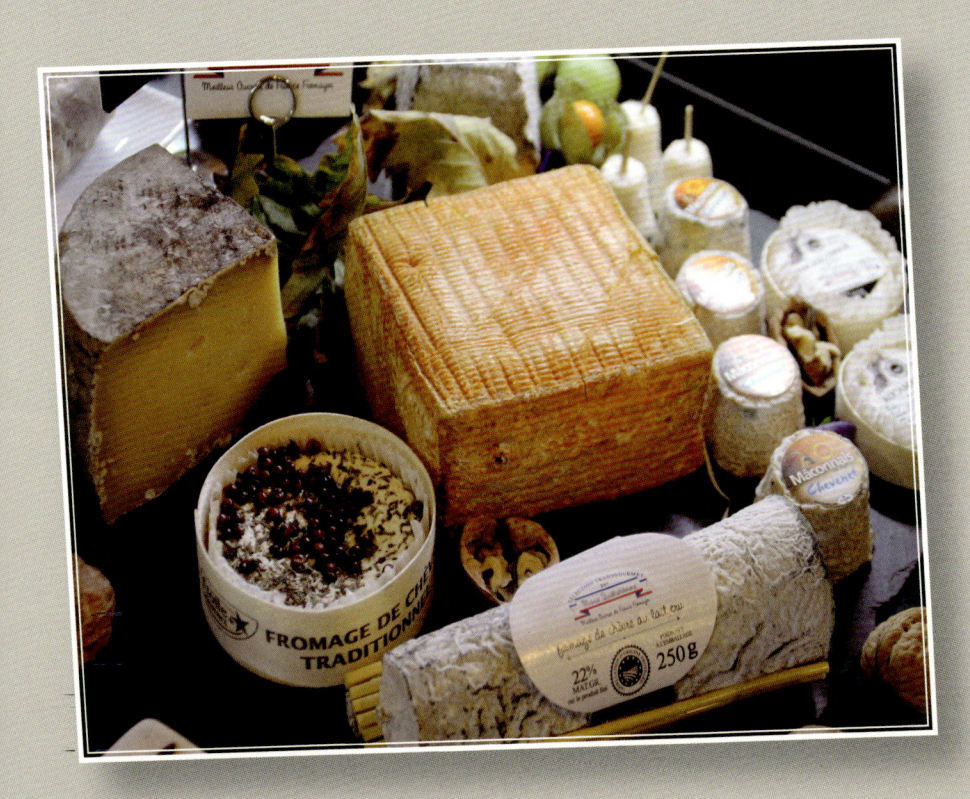

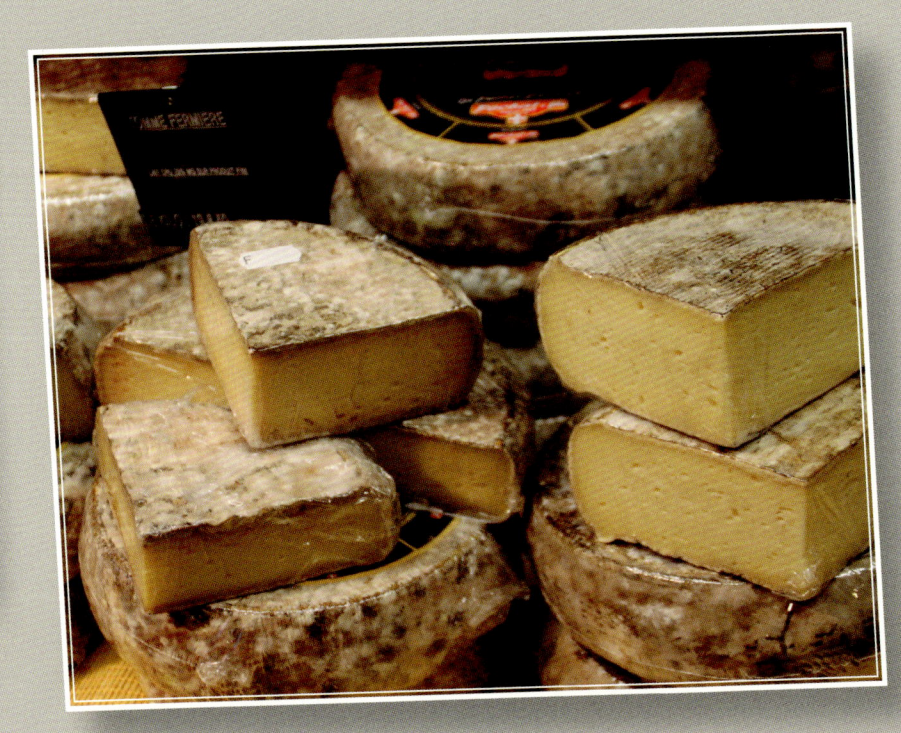

Bread

Back in history, bread was life for the peasants of France, and its high price and shortage of supply were contributing factors which lead to the 1789 Revolution.

Today, it is still very much part of French culture and gastronomy, being bought fresh every morning by the majority of the population, and eaten with most, if not all, meals.

The French mostly appreciate it just out of the oven, still warm, with a crusty, crispy exterior and a soft interior.

There is a *boulangerie* in every town and village and the sight of a Frenchman carrying a *baguette* tucked under his arm has become a symbol of France!

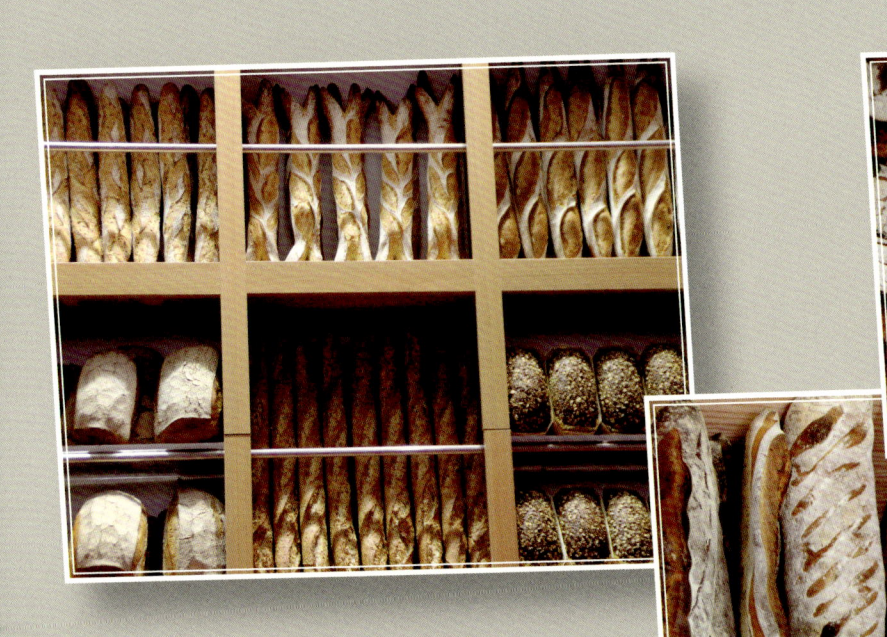

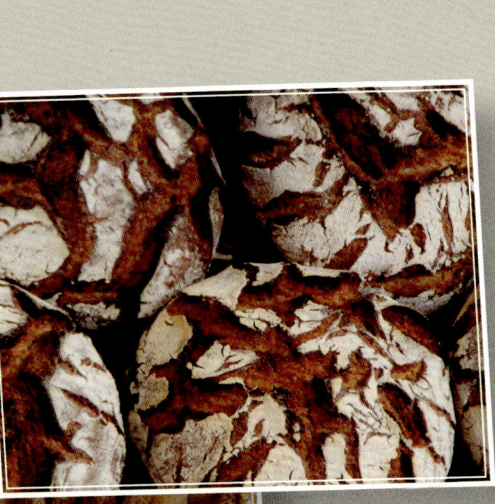

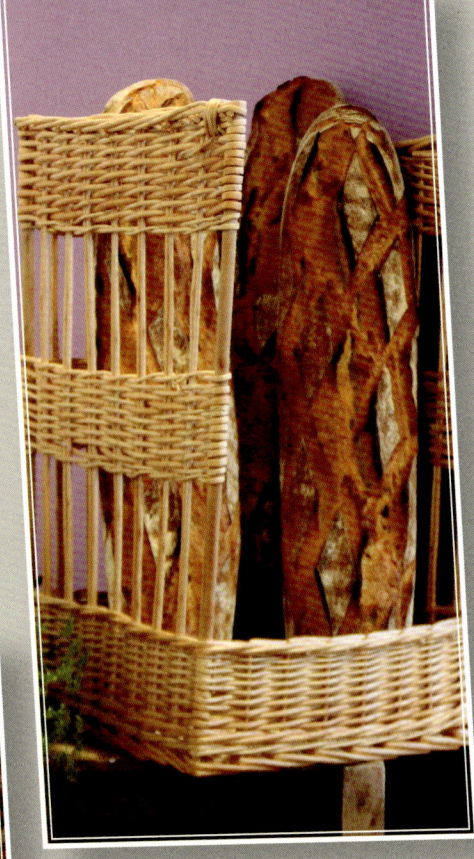

French gastronomy

Pâtisserie

Sweet foods are the delightful indulgence of the French! *Pâtisserie* is the art of making sweets and desserts. Unlike the main course, these treats are not exactly meant for nourishment—they are eaten for pleasure, at the end of a meal.

Pâtisserie has become the greatest skill in French gastronomy, requiring years of training and practice.

Foreigners stand in front of the shop windows of *boulangeries-pâtisseries*, amazed at the incredible vast selection on display. *Pâtissiers* present their creations as works of art; charming with their shimmering colours, amazing shapes and explosive flavours.

They add a touch of modernity and novelty to *grand-mère's* original recipes, creating a desire to rediscover these desserts.

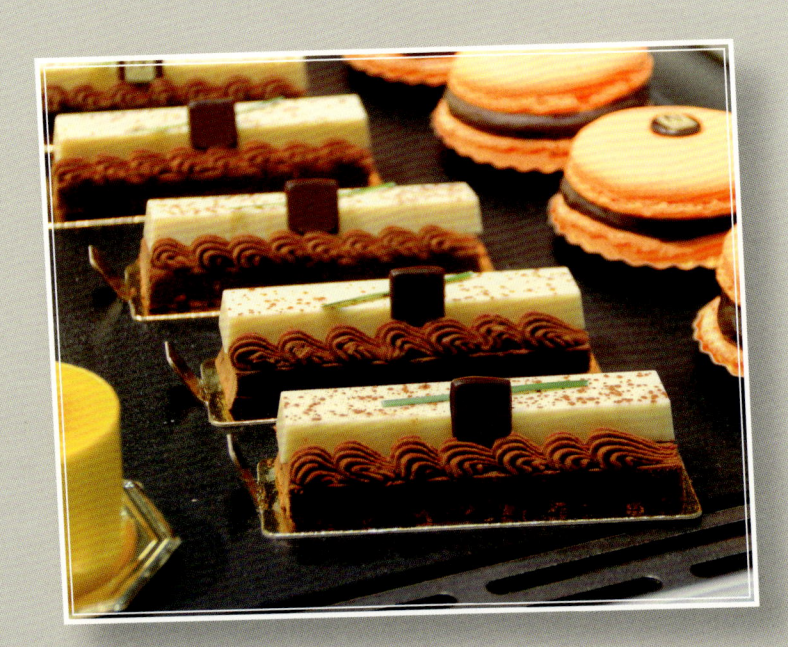

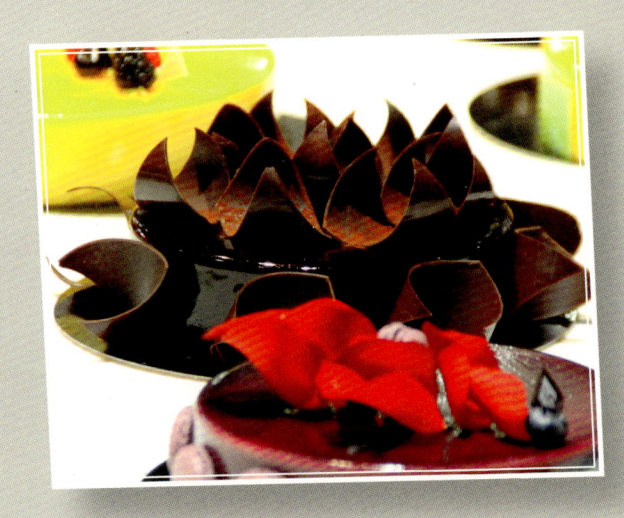

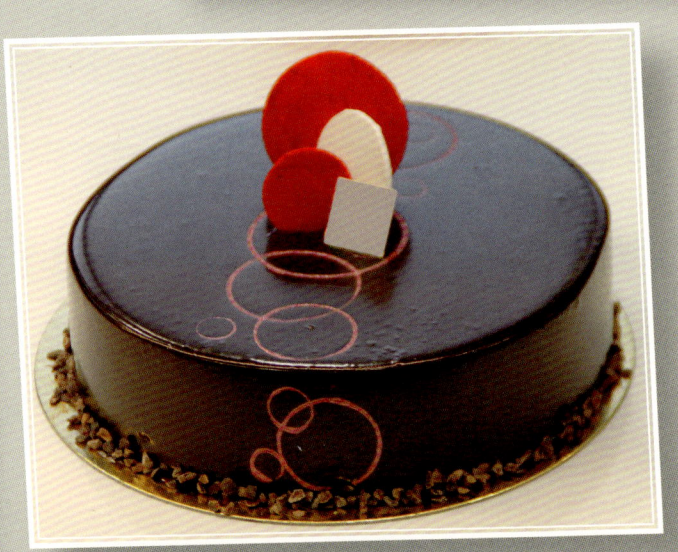

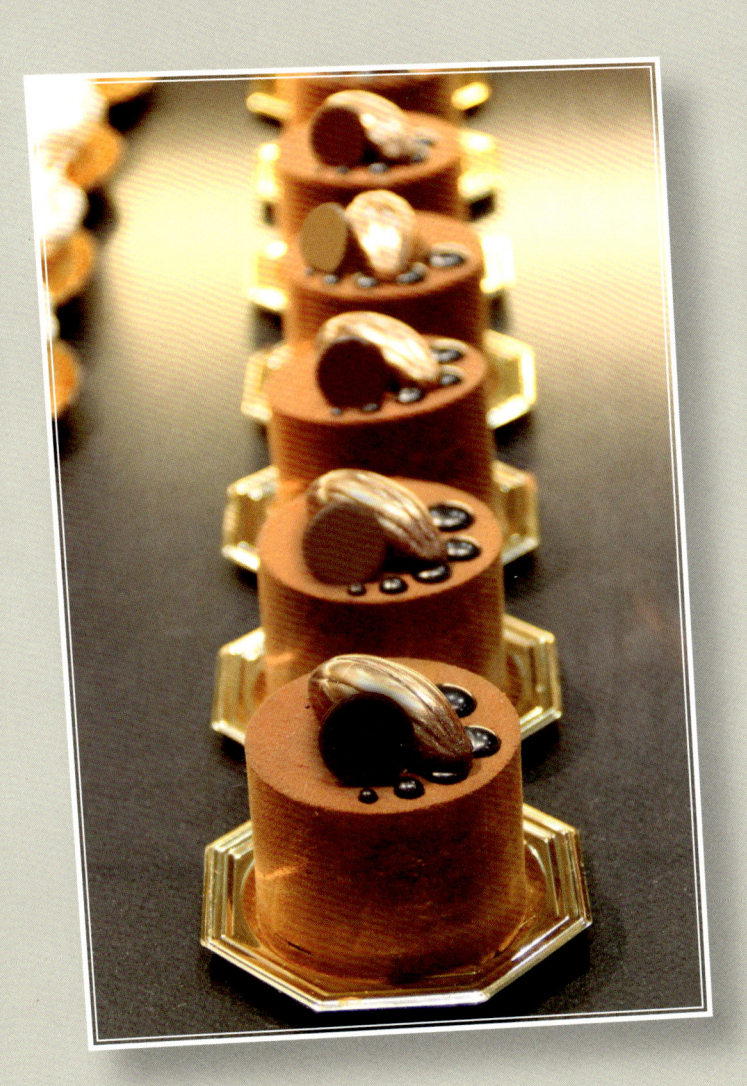

Many famous *pâtisseries*, known around the world, such as *Paris-Brest, Saint-Honoré, religieuses, macarons, éclairs*... are heirs of past innovative and artistic expertise. Today, famous *pâtissiers*, such as Pierre Hermé, Philippe Andrieu, Christophe Michalak, Christophe Felder and Philippe Conticini, prefer to recreate some of the original classics by introducing exotic colours and flavours, and then display their creations all over the world.

Macarons flavoured with rose petals; caramel salted butter; liquorice; basil and lime; sour cherry with amaretto; hazelnut and white truffle or olive oil and vanilla are just some of the new creations.

Students from all over the world come to study *pâtisserie* in centres such as *L'Ecole Nationale Supérieure de la Pâtisserie* in Yssingeaux (Haute-Loire).

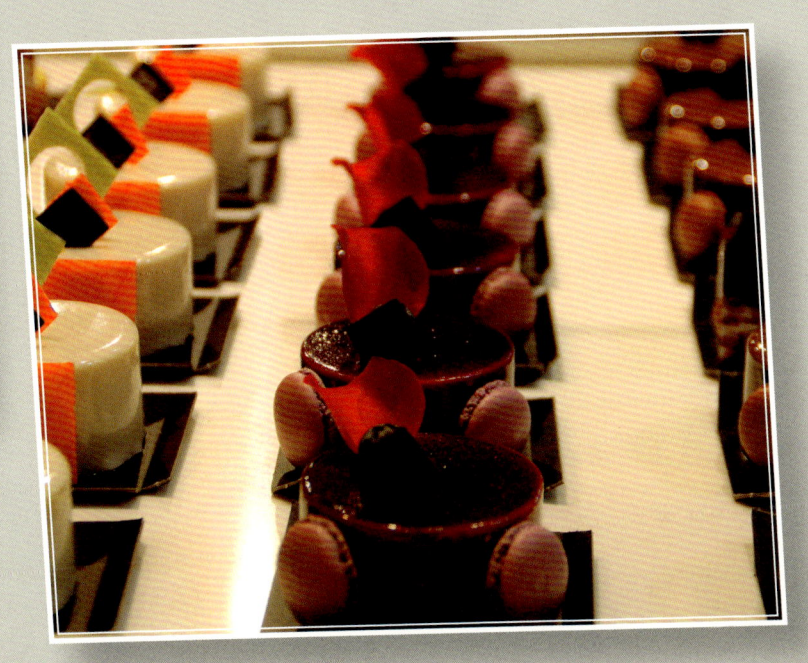

French gastronomy

Honey

Although perhaps not recognised as specialities peculiar to France, the many varieties of honey are certainly worthy of mention. There are more than 40 varieties produced and, perhaps because of some underlying knowledge of its benefits, the French are the biggest consumers of honey in Europe.

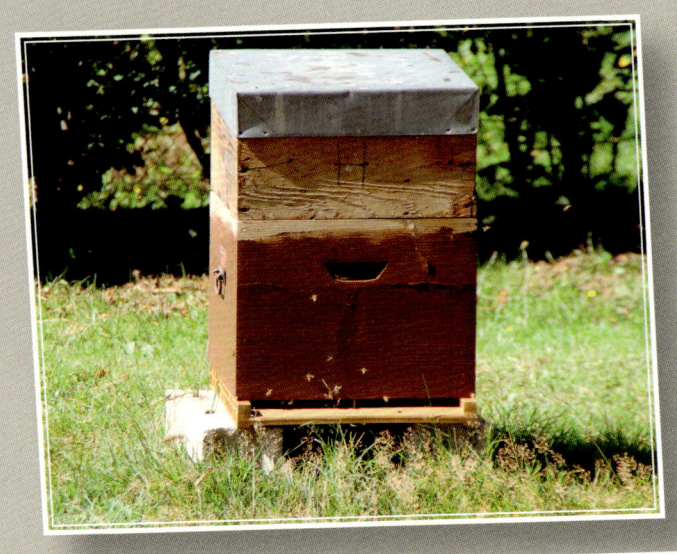

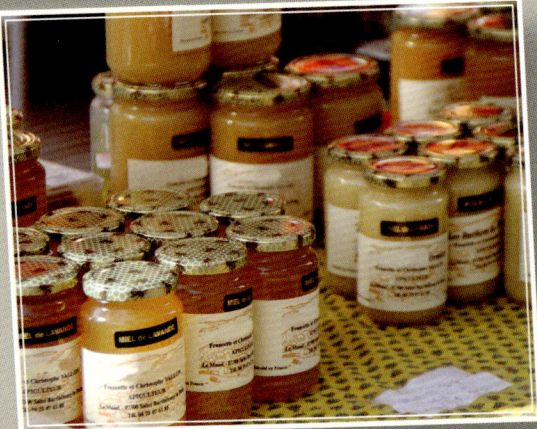

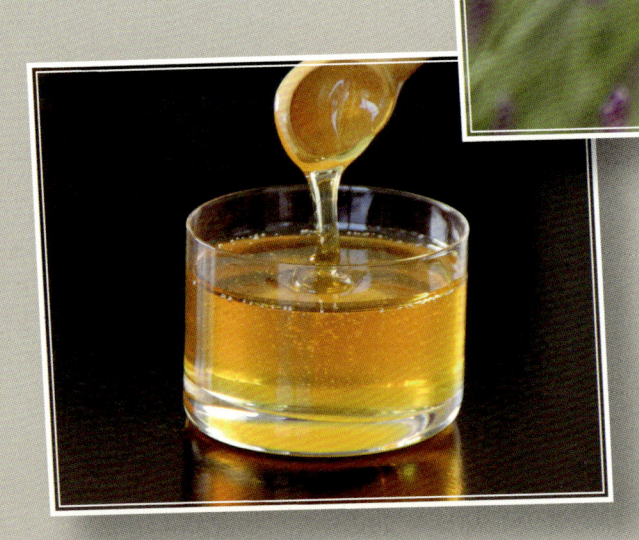

From mountainous landscapes, pine forests, green fields and Mediterranean terrain, vast differences in colour, texture and flavour are found in the many varieties of honey: *miel d'acacia* (acacia honey), *miel de châtaignier* (chestnut honey), *miel de tilleul* (lime blossom honey), *miel de lavande* (lavender honey), *miel de tournesol* (sunflower honey)...

These are just some of the well-known types sold.

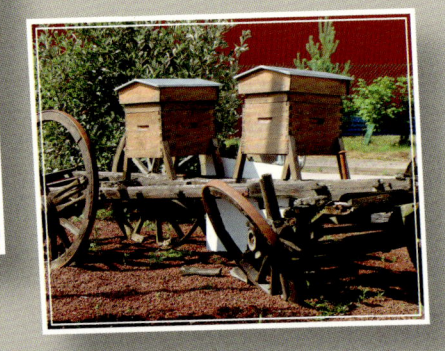

FRENCH WINES & SPIRITS

Overview

The production of alcoholic drinks in France is rich in varieties of wines and spirits. Approximately 1.7% of the land is dedicated for the production of wine, and has become recognised throughout the world as an integral part of French culture. With such a variety of soils and climate, there is a range of different types of wines for everybody's taste.

Brandy, often known as *eau-de-vie*, is a spirit produced by distilling wine.

French brandies

Armagnac and Cognac are traditional French brandies produced in geographically different production areas and are among the best brandies is the world.

Cognac, often called the 'king of alcohol', is manufactured in Charentes, close to the Atlantic coast. It must meet certain legal requirements before it can bear the distinguished name of Cognac. Its development has 4 phases: vinification, distillation, ageing, and mixing. At the time of mixing, the *eaux-de-vie* is mixed with other *eaux-de-vie* of previous years.

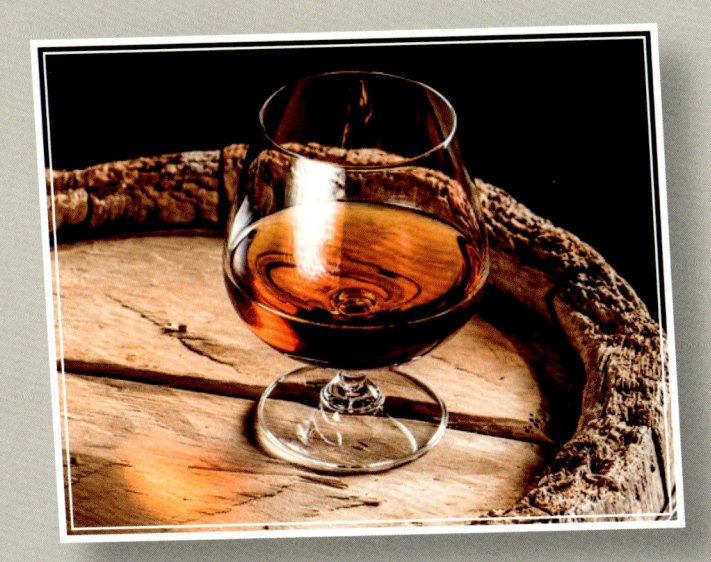

Cognac has to be left to age in oak casks for a certain number of years. Special marks on the bottle refer to how long they have been left to mature. The age refers to the period during which it rested in oak casks and will always be the age of the youngest *eau-de-vie* in the blend. Unlike wine, a Cognac will always be the same age it was when bottled.

VS (Very Special) or ***	a minimum of 2 years.
VSOP (Very Superior Old Pale)	a minimum of 4 years.
XO, Napoleon or *Hors d'Age*	a minimum of 6 years.

Most Cognacs however, are aged considerably longer than the minimum legal requirement. *Hors d'age* is officially equal to XO, but marked to present a very high quality product that is beyond the official age.

French gastronomy

Armagnac is a fragrant, flavoursome kind of brandy produced in Armagnac in *Gascogne* and is the oldest *eaux-de-vie* from French wine produced since the Middle Ages. Even though it is sometimes confused with Cognac, they are very different in many respects. Indeed, France's two finest brandies are not very similar at all.

Armagnac's best grapes are grown in mainly warm temperatures on sandy soil whereas Cognac's grapes are grown on chalky soil with milder temperatures. Traditional Cognac is produced from wine made from 98% *Ugni blanc* grapes, but Armagnac is distilled from wine using a blend of grapes such as *Ugni blanc, Folle blanche, Colombard* and *Bacco,* and is traditionally singled-distilled in a mobile still rather than distilled twice in a pot still as for Cognac.

As it is made by smaller producers, the volume of production is far smaller than Cognac and is therefore not so well known outside Europe.

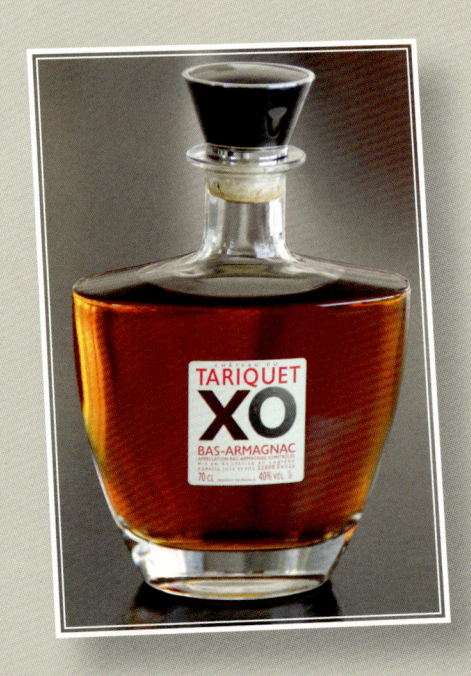

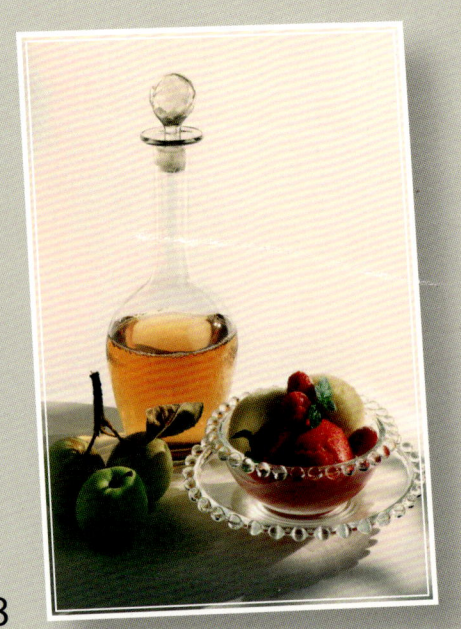

A *trou normand* is an unusual tradition originating from Normandy consisting of a little glass of brandy, after the main course and before the cheese and dessert. (This is intended to settle the stomach and reawaken the palate therefore creating a hole in the stomach in order to regain the appetite for the next course!)

Originally, this consisted of a little glass of Calvados (a brandy made in Normandy). In more recent years, a lighter *trou normand* has been invented where an apple sorbet is watered over with a little Calvados. Since then, other regions have developed the idea by changing the contents. For example, in *Gascogne* a *trou gascon* consists of a sorbet watered with Cognac or Armagnac, or in *Lorraine,* a Mirabelle sorbet is watered with Mirabelle brandy.

FRENCH CUISINE, AN ART OR A WAY OF LIFE?

Within a country possessing such differences in landscapes and climate, the wealth of natural food resources is understandable. From the majestic snowy peaks of the Alps to the balmy Mediterranean seaside resorts and across the rolling lush fields of Brittany, there is always more to explore and discover.

Whereas the rest of the world enjoys French cuisine—indeed much of the world's cuisine originates from France—the French themselves are hesitant to take on foreign ideas and techniques. So, although there are vast diversities in cuisine within the country (like the landscape itself), many customs and habits remain unchanged.

Some would say that cuisine in France is not so much an art but a way of life; a culture where simplicity and flavour are the signs of perfection.

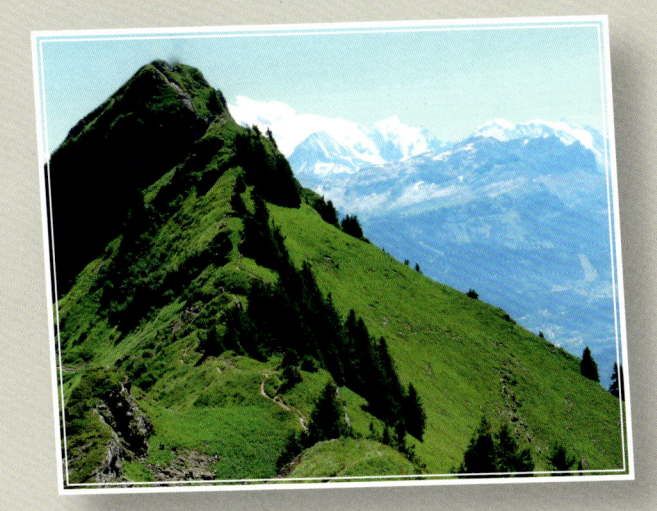

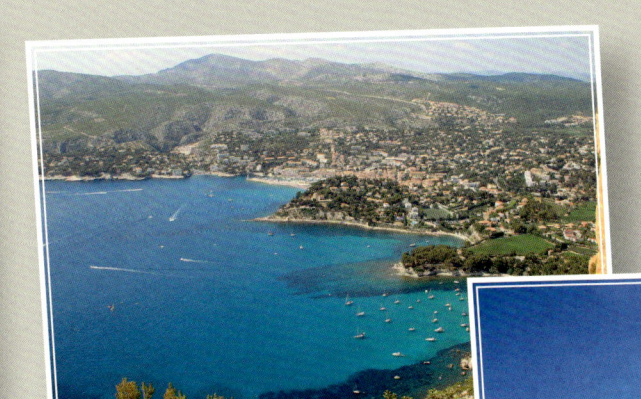

Others would argue that with such a deep-rooted history of patriotic gastronomy, it is an opportunity to flaunt contemporary talents and a challenge to the skill and success of any practising chef.

Whichever is true, and in many ways both are, France is certainly distinguished for its culture in culinary genius and success.

French gastronomy

REGIONS OF FRANCE

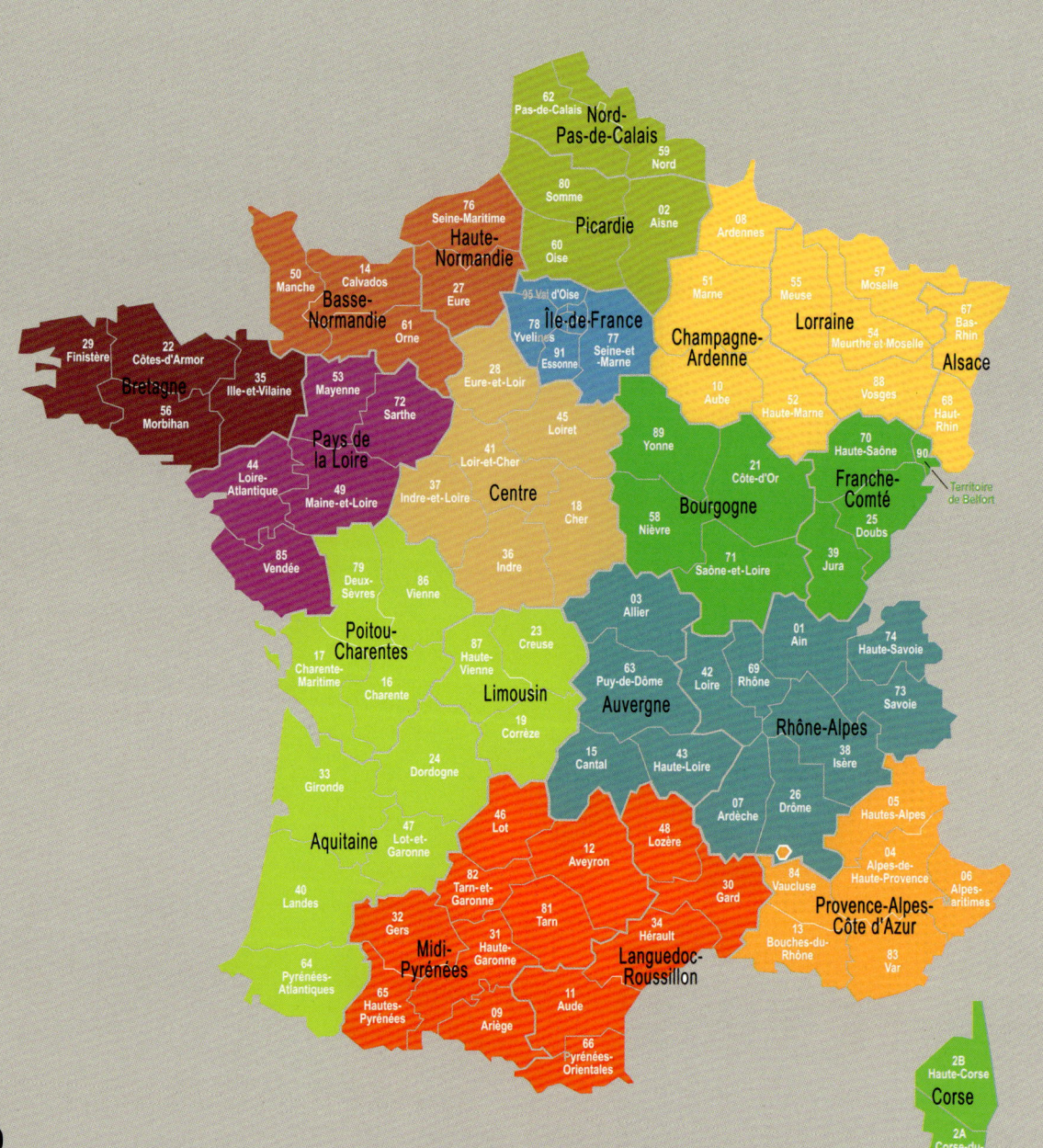

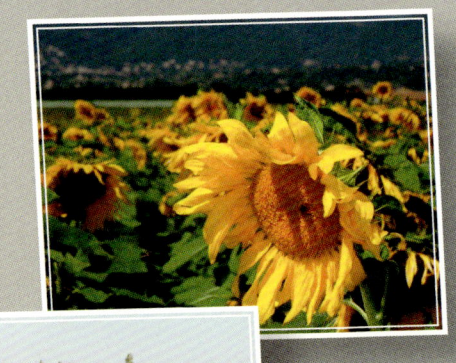

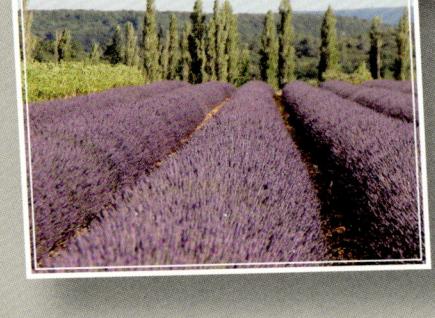

The richness of French cuisine is largely due to the diversity of the country's climate and vegetation across the different regions. By exploiting nature and using what was available, recipes have been created in each region over the years initiating strong culinary traditions.

Due to the vast number of specialities found across France, only a selection has been mentioned.

ALSACE-LORRAINE/CHAMPAGNE-ARDENNE

Constituent Departments—*Ardennes* (08), *Aube* (10), *Bas-Rhin* (67), *Haute-Marne* (52), *Haut-Rhin* (68), *Marnes* (51), *Meurthe-et-Moselle* (54), *Meuse* (55), *Moselle* (57), *Vosges* (88)

Alsace is situated on a fertile plain between the Vosges mountain range and the Black Forest with the River Rhine on the east. Half-timbered houses, built around Romanesque churches lend a picturesque charm to Alsatian villages. Having been under German occupation several times, it has left a very strong Germanic influence including its traditional cuisine. This area benefits from a special climate which allows the production of **excellent wines** and is known to be one of the most exceptional winegrowing areas of France. **Cabbages, potatoes and asparagus** are grown in large quantities in this region.

Lorraine has vast geographic diversities—plains, lakes, mountains and forests.

Champagne-Ardenne has a cooler climate than its *Bourgogne* neighbour thus producing grapes that are not so sweet but more suitable for champagne production. From the chalky grounds of this region, between the towns of *Reims, Epernay* and *Châlons* there are over 30,000 hectares of vineyards producing grapes for **champagne.**

CULINARY SPECIALITIES

The gastronomy from **Alsace** is rich in local specialities with its wine enriched tarts, the famous **choucroute** (sauerkraut), **potée** (hotpot of pork and cabbage), **jambonneau à l'os** (knuckle of ham on the bone) or **baeckeofe** (hotpot of a blend of three meats—lamb, beef and pork—and potatoes).

Dragées de Verdun (sugared almonds) were once just a local speciality of Verdun but very quickly became an emblem of marriages in France. Wrapped in little parcels, they are given away at weddings and other special occasions, to keep as souvenirs.

Champagne-Ardennes also provides a number of regional specialities such as **jambon de Reims** (pork shoulder seasoned with champagne).

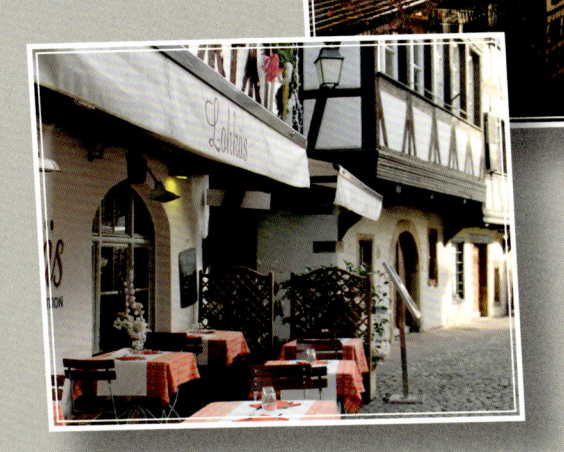

REGIONAL CHEESES

Alsace-Lorraine: Munster, Munster-Guéromé.
Champagne-Ardennes: Brie de Meaux, Brie de Melun, Chaource, Langres, Maroilles

LOCAL WINES

Alsace: Alsace chasselat ou gutedel, Alsace Gewurztraminer, Alsace klevener-de-heiligenstein, Alsace Pinot noir, Alsace Reisling, Alsace Edelzwicker, Alsace Grand cru, Alsace Muscat, Alsace Pinot gris, Alsace Pinot ou Klevner, Alsace Sylvaner
Lorraine: Côtes de Toul
Champagne: Sparkling wine: Champagne
Still wine: Coteaux-champenois, Rosé des Riceys

OTHER SIGNIFICANT LIQUORS

Cerises à l'eau-de-vie (cherries in brandy) and other white eaux-de-vies: Mirabelle, kirsch, poire, quetsche, framboise
Bière blonde d'Alsace, bière blonde de Lorraine
Marc de Champagne

NOTABLE THREE STAR RESTAURANTS

AUBERGE DE L'ILL, 68970 Illhaeusern – chef Marc Haeberlin
L'ASSIETTE CHAMPENOISE, 51430 Tinqueux – chef Arnaud Lallement

French gastronomy

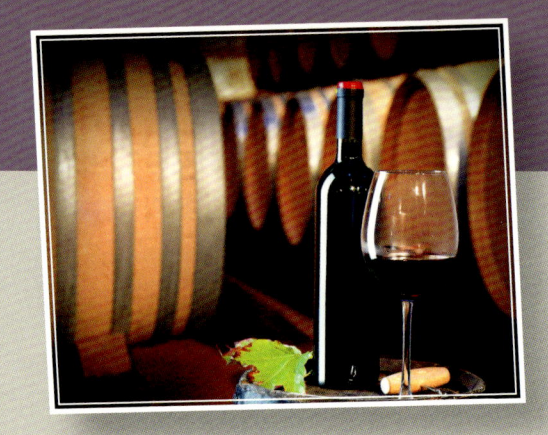

AQUITAINE/LIMOUSIN/POITOU-CHARENTES

Constituent Departments—*Charente* (16), *Charente-Maritime* (17), *Corrèze* (19), *Creuse* (23), *Deux-Sèvres* (79), *Dordogne* (24), *Gironde* (33), *Haute-Vienne* (87), *Landes* (40), *Lot-et-Garonne* (47), *Pyrénées-Atlantiques* (64), *Vienne* (86).

With hundreds of kilometres of Atlantic coastline, it provides delicious seafood, including **moules de Bouchot** (mussels), and the famous **huitres d'Arcachon** (oysters). It is the most productive place in France for these seafoods.

Aquitaine is known for its **foie gras**, and **truffes** (truffles), but also for its quality and quantity of **wine**—especially *Bordeaux*. Gastronomy here is often regarded as the best.

Poitou-Charentes is well-known for its excellent **butter** and *Charentes* has become famous for its production of **Cognac**.

Cuisine in *Limousin* is renowned for its exceptional **quality meat**, **sweet chestnuts** and **wild mushrooms**. In 1736, the first production of **earthenware and porcelain** began at Limoges, bringing prosperity to the region, and this type of porcelain can still be seen in the homes and on restaurant tables today worldwide.

CULINARY SPECIALITIES

This region is mostly famous for its production of **jambon de Bayonne** (cured ham), **piment d'Espelette**, **foie gras** and **truffes du Périgord**. **Pruneaux d'Agen** (prunes) and walnut oil are also a speciality from here.

Limousin **meat** (especially *Limousin* beef) is predominant here. **Pommes du Limousin** (apples), are the only apples to have obtained an *Appellation d'Origine Protégée* (AOP).

Poitou-Charentes is well-known for **huîtres de Marrennes-Oléron** (oysters) and **beurre de Charentes-Poitou** which is probably one of the best butters produced in France. **Melon charentais** are grown in this area.

• REGIONAL CHEESES
Aquitaine: *Ossau-Iraty, Rocamadour*
Poitou-Charentes: *Chabichou*

• NOTABLE THREE STAR RESTAURANTS
LES PRÉS D'EUGÉNIE – MICHEL GUÉRARD, 40320 Eugénie-les-Bains – chef Michel Guérard

• LOCAL WINES

Bordeaux:
Entre-Deux-Mers: Bordeaux-Haut-Benauge, Cadillac-Côtes-de-Bordeaux, Entre-deux-mers, Loupiac, Premières-Côtes-de-Bordeaux, Sainte-Croix-du-Mont, Sainte-Foy-Bordeaux
Graves: Graves, Graves Supèrieur, Pessac-Léognan
Médoc: Haut-Médoc, Listrac-Médoc, Margaux, Médoc, Moulis-en-Médoc, Pauillac, Saint-Estèphe, Saint-Julien
Rives Droite: Blaye – Côtes de Bordeaux, Canon-Fronsac, Castillon – Côtes de Bordeaux, Côtes-de-Blaye, Côtes-de-Bourg, Francs – Côtes de Bordeaux, Fronsac, Lalande-de-Pomerol, Lussac-Saint-Emilion, Montagne-Saint-Emilion, Pomerol, Puisseguin-Saint-Emilion, Saint-Emilion, Saint-Emilion Grand Cru, Saint-Georges-Saint-Emilion
Sauternais: Barsac, Cadillac, Cérons, Loupiac, Sainte-Croix-du-Mont and *Sauternes* are sweet, full-bodied dessert white wines.

Sud-Ouest:
Bergeracois et Duras: Bergerac, Pécharmant, Montravel, Côtes de Duras
Light sweet wines: Monbazillac, Saussignac, Rosette
Rich sweet wines: Haut-Montravel
Moyenne Garonne: Buzet, Côtes-du-Brulhois
Pièmont Pyrénéen: Irouléguy, Jurançon, Madiran, Pacherenc du Vic-Bilh

Poitou-Charentes: Pineau des Charentes (a fortified sweet wine)

• OTHER SIGNIFICANT LIQUORS
Cognac, Armagnac, *Cidre du Limousin*

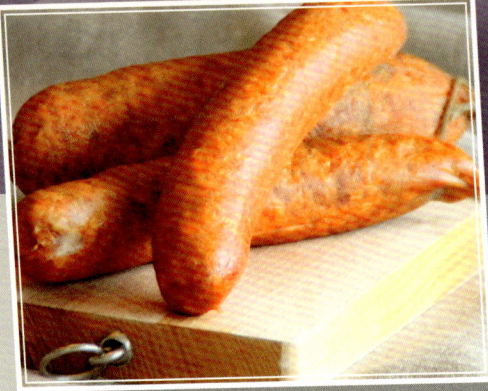

BOURGOGNE/FRANCHE-COMTE

Constituent Departments— *Côte-d'Or* (21), *Doubs* (25), *Haute-Saône* (70), *Jura* (39), *Nièvre* (58), *Saône-et-Loire* (71), *Territoire De Belfort* (90), *Yonne* (89)

Gastronomies from **Bourgogne** and **Franche-Comté** are quite diverse from each other including their respective wines: the **grands crus** of *Bourgogne* and the **vin jaune** (yellow wine) from *Franche-Comté*.

Bourgogne has a variety of dishes which have become recognised worldwide such as the famous *boeuf bourguignon*, *coq au vin* or *escargots de Bourgogne* (snails cooked in garlic butter).

Franche-Comté is situated between mountains, forest and pastureland, not prominent in agriculture but provides good pasture for cattle and a lot of dairy farming. The Jura vineyards are probably the oldest in France where the *vin jaune* (yellow wine) is produced.

CULINARY SPECIALITIES

Dijon is France's capital for **pain d'épices** and **mustard**.
Crème de Cassis was promoted by the Canon Kir, deputy mayor of Dijon, who used it to soften the acidity of white wine.

Kir is an *apéritif* which consists of mixing the *crème de cassis de Dijon* with a white *aligoté* wine. Today, there are several varieties: *Kir royal*—with sparkling white wine, *Kir lorrain*—with plum liqueur, *Kir ardéchoise*—with *crème de châtaigne* (chestnut) or *Kir breton*—with cider or other *crème de fruits*.

This region provides **Charolais beef**—a race easily identified by its white or ivory hide—and its aptitude for fattening has led it to become the preferred breed of beef cattle in France.
Franche-comté is famous for its varieties of sausages such as **saucisse de Morteau** and **saucisse de Montbéliard**.

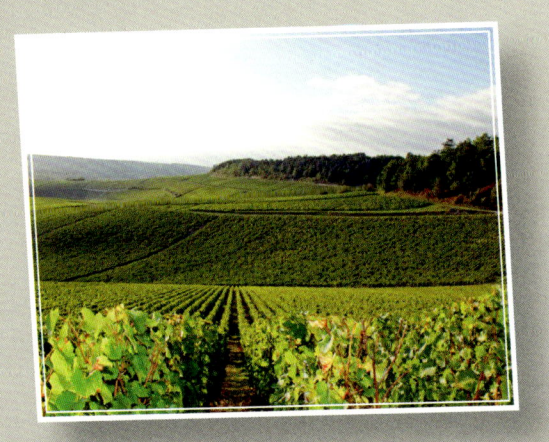

• **REGIONAL CHEESES**
Bourgogne: Epoisses, Mâconnais, Chaource, Langres, Brillat-Savarin
Franche-Comté: Mont d'Or, Comté, Gruyère français, Bleu de Gex, Morbier, Cancoillotte

• **LOCAL WINES**
Bourgogne:
Côte Chalonnaise: Bouzeron, Givry, Montagny, Mercurey, Rully
Mâconnais: Pouilly-Fuissé, Pouilly-Loché, Pouilly-Vinzelles, Saint-Véran, Viré-Clessé
Chablisien: Bourgogne, Petit Chablis, Chablis, Chablis premier cru, Chablis grand cru, Irancy, Saint-Bris
Côte de nuits: Chambertin, Clos-de-Vougeot, Clos-des-Lambrays, Fixin, Nuits-Saint-Georges, Musigny, Romanée-Conti
Côte de Beaune: Corton, Corton-Charlemagne, Côte-de-Beaune-Villages, Meursault

Beaujolais: Côte-de-brouilly, Saint-amour, Chénas, Juliénas, Moulin-à-vent
Jura is renowned for its famous *vin jaune* and *vin de paille* : Arbois, Château-Châlon, Côtes-du-Jura

• **OTHER SIGNIFICANT LIQUORS**
Crème de cassis (blackcurrant liqueur)

• **NOTABLE THREE STAR RESTAURANTS**
LE RELAIS BERNARD LOISEAU, 21210 Saulieu – chef Patrick Bertron
MAISON LAMELOISE, 71150 Chagny – chef Eric Pras

French gastronomy

BRETAGNE

Constituent Departments— *Côtes d'Armor* (22), *Finistère* (29), *Ille-et-Vilaine* (35), *Morbihan* (56)

Bretagne is situated in the North-West of France and is a place of traditions and folklore, preserving traditional specialities characterised by typical dishes. Possessing approximately 3,000 kilometres of diverse coastline, this region provides great varieties of **fish and shellfish**. It has an oceanic climate with regular rainfall and is known for its **quality vegetables**.

CULINARY SPECIALITIES

Artichokes and **cauliflowers** are local emblems and are cultivated with other vegetables such as potatoes and **oignons de Roscoff** (onions).

Crêpes de froment (wheat crêpes) are a speciality in *Basse Bretagne* and **galettes de sarrasin** (buckwheat pancakes) are a speciality in *Haute Bretagne*. Galettes de sarrazin are eaten as a savoury, whereas *crêpes de froment* are served as a sweet.

Oysters are the most popular shellfish in this region and are often eaten raw, although some restaurants serve them hot.

Several sweet recipes originate from here such as: **crêpes dentelle de Quimper** (rolled, light, thin crispy biscuits, prepared using the same basic ingredients as crêpes), **Far Breton** (a sweet flan) and **kouign-amann** (a yeast cake containing layers of butter and sugar folded in).

• **REGIONAL CHEESES**
Saint Paulin

• **OTHER SIGNIFICANT LIQUORS**
Cidre de Bretagne

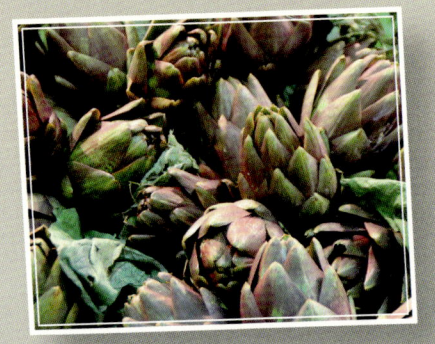

CENTRE

Constituent Departments— *Cher* (18), *Eure-et-Loir* (28), *Indre* (36), *Indre-et-Loire* (37), *Loiret* (45), *Loir-et-Cher* (41)

South of Paris, geographically this region is in the centre of France where there are beautiful **châteaux** and vineyards along the Loire Valley which, amongst other wines, produce **excellent dry and sweet white wines**. Often known as the 'garden of France', it has a moderate climate.

This region, abundant in forests, lakes and cereal plains, also offers a **selection of meats** such as poultry from Orléans, or wild boar and other game from the *Sologne* forests. These used to be enjoyed by the French kings and nobles and are still appreciated today.

CULINARY SPECIALITIES

Charcuterie selection such as **rillettes de Tours**, or **pâté de Chartres**.

Orléans once known as the 'city of vinegars' became famous, thanks to its vinegar manufacturing since the Middle Ages.

• **REGIONAL CHEESES**
Crottin de Chavignol, Pouligny Saint-Pierre, Sainte-Maure de Touraine, Selles-sur-Cher, Valençay

• **LOCAL WINES**
Vallée de la Loire:
Centre: Sancerre, Quincy, Reuilly, Menetou-Salon
Touraine: Bourgueil, Cheverny, Chinon, Touraine, Vouvray

CORSE

Constituent Departments—*Corse-du-Sud* (2A), *Haute Corse* (2B)

Corse is a Mediterranean island of beautiful beaches, mountains and historic monuments. With significant slopes, a unique climate of sunshine—approximately 3,000 hours of sunshine per year—abundant rainfall, strong winds and mild winters, *Corse* is an excellent situation for vineyards. It is probably best known in gastronomy for its production of **wines**, **charcuterie**, **sheep** or **goat's cheeses**, as well as being the paradise of **citrus fruits**.

Although geographically it is very near to Italy, *Corse* has belonged to France since 1769.

CULINARY SPECIALITIES

Charcuterie is exceptional due to the local *cochons noirs* (black pigs) who are allowed to roam loose and feed from Corsican scrub, giving the meat a subtle, unique flavour and an undeniable quality. Charcuterie includes **prisuttu, coppa, lonzu, figatellu, salamu** and **salsiccia**.

Fish and **seafood** have become part of its gastronomic heritage.

Thanks to plenty of sunshine and hilly terrain, **citrus fruits** such as oranges, clementines, mandarins, lemons and kiwis grow in abundance.

Corsican honey is the only French honey to benefit from a Label of Controlled Origin.

• REGIONAL CHEESES
Bastelicacciu, Brocciu

• LOCAL WINES
Ajaccio, Patrimonio, Vin-de-Corse
Sweet wine : *Muscat-du-Cap-Corse*

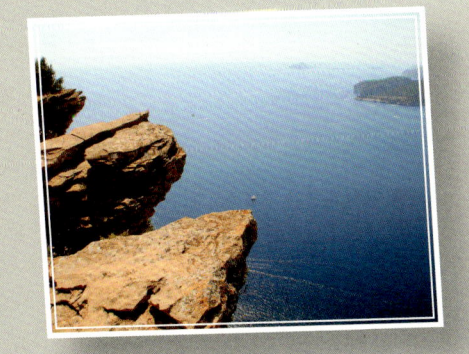

HAUTE-NORMANDIE/BASSE-NORMANDIE

Constituent Departments—*Calvados* (14), *Eure* (27), *Manche* (50), *Orne* (61), *Seine-Maritime* (76)

Normandie is situated in the North of France with its borders on the English Channel, providing numerous **crustaceans** such as *Saint Jacques*, prawns or lobsters. With a mild, wet, oceanic climate, **dairy produce** and **apples** are produced in abundance and this region is best known for being the place of **cream**, **butter** and **cider**.

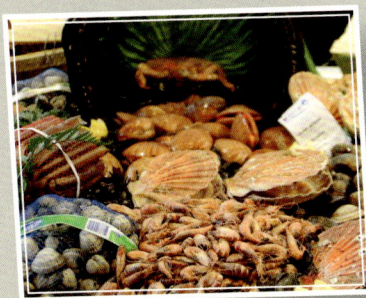

CULINARY SPECIALITIES

Vast quantities and varieties of freshly-caught fish are sold by auction in the fish markets by local fishermen. *Normandie* is France's number one region for **coquilles st. Jacques** (scallops), which are distinguished by a large meaty nut and a beautiful coral.

Normandie is renowned for its excellent dairy products especially its creams such as *crème d'Isigny*. In addition to this is the varied and delicious cheese platter.
Apples from here are often used in desserts, tarts and cakes, but also for making cider and **calvados**.

A *trou normand* originally consisted of a little glass of calvados served between two courses to stimulate the guests' appetite. Today, a *trou normand* is generally served as a sorbet with calvados watered over.

• REGIONAL CHEESES
Camembert, Livarot, Pont l'Evêque, Cœur de Neufchâtel

• OTHER SIGNIFICANT LIQUORS
Cider and Calvados, a distilled cider are produced here. It is said that cider is drunk in *Normandie* as wine is drunk elsewhere in France!

Bénédictine, a herbal liqueur, was originally distilled by *Bénédictine* monks.

French gastronomy

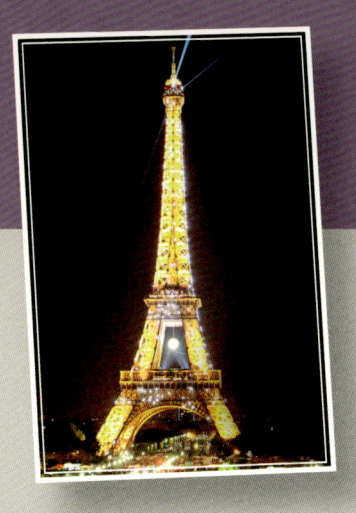

ILE-DE-FRANCE

Constituent Departments—*Essonne* (91), *Seine-et-Marne* (77), *Seine-Saint-Denis* (93), *Val de Marne* (94), *Val-d'Oise* (95), *Yvelines* (78)

Ile-de-France is the root of traditional gastronomy and French cuisine. This region combines and **concentrates all the cuisine around France** and the best products from all over the country are found here, allowing chefs to express their creativity!

In **Paris** and its suburbs, there are more than 10 million inhabitants and are over 9,000 restaurants, displaying the cultural, historical and exceptional gastronomic heritage, known worldwide.

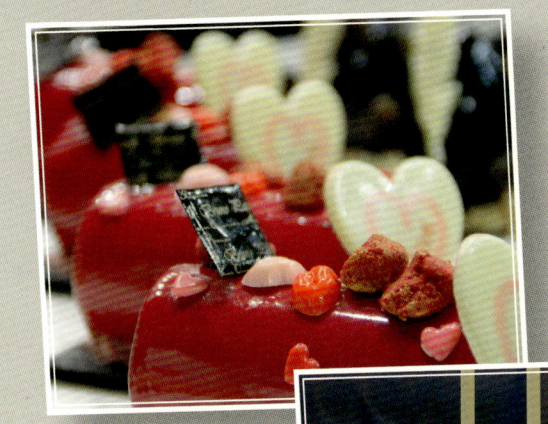

CULINARY SPECIALITIES

Many products sold in grocery stores and markets of the city grow in the cultivated land surrounding the capital. The exceptional *Ile-de-France* speciality list is long: *baguette*, croissants, *macarons*, Paris-Brest, *galette des rois parisienne*, *brioche de Nanterre*, *tarte Bourdaloue* (pear and almond tart), *opéra*, *millefeuille*, savarin, *chouquette*...

• REGIONAL CHEESES
Brie de Meaux, Brie de Melun, Coulommiers

• LOCAL WINES
Vin de Pays de Seine et Marne

• OTHER SIGNIFICANT LIQUORS
Grand Marnier, Noyau de Poissy

• NOTABLE THREE STAR RESTAURANTS
L'AMBROISIE, 75004 Paris 04 – chef Bernard Pacaud
LE MEURICE ALAIN DUCASSE, 75001 Paris 01 – chefs Alain Ducasse et Jocelyn Herland
LE PRÉ CATELAN, 75016 Paris 16 – chef Frédéric Anton
PIERRE GAGNAIRE, 75008 Paris 08 – chef Pierre Gagnaire
EPICURE AU BRISTOL, 75008 Paris 08 – chef Eric Frechon
ALLÉNO PARIS – PAVILLON LEDOYEN, 75008 Paris 08 – chef Yannick Alléno
GUY SAVOY, 75006 Paris 06 – chef Guy Savoy
ASTRANCE, 75016 Paris 16 – chef Pascal Barbot

LANGUEDOC-ROUSSILLON/MIDI -PYRENEES

Constituent Departments—*Ariège* (09), *Aude* (11), *Aveyron* (12), *Gard* (30), *Gers* (32), *Haute-Garonne* (31), *Hautes-Pyrénées* (65), *Hérault* (34), *Lot* (46), *Lozère* (48), *Pyrénées-Orientales* (66), *Tarn* (81), *Tarn-et-Garonne* (82)

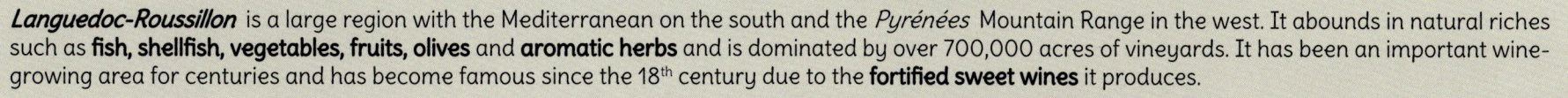

Languedoc-Roussillon is a large region with the Mediterranean on the south and the *Pyrénées* Mountain Range in the west. It abounds in natural riches such as **fish, shellfish, vegetables, fruits, olives** and **aromatic herbs** and is dominated by over 700,000 acres of vineyards. It has been an important wine-growing area for centuries and has become famous since the 18th century due to the **fortified sweet wines** it produces.

Traditional gastronomy in *Midi Pyrénées* is portrayed by France's most luxurious products such as **foie gras, truffe noir** and **Roquefort**—specialities exploited by talented chefs in restaurants around this region.

CULINARY SPECIALITIES

Les salins du Midi has the biggest sea salt production in France.

Foie gras, produced from the livers of maize-fattened ducks and geese—an icon of French gastronomy!

Truffe noir (black truffle), found exclusively in the Lot Department, is one of the highlights of French *haute cuisine*. It has become a distinctive symbol of *Midi-Pyrénées* gastronomy.

Anchois de Collioure (anchovies)—popular in Collioure, a fishing village on the French Catalan coast, traditionally known as 'the anchovy capital of France'.

Midi Pyrénées provides more than half of the garlic production in France.

Cassoulet (meat and bean casserole)—a traditional speciality.

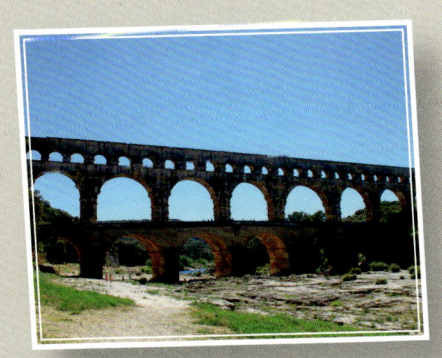

• REGIONAL CHEESES
Languedoc-Roussillon: Pélardon
Midi-Pyrénées: Bleu des Causses, Rocamadour, Roquefort, Laguiole

• LOCAL WINES
Vallée du Rhône: Côtes-du-Rhône Village, Lirac, Tavel
Languedoc-Roussillon: Cabardès, Corbières, Languedoc, Malepère, Minervois, Saint-Chinian, Collioure, Côtes-du-Roussillon
Sparkling wine: Blanquette-de-Limoux
Fortified sweet wines: Banuyls, Muscat de Rivesaltes, Rivesaltes, Maury
Sud-Ouest:
Pièmont Massif Central: Cahors, Gaillac, Marcillac, Fronton, Lavilledieu
Pièmont Pyrénéen: Madiran, Pacherenc du Vic-Bilh

• OTHER SIGNIFICANT LIQUORS
Armagnac

• NOTABLE THREE STAR RESTAURANTS
BRAS, 12210 Laguiole – chefs Michel et Sébastien Bras
AUBERGE DU VIEUX PUITS, 11360 Fontjoncouse – chef Gilles Goujon

37

French gastronomy

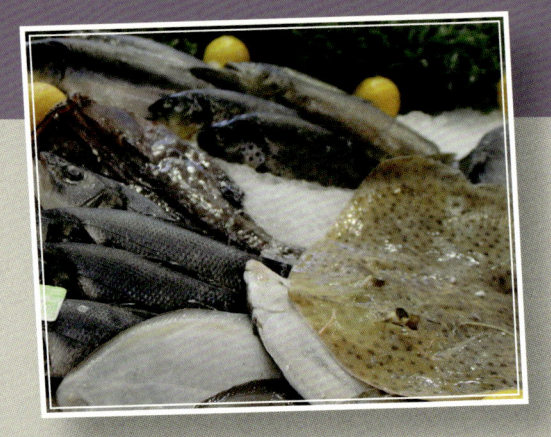

NORD-PAS-DE-CALAIS/PICARDIE

Constituent Departments-*Aisne* (02), *Nord* (59), *Oise* (60), *Pas-de-Calais* (62), *Somme* (80)

There are many traditional breweries in *Nord-Pas-De-Calais* and *Picardie*, producing **good quality beer** which has an influence on the gastronomy in this region—beer is used in cooking rather than wine and since the last century, each village has a local bar which serves their own brand of beer.

Nord-Pas-De-Calais is situated on the Belgium border and much of its cuisine has been inherited from Flanders. It has wild coastal borders including the largest fishing port in France—Boulogne. Nearly every coastal village has their own local **fish market**. Large areas of agricultural land produce **wheat, beets** and **chicories**, and grazing land for **dairy cattle**.

Picardie is often known as **France's market garden** and its cuisine benefits much from the local produce such as **freshwater fish,** *agneau de pré-salé* (salt meadow lamb) and delicious **dairy products**.

CULINARY SPECIALITIES

The North of France is an area which cultivates **excellent quality vegetables**.

Bêtises de Cambrai, a popular sweet among French, traditionally mint flavoured. This delicacy was named a '*bêtise*'—meaning blunder in English—as it was said to have been invented accidently in the 19th century by a young apprentice in this area.

- **REGIONAL CHEESES**

Dauphin, Boulette d'Avesnes, Maroilles (one of the oldest cheeses in France, has been produced in this region since the 7th century), *Mimolette, Rollot de Picardie*

- **OTHER SIGNIFICANT LIQUORS**

Beers: *Ch'Ti, Amadeus, Jenlain, Saint Landelin, Septante-5, Gayant, Grain d'Orge, Sebourg, Gavroche, Saint-Poloise, Ambre des Flandres, Belzebuth, bière de Garde, Pot Flamand*, etc.

PAYS DE LA LOIRE

Constituent Departments-*Loire-Atlantique* (44), *Maine-et-Loire* (49), *Mayenne* (53), *Sarthe* (72), *Vendée* (85)

Pays de la Loire benefits from a mild climate making it an ideal region for **agricultural production** and **vineyards**. The Atlantic coast here supplies a range of **fresh fish** and **shellfish**.

CULINARY SPECIALITIES

Cuisine in *Pays de la Loire* is mostly distinguished by its quality of regional products: **champignons de Paris** (button mushrooms), **pommes de terre nouvelles de Noirmoutier** (new potatoes) and provides 85% of *mâche* (lamb's lettuce) in France. This area is the top ranking region for certified organic produce.

The famous *sel de Guérande* (salt) is produced using 1,000 year old traditional methods.

- **REGIONAL CHEESES**

Curé Nantais, Saint Paulin

- **LOCAL WINES**

Vallée de la Loire:
Anjou-Saumur: Anjou, Cabernet d'Anjou, Jasnières, Savennières, Côteaux du Layon, Saumur, Saumur-Champigny, Quarts-de-Chaume
Nantes: Muscadet-Sèvres-et-Maine, Muscadet-Côteaux-de-la-Loire, Muscadet-Côtes-de-Granlieu

- **OTHER SIGNIFICANT LIQUORS**

Cointreau, Guignolet, Cidre de Mayenne

PROVENCE-ALPES-COTE D'AZUR (PACA)

Constituent Departments—*Alpes-de-Haute-Provence* (04), *Alpes-Maritimes* (06), *Bouches-du-Rhône* (13), *Hautes-Alpes* (05), *Var* (83), *Vaucluse* (84)

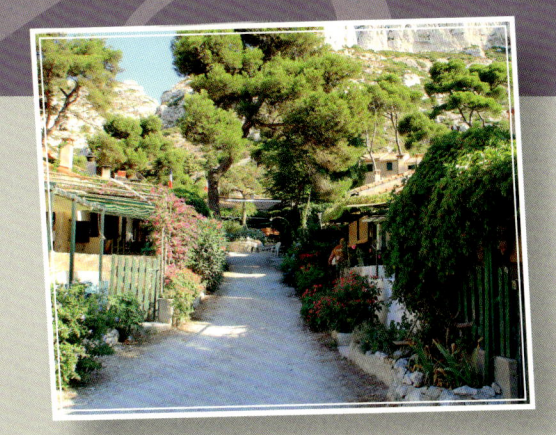

Situated in the South-East of France, **PACA** has the Mediterranean in the south, the Italian border in the east and the *Massif Alpins* (Alpine Mountain Range) in the north. Traditional cuisine is created around local produce—**olive oil, aromatic herbs, garlic, vegetables**, etc., and is a reflection of the region itself—bright, sun-soaked, colourful and with plenty of fragrances and flavours. Its reputation as a healthy diet has spread throughout the world.

CULINARY SPECIALITIES

Lavender, olives and **olive oil** are symbolic products in this region.

La Camargue is famous for its **rice** which has been cultivated since 1830 and is the most northerly rice-growing area in Europe.

The sea provides a rich resource of fish which are used in traditional dishes such as the famous **bouillabaisse**, a fish soup served with croutons rubbed in garlic, *rouille* (a spicy Provençal sauce) and whole fish.

Calissons d'Aix are a speciality from Aix en Provence. These sweets are made from a thin layer of candied melon and ground almonds, topped with royal icing and put on an unleavened bread base.

• **REGIONAL CHEESES**
Le Banon

• **LOCAL WINES**
Vallée du Rhône: *Rasteau sec, Gigondas, Beaumes-de-Venise, Vacqueyrus, Châteauneuf-du-Pape, Côtes-du-Rhône, Côtes-du-Rhône Village, Luberon, Ventoux*
Fortified sweet wines: *Rasteau, Muscat de Beaumes-de-Venise*
Provence: *Bandol, Bellet, Cassis, Coteaux-d'Aix-en-Provence, Côtes-de-Provence, Les Baux-de-Provence*

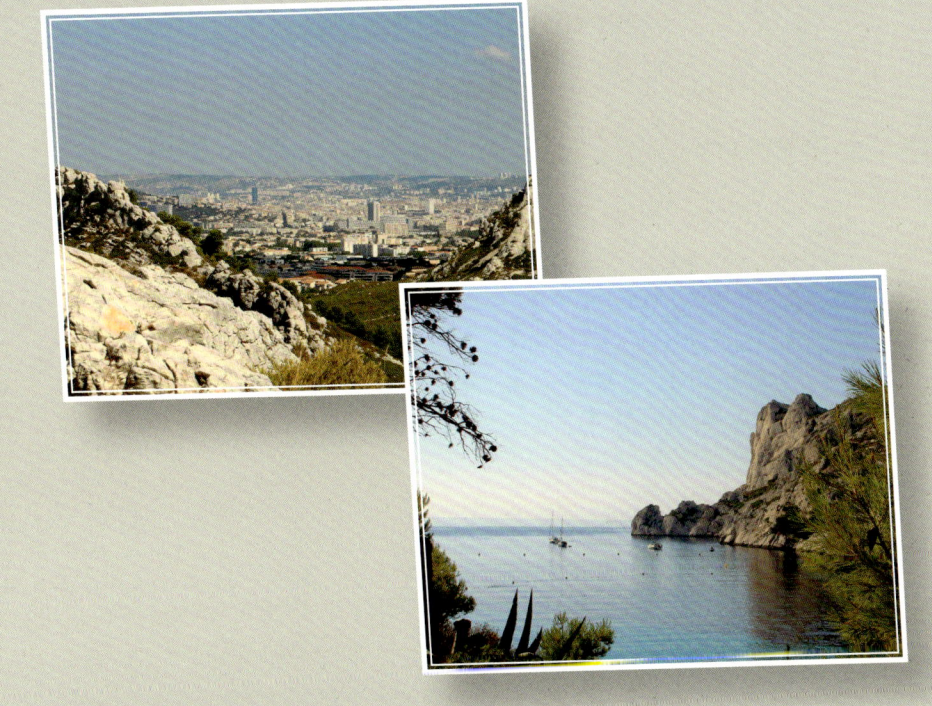

• **NOTABLE THREE STAR RESTAURANTS**
LE PETIT NICE, 13007 Marseille 07 – chef Gérald Passédat
RÉSIDENCE DE LA PINÈDE – LA VAGUE D'OR, 83990 St-Tropez – chef Arnaud Donckele

• **OTHER SIGNIFICANT LIQUORS**
Pastis

French gastronomy

RHÔNE-ALPES/AUVERGNE

Constituent Departments—*Ain* (01), *Allier* (03), *Ardèche* (07), *Cantal* (15), *Drôme* (26), *Haute-Loire* (43), *Haute-Savoie* (74), *Isère* (38), *Loire* (42), *Puy-de-Dôme* (63), *Rhône* (69), *Savoie* (73)

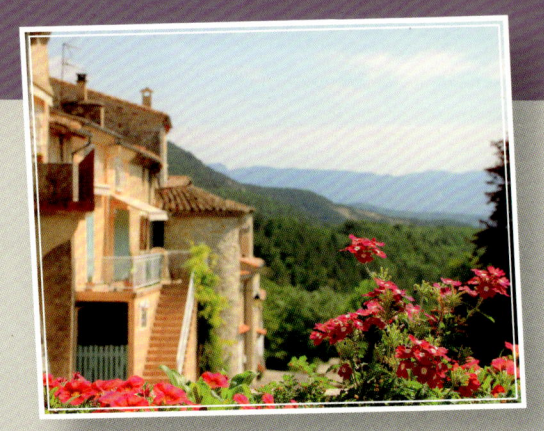

Rhône-Alpes is a beautiful region with a vast diversity of landscapes. It is situated on three mountain ranges: the Alps in the west where stands *Mont Blanc* (4808 metres)—the highest peak in Europe—the Jura Mountain Range in the north-east and the *Massif Central* to the west. This region is often regarded as the centre of gastronomy due to the wealth of produce within its borders and has provided a solid foundation of regional cooking from *Savoie, Ardèche, Dauphiné* and *Auvergne*.

Savoie has a very old cheese-making tradition probably dating back to the 15th century thanks to the vast areas of quality pastureland. Gastronomy here is predominately based on local grown produce adapted to the harsh mountainous climate, and includes **potatoes** and *Savoie* **cheeses**.

For many years, **chestnuts** have been an essential ingredient in *Ardèche* cuisine.

Dauphiné gastronomy is as varied as the land itself! It is a mixture of *Provence* and *Savoie,* for example, in the use of olive oil or walnuts.

Auvergne is a rural and mountainous region and has taken the lead—globally—in **regional French cheeses**, both in quality and variety, since the Gallo-Roman period. Typical cuisine in this part is simple, nourishing and wholesome, and has a peasant-style origin.

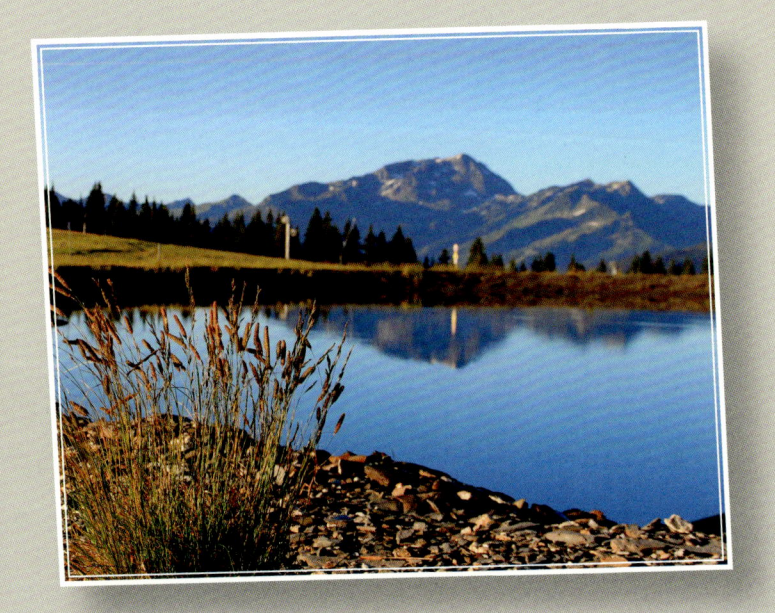

CULINARY SPECIALITIES

Lyon is considered by many as the 'capital of gastronomy' and has one of the most renowned traditional types of cuisine. It is famous for its selection of **charcuterie** such as: *rosette de Lyon* (type of slicing sausage), *rillettes, pâtés de campagne* (farmhouse pâté) and *cervelat*.

Le Puy in *Haute-Loire* is where the traditional **green lentils** *du Puy* are grown, cultivated without added fertiliser, covering 88 communes.

Auvergne has over 100 sources of **natural volcanic mineral water** such as *Volvic, Saint-Yorre, Vichy Célestins, Rozana, Mont Dore* and *Chateldon*.

- **REGIONAL CHEESES**

Rhône-Alpes: Picodon de l'Ardèche et de la Drôme, Saint-Félicien, Saint-Marcellin, Abondance, Beaufort, Chevrotin, Emmental de Savoie, Reblochon, Tomme de Savoie

Auvergne: Bleu d'Auvergne, Cantal, Fourme d'Ambert, Fourme de Montbrison, Saint-nectaire, Salers

- **LOCAL WINES**

Beaujolais: Brouilly, Régnié, Chiroubles, Fleurie, Chénas, Juliénas, Morgon, Moulin-à-vent, Beaujolais, Beaujolais village, Beaujolais supérieur

Beaujolais Nouveau is the only wine that can be legally consumed in the year of its production— released annually on the third week in November.

Vallée du Rhône: Côte-rôtie, Condrieu, Château-grillet, Saint-Joseph, Cornas, Saint-Péray, Crozes-hermitage, Hermitage, Vinsobres, Côtes-du-Rhône, Côtes-du-Rhône Village

Sparkling white wine: *Clairette de Die*

Savoie: Crépy, Roussette de Savoie, Seyssel, Vin de Savoie

Vallée de la Loire: Côte-Roannaise, Côte-du-Forez

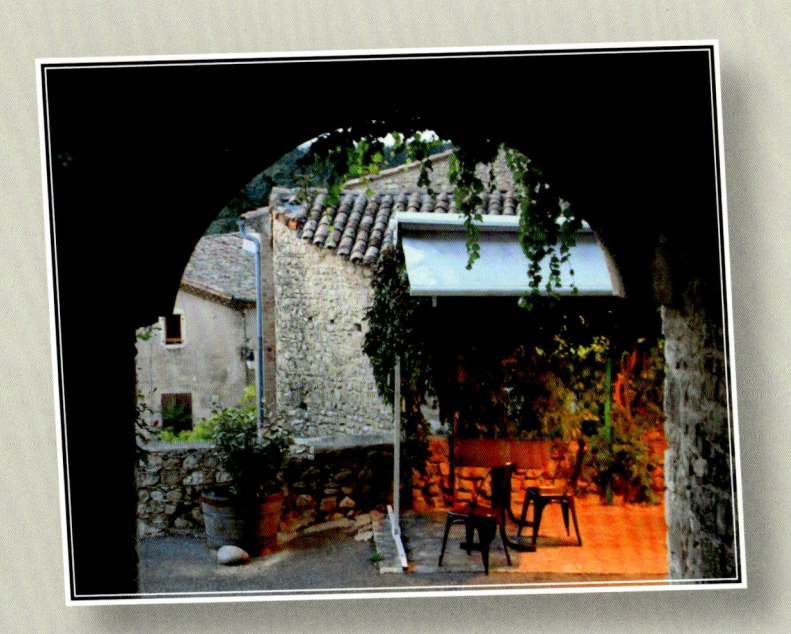

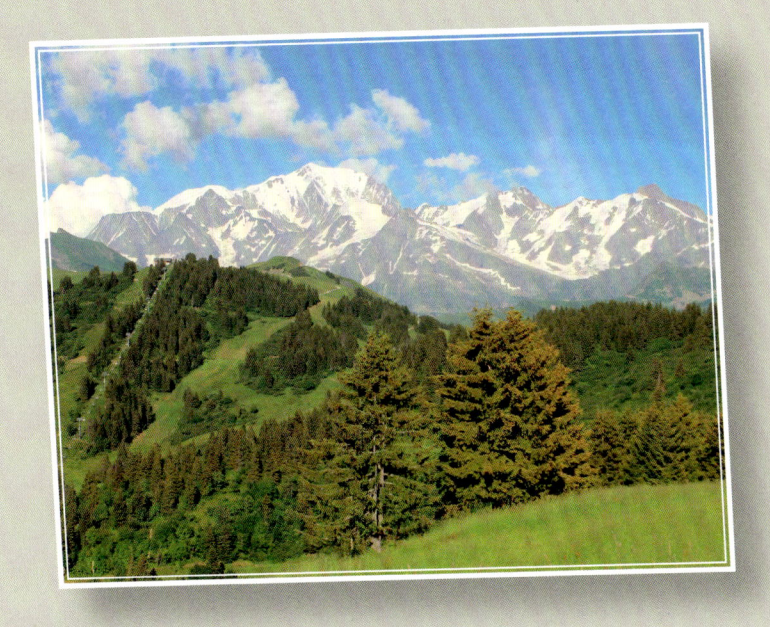

- **OTHER SIGNIFICANT LIQUORS**

Chartreuse, *Génépi des Alpes, Verveine du Velay*

NOTABLE THREE STAR RESTAURANTS

PAUL BOCUSE, 69660 Collonges- au-Mont-d'Or - chef Paul Bocuse
TROISGROS, 42300 Roanne – chef Michel Troisgros
GEORGES BLANC, 01540 Vonnas – chef Georges Blanc
PIC, 26000 Valence – chef Anne-Sophie Pic
RÉGIS ET JACQUES MARCON, 43290 St. Bonnet-le-Froid – chefs Régis et Jacques Marcon
LA BOUITTE, 73440 St Marcel – chefs René et Maxime Meilleur
FLOCONS DE SEL, 74120 Megève – chef Emmanuel Renaut

Soups
Soupes

46   Vegetable soup
Potage de légumes

48   French onion soup
Soupe à l'oignon gratinée

50   Carrot soup
Soupe à la carotte

52   Cream of mushroom soup
Velouté de champignons

54   Cream of courgette soup
Velouté de courgettes

56   Cream of pumpkin soup
Velouté de potiron

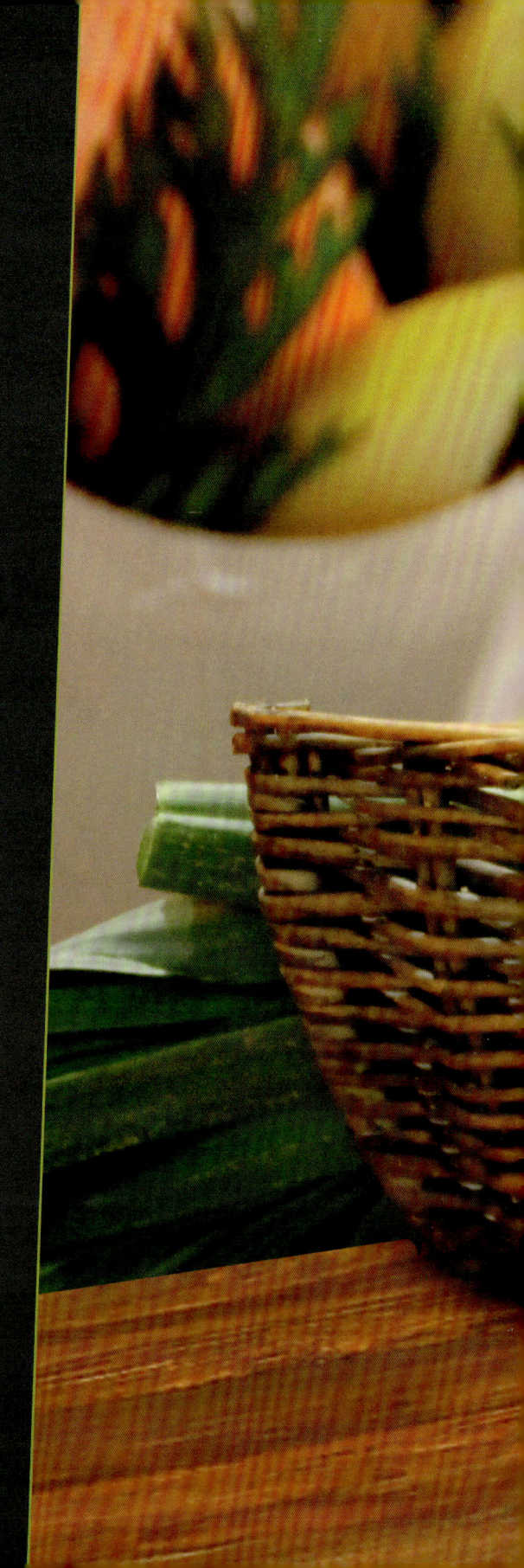

Soups *Soupes*

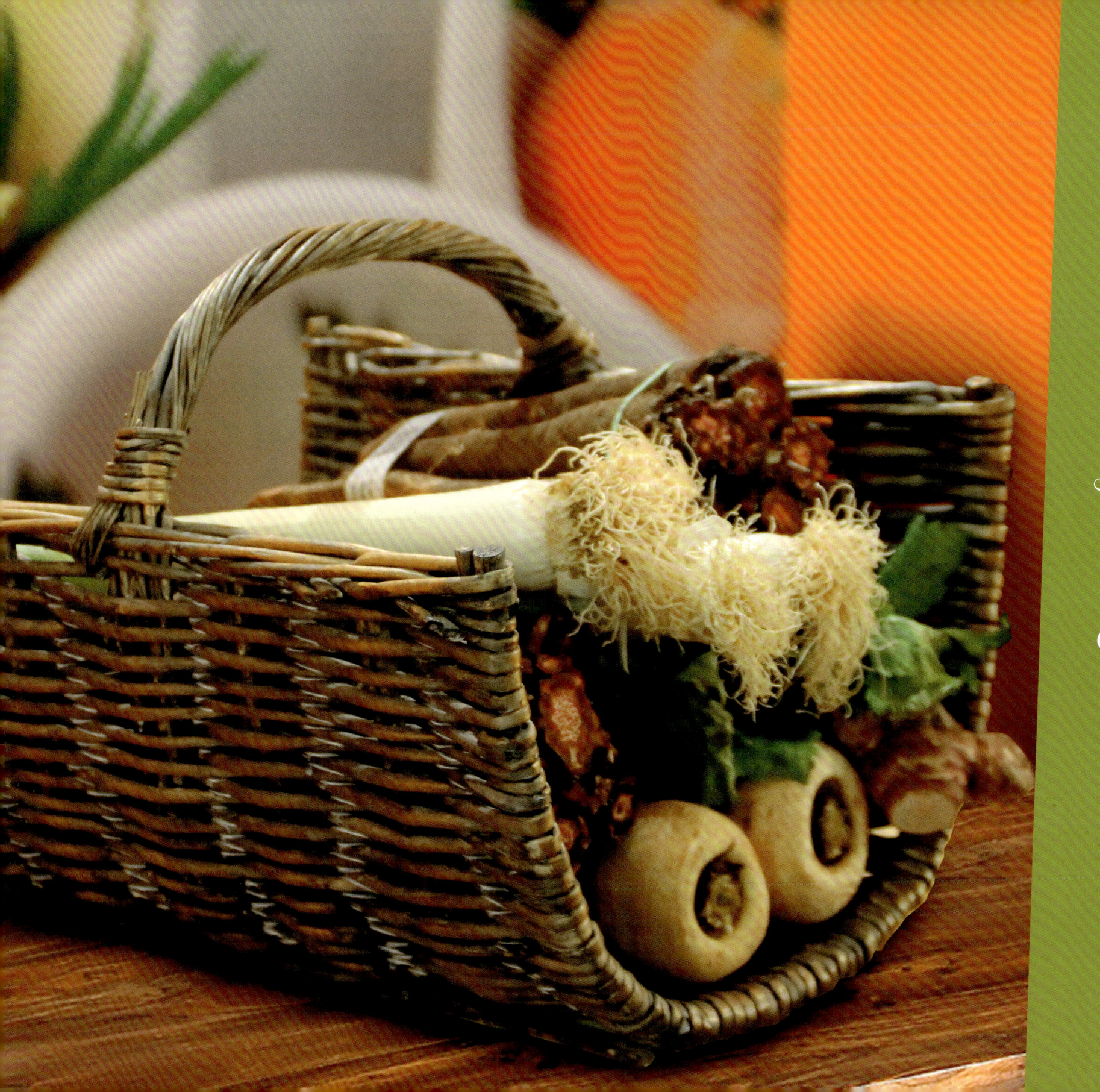

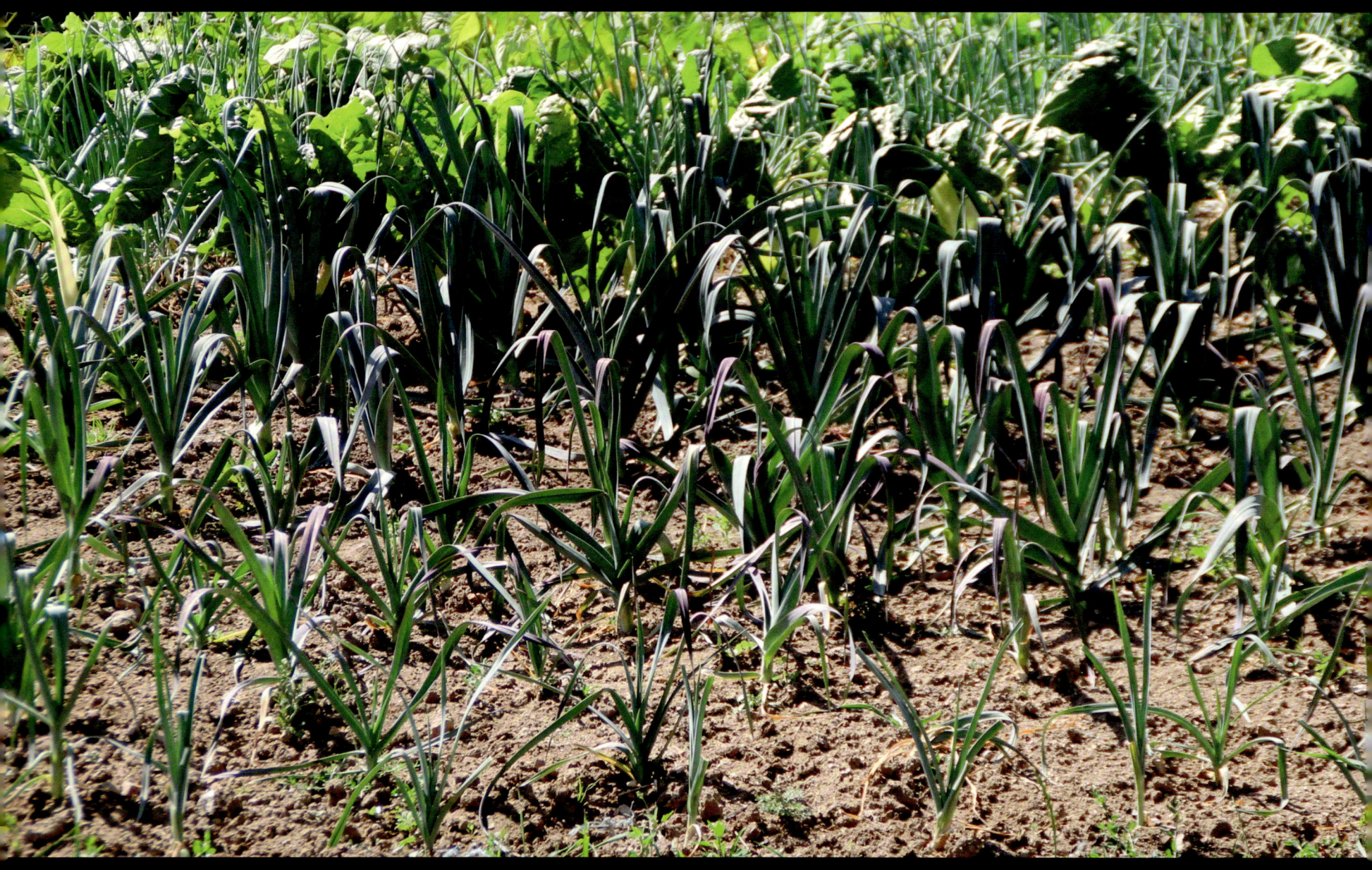

For a nourishing appetiser...

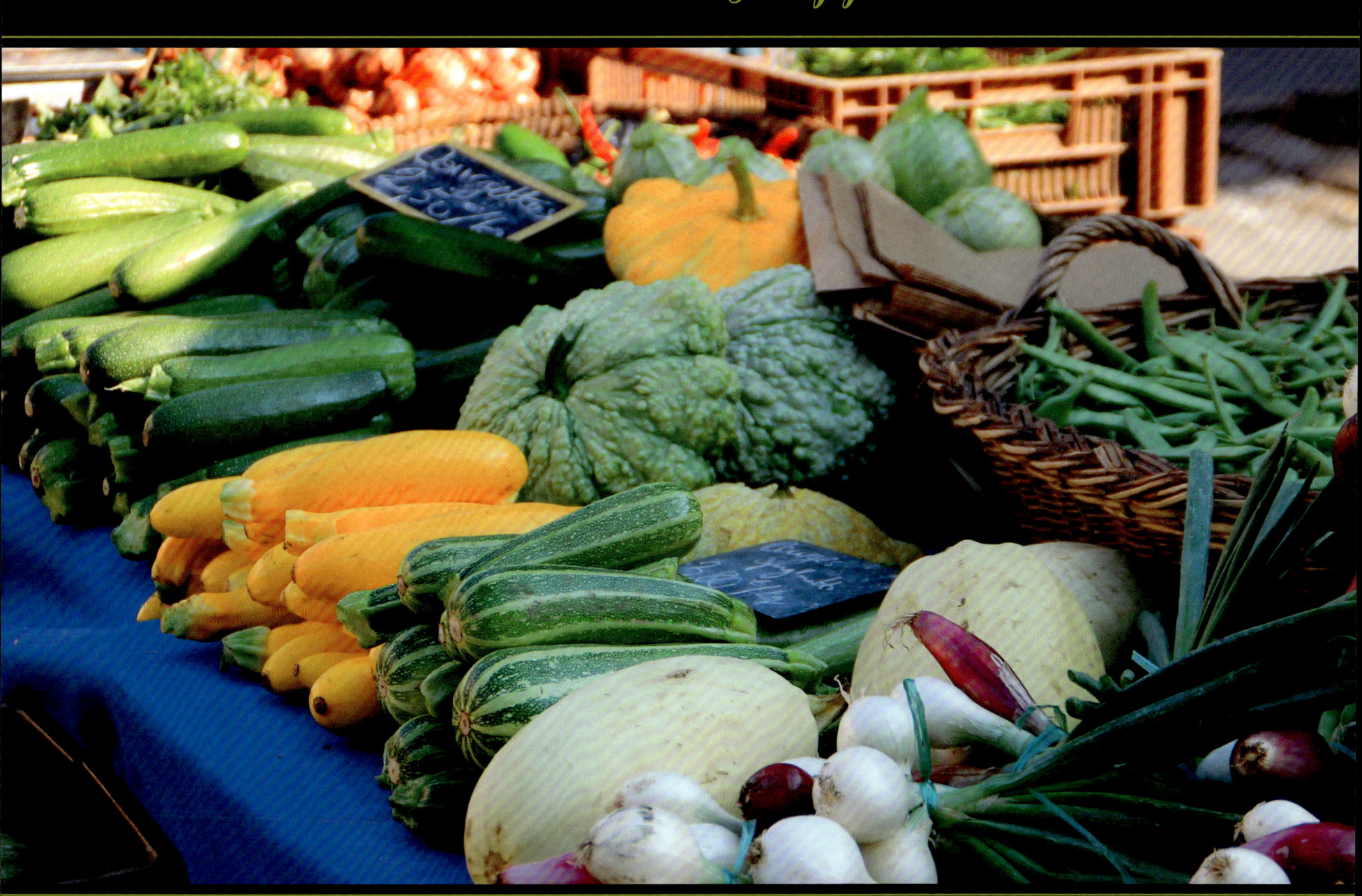

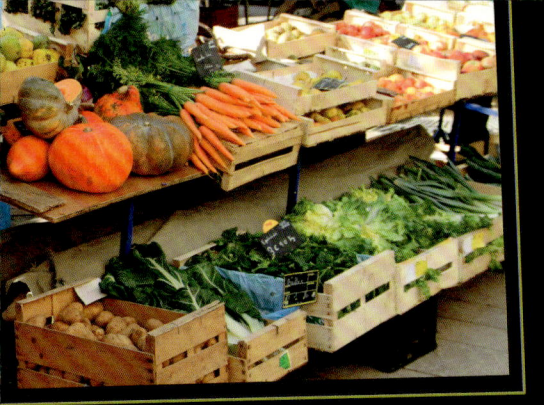

Vegetable soup
Potage de légumes

Peel the carrots and potatoes. Wash and cut all the vegetables into small pieces. Peel and finely chop the onion.

Heat the olive oil in a pressure cooker and lightly fry the onion, leeks and celery (leaving aside the leaves) for 5 minutes on a medium heat, stirring from time to time.

Add the carrots, potatoes, garlic clove and celery leaves. Cover with water. Season with salt and pepper.

Shut the lid and cook for 10 minutes once it has come up to pressure.

Blend the cooked vegetables in their cooking water.

Serve hot.

For a quicker option: cook the vegetables without frying the onions, leek and celery first.

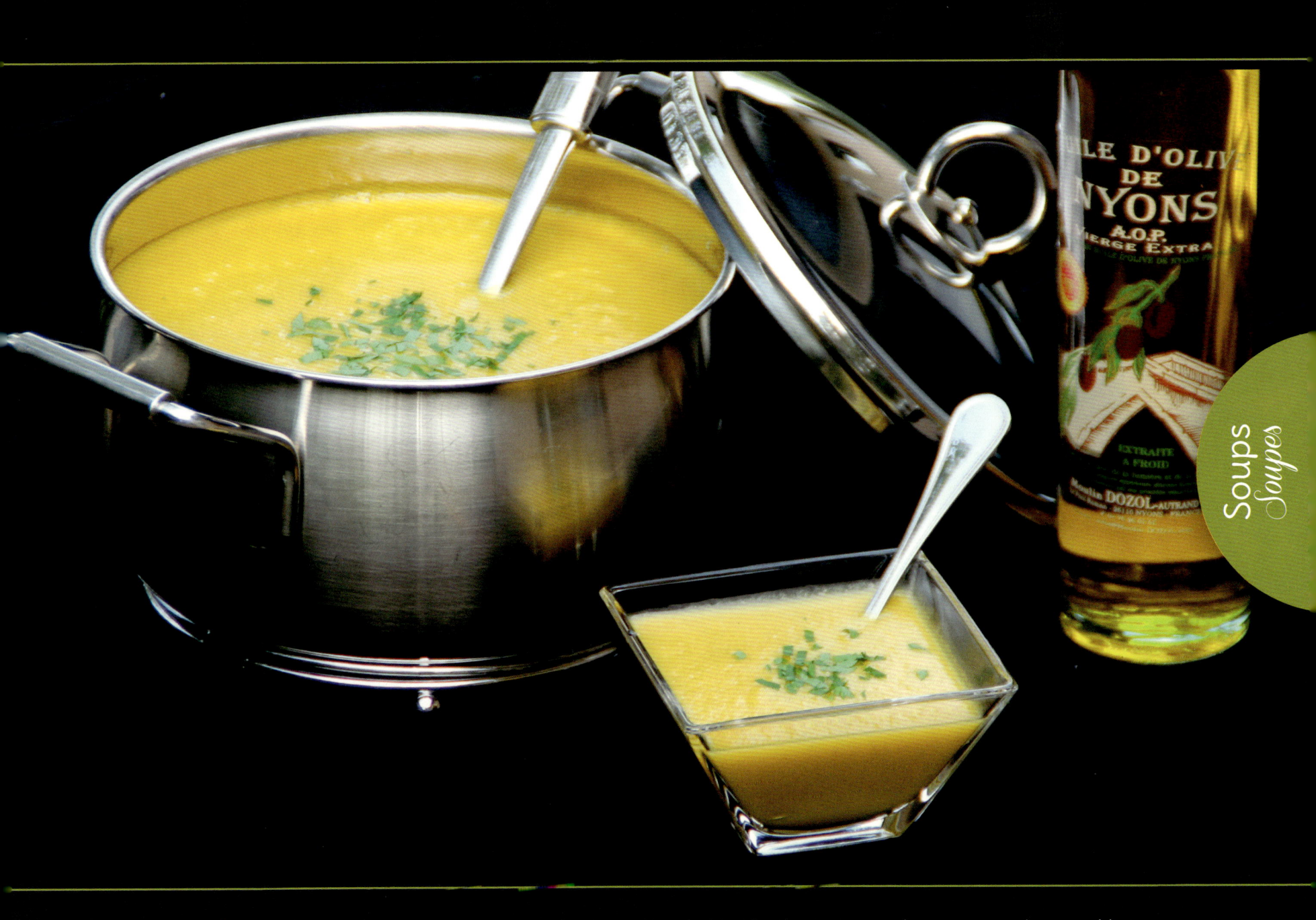

This is a good 'all-round' soup and can even be poured into babies' bottles to ensure they get enough vegetables.

Soups *Soupes*

47

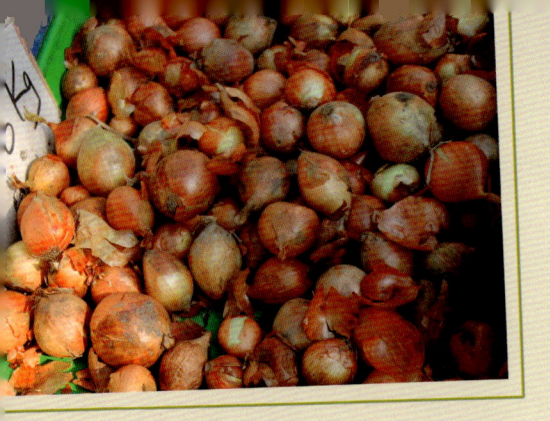

French onion soup
Soupe à l'oignon gratinée

Heat the olive oil in a saucepan, add the onions and garlic. Sauté over a low heat for about 30 minutes or until the onions are soft and lightly golden, stirring from time to time.

Sprinkle the cooked onions with the flour, salt and pepper.

Add the wine. Leave to cook on a moderate heat for about 10 minutes.

Bring the meat stock to the boil in another saucepan and then pour over the onion mix. Add the bay leaf.

Simmer for about 15 minutes. Remove the bay leaf.

Toast the bread on a baking sheet.

Pour the soup into individual ovenproof soup bowls, sprinkle with the toast and grated cheese. Season with pepper, and grill for approximately 5 - 10 minutes or until the cheese melts.

Oven: 220°C

- 4 tablespoons olive oil, or butter
- 400 g onions, sliced
- 1 garlic clove, crushed
- 1 tablespoon plain flour
- 100 ml dry white wine
- 1½ litres chicken or beef stock
- 1 bay leaf
- 250 g bread, cubed
- 80 g cheese, grated (*emmental* and *comté*)
- Salt and pepper

Soups
Soupes

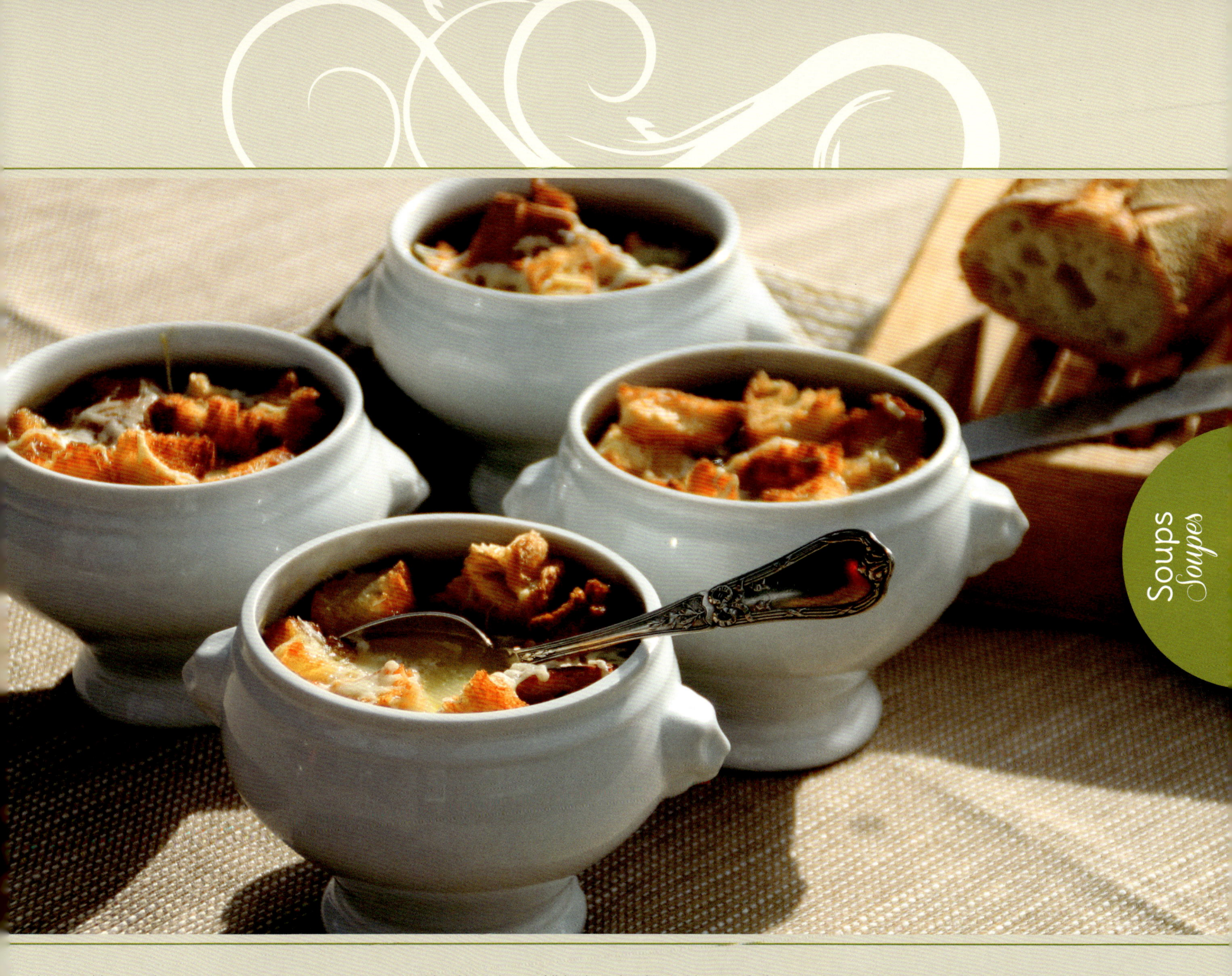

Legend has it that this great classic was invented by King Louis XV when he found himself alone in his huntsman's lodge with nothing to eat apart from onions, butter and champagne. He cooked all three together and thus the first French onion soup was created!

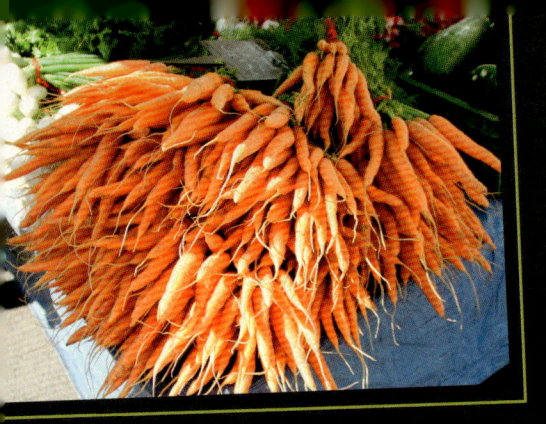

Carrot soup
Soupe à la carotte

Fry the bacon and onion together in a large saucepan for about 10 minutes, or until the onion begins to turn transparent.

Peel and slice the carrots and add to the pan. Cook for another 10 minutes.

Add the stock. Cover and simmer for about 1 hour.

Blend until smooth. Return to the heat adding the cream and season with salt and pepper.

Whisk before serving.

- 1 kg carrots
- 1 onion, chopped
- 100 g smoked bacon, chopped
- 2 ¼ litres vegetable stock
- 150 ml double cream
- Salt and pepper

Soups / *Soupes*

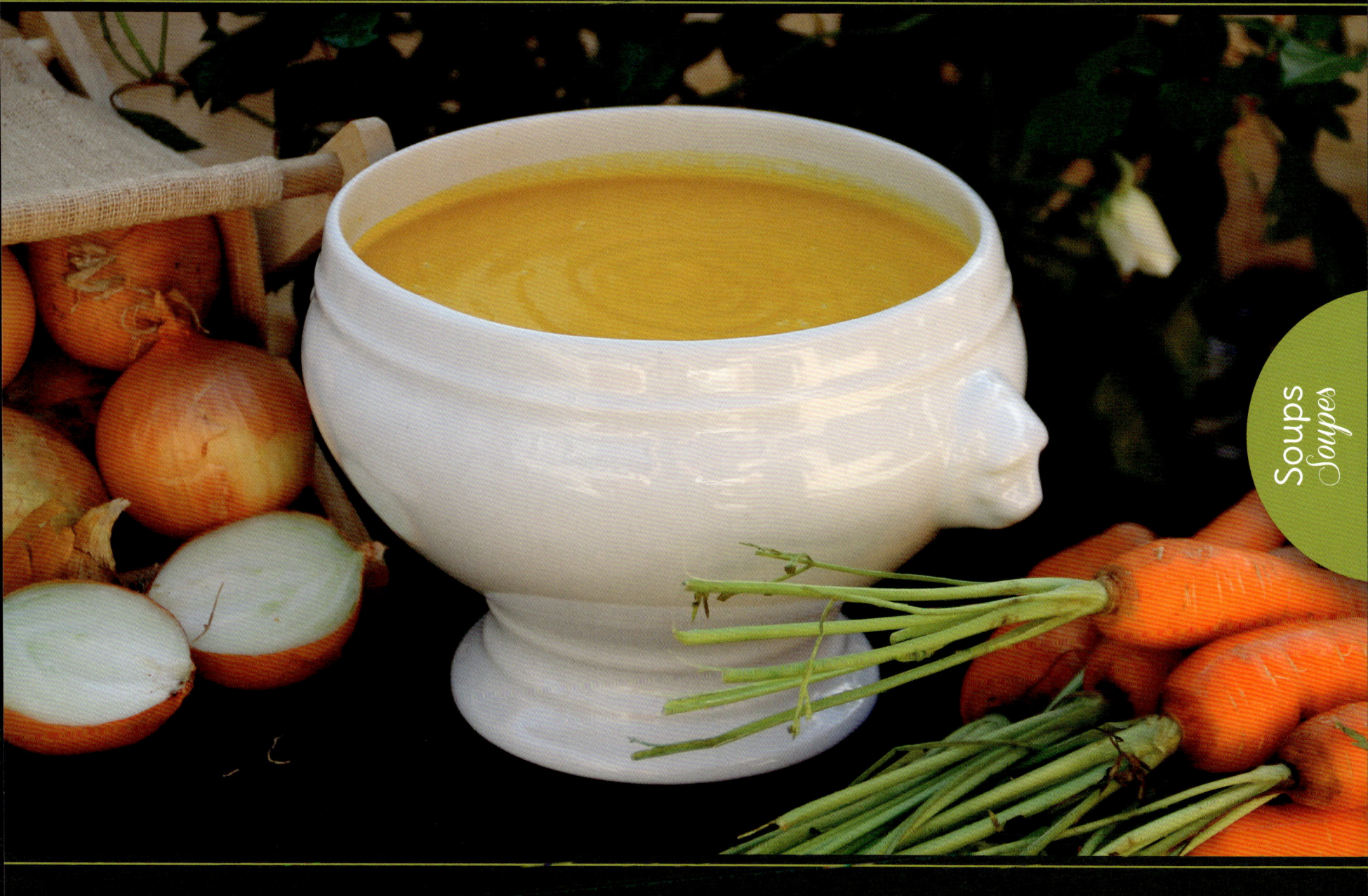

A delicious, nutritious, creamy soup with a hint of bacon.
This recipe is sometimes known as *soupe de Crécy*—Crécy is a town in the north of France famous for its carrots.

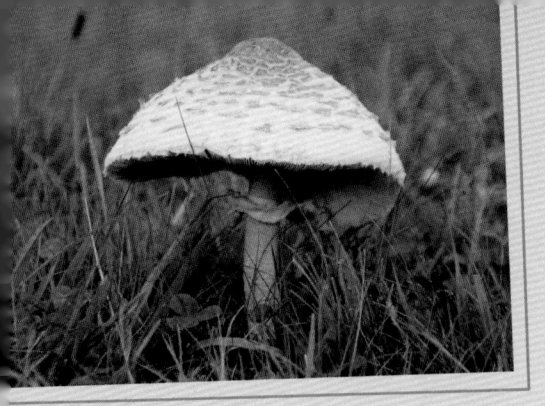

Cream of mushroom soup
Velouté de champignons

Heat some olive oil in a heavy-based saucepan and fry the onion and garlic for about 5 minutes. Add the mushrooms and fry until they are soft and the liquid absorbed.

Crumble the stock cube into the water, add to the mushroom mix and bring to the boil. Leave to simmer on a low heat for about 30 minutes.

Dissolve the cornflour in a little water and stir into the soup. Cook for another 5 minutes.

Blend until smooth, add the chives and parsley. *If preferred, add the herbs before blending for a smoother result with no decorative herbs visible.*

Return to the heat before serving and carefully stir in the cream. *Do not allow to boil.*

Season with salt and pepper, if necessary.

Pour into warm serving bowls and serve with a swirl of *crème fraîche* on top.

- 500 g fresh mushrooms, sliced
- 1 onion, chopped
- 2 garlic cloves, crushed
- Olive oil
- 1 stock cube
- 1 litre water
- 1 tablespoon cornflour
- 4 tablespoons double cream
- Salt and pepper
- A few chives, finely chopped
- A few sprigs of parsley, finely chopped
- *Crème fraîche* (optional)

Soups *Soupes*

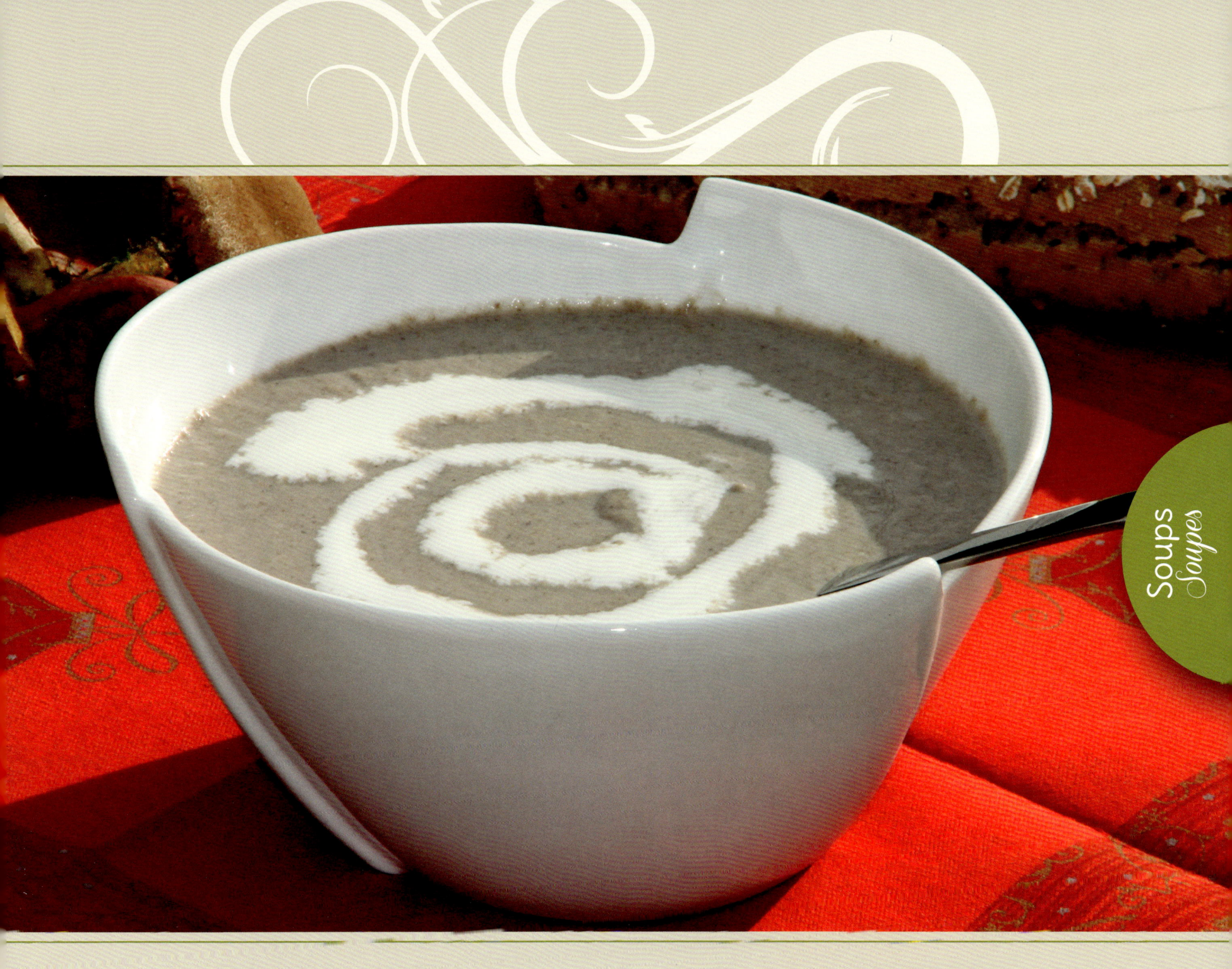

A delicious and simple soup to prepare. Enjoy in the autumn when mushrooms are in abundance. Alternatively, use *champignons de Paris* (button mushrooms), which can be found all year round.

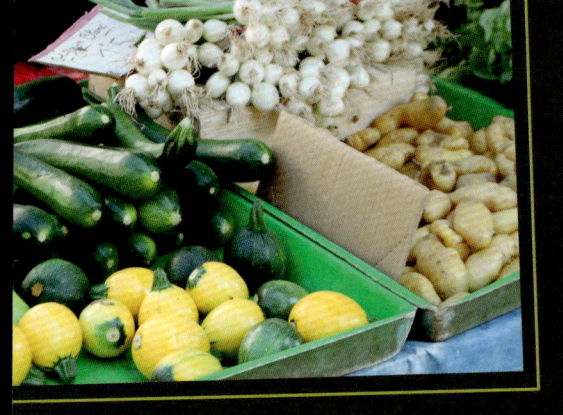

Cream of courgette soup
Velouté de courgettes

Wash and slice the courgettes.

Heat the olive oil in a large saucepan. Add the onion and garlic and fry until lightly coloured. Add the courgettes and continue cooking on a moderate heat for about 3 minutes. Do not allow the courgettes to colour.

Stir in the flour. Add the chicken stock, bring to the boil and simmer for about 20 minutes, stirring from time to time.

Add *La vache qui rit* ® and blend in a liquidiser. Season with salt and pepper.

Return to the saucepan and heat slightly.

Serve warm.

- 700 g courgettes *(zucchini)*
- 3 tablespoons olive oil
- 1 large onion, chopped
- 1 garlic clove, crushed
- 1 level tablespoon plain flour or cornflour
- 1 litre chicken stock
- 50 g *La vache qui rit* ® cheese
- Salt and pepper

For a variation, replace *La vache qui rit* ® cheese with a soft cheese like *Garlic and Herbs Boursin* ® cheese or a fresh goat's cheese.

Soups *Soupes*

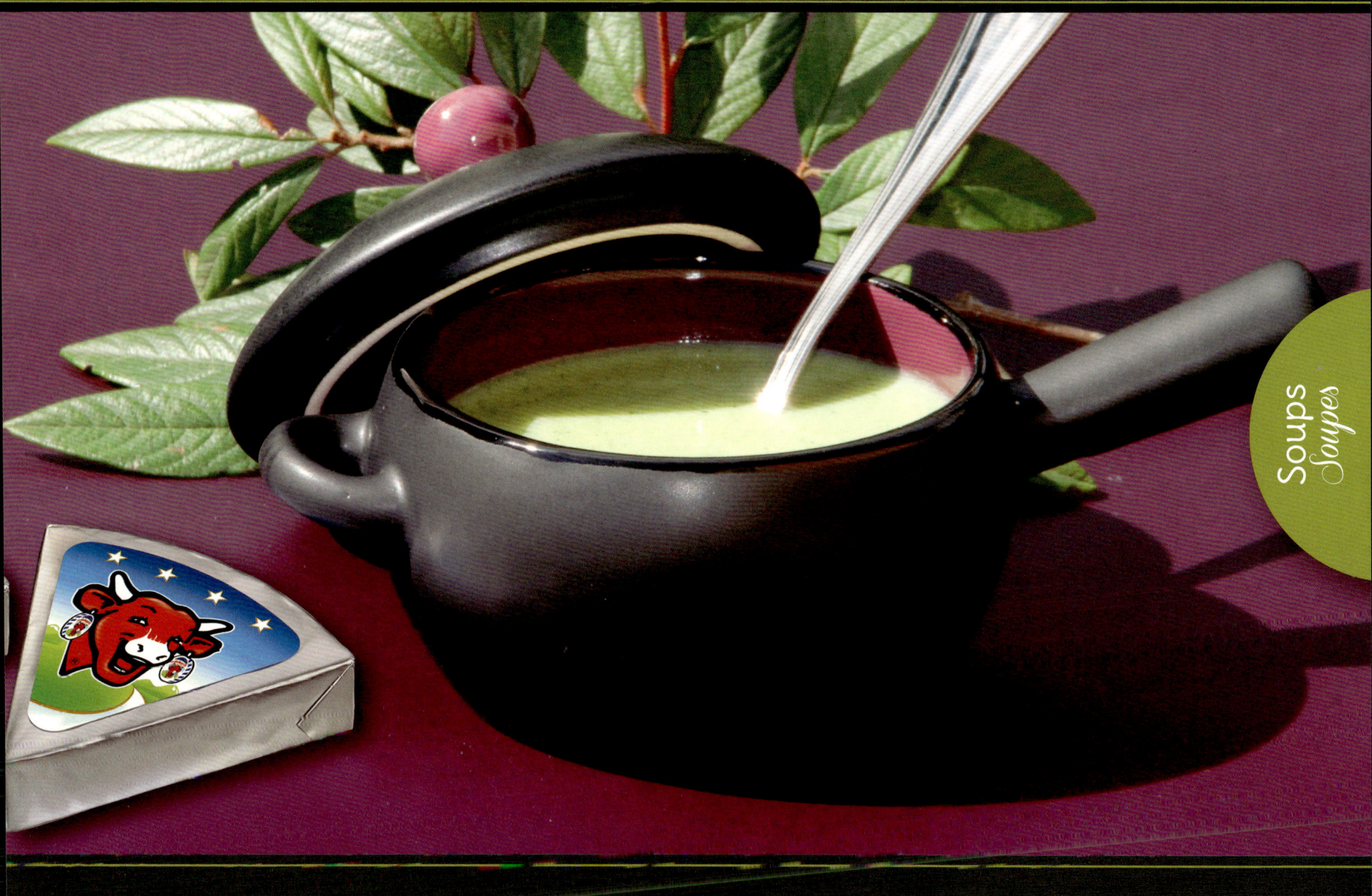

La vache qui rit ® is a processed cheese that was first produced in France in 1921, by Léon Bel.
Over 90 years later, it is still being enjoyed in more than 120 different countries.
Known as The laughing cow ® (in English), *Die lachende kuh* ®(in German), *Den skrattande kon* ® (in Swedish) or *La vaca que rie* ® (in Spanish).

55

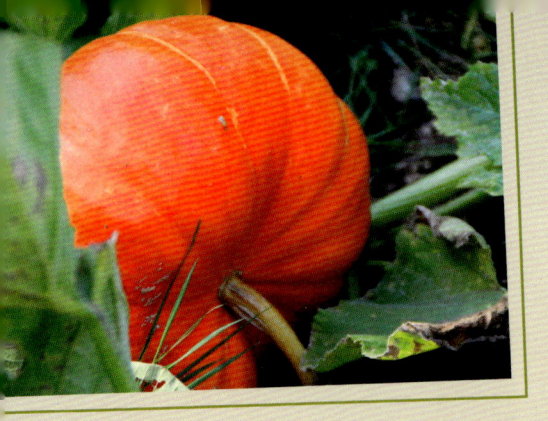

Cream of pumpkin soup
Velouté de potiron

Cut the leek in half lengthways, wash and slice.

Heat the olive oil in a pressure cooker and lightly fry the leek. Dissolve the stock cube in water, add to the leek with all the remaining ingredients (except cream).

Add the water with the chicken stock cube. Season with salt.

Close the lid and bring to pressure. Cook for 8 minutes once it is up to pressure.

Add the cream and blend.

Serve hot with grilled croûtons.

- 1 kg pumpkin, peeled and chopped
- 2 tablespoons olive oil
- 1 large leek - white part only
- 3 carrots (250 g), peeled and chopped
- 1 garlic clove, cut in half
- Leaves from 1 celery stalk
- 2 level teaspoons nutmeg
- 2 pinches curry powder
- 1 litre water
- 1 chicken stock cube
- 2 teaspoons salt
- 2 tablespoons double cream

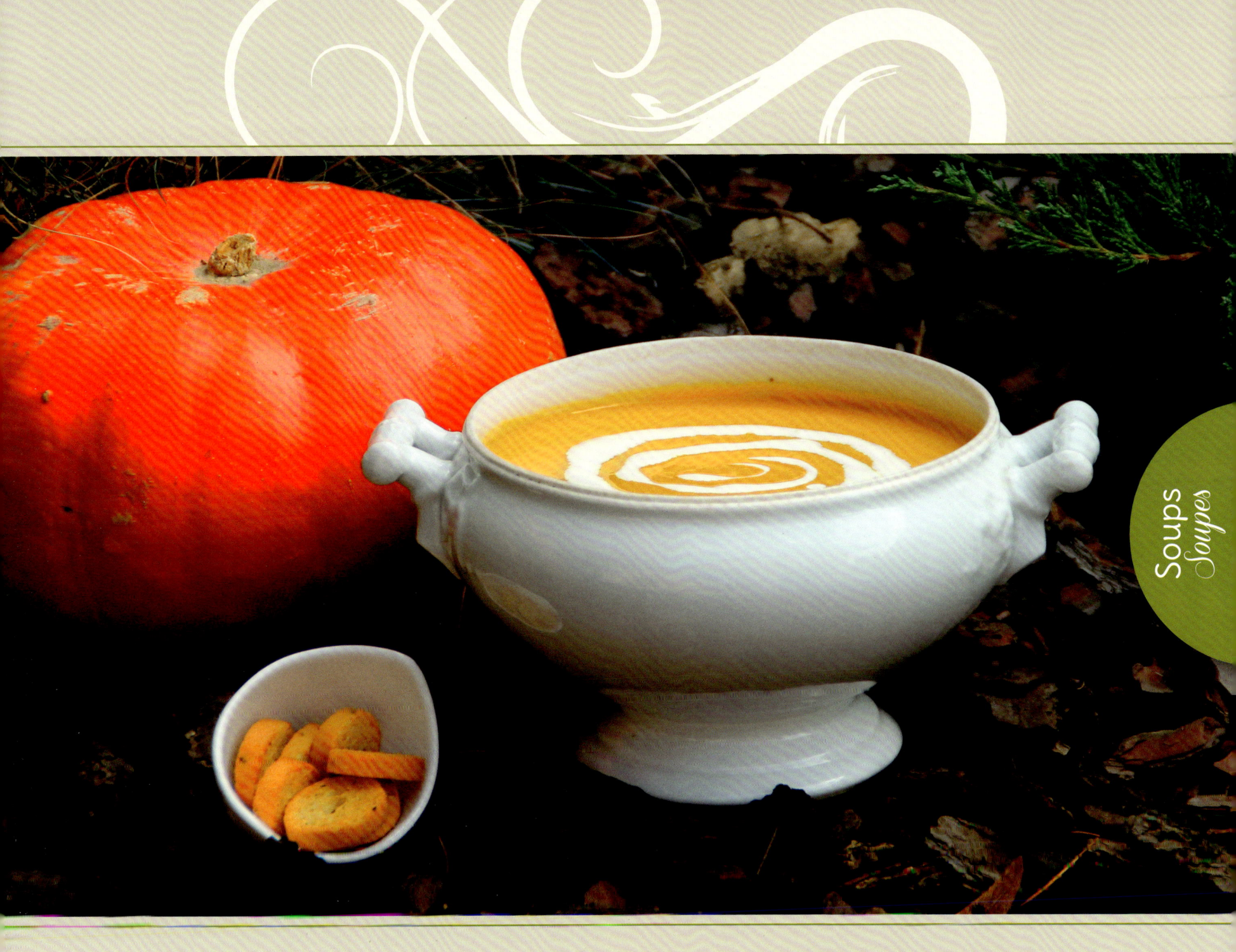

Delicious! For a winter's evening meal this thick, orange-coloured soup is very tempting—even the children enjoy it.

Soups *Soupes*

57

Salads
Salades

62 Walnut salad
Salade aux noix

64 Chicory salad
Salade d'endives

66 French bean salad
Salade de haricots verts

68 Lentil salad with bacon and tomatoes
Salade de lentilles aux lardons et tomates

68 Lentil salad with broccoli
Salade de lentilles au brocoli

70 Dandelion and bacon salad
Salade de pissenlits aux lardons

72 Lamb's lettuce with *ravioles* and walnuts
Salade de mâche aux ravioles et noix

74 Niçoise salad
Salade niçoise

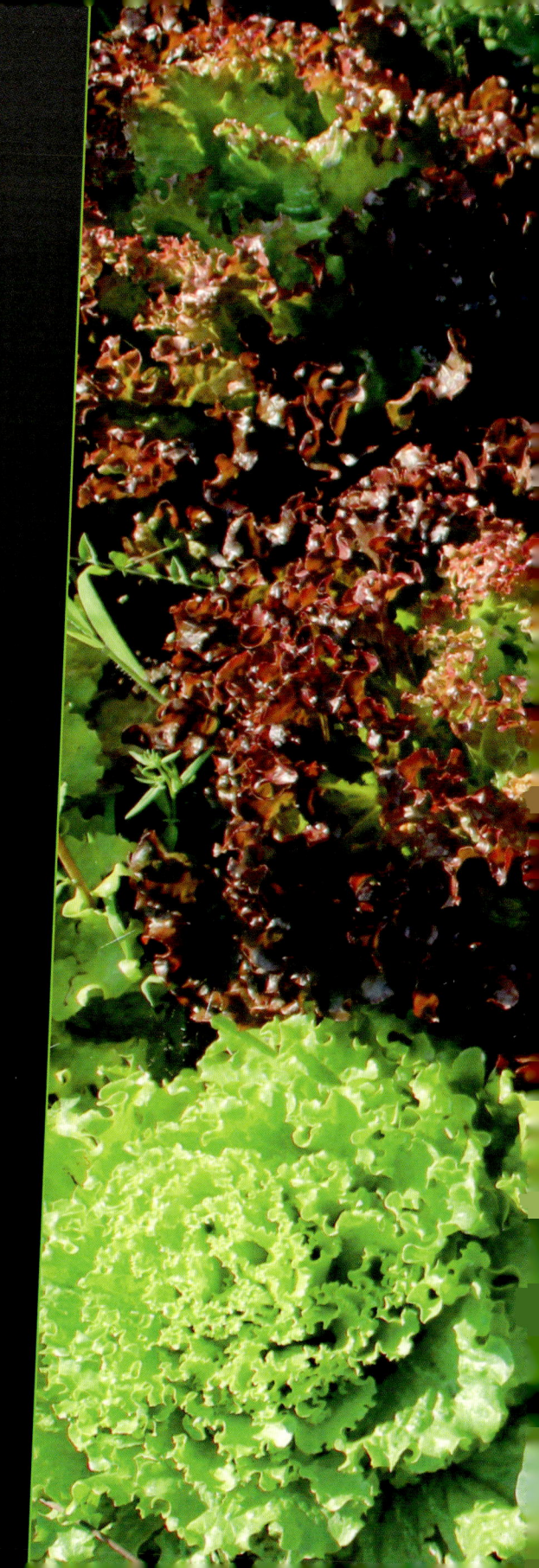

Salads *Salades*

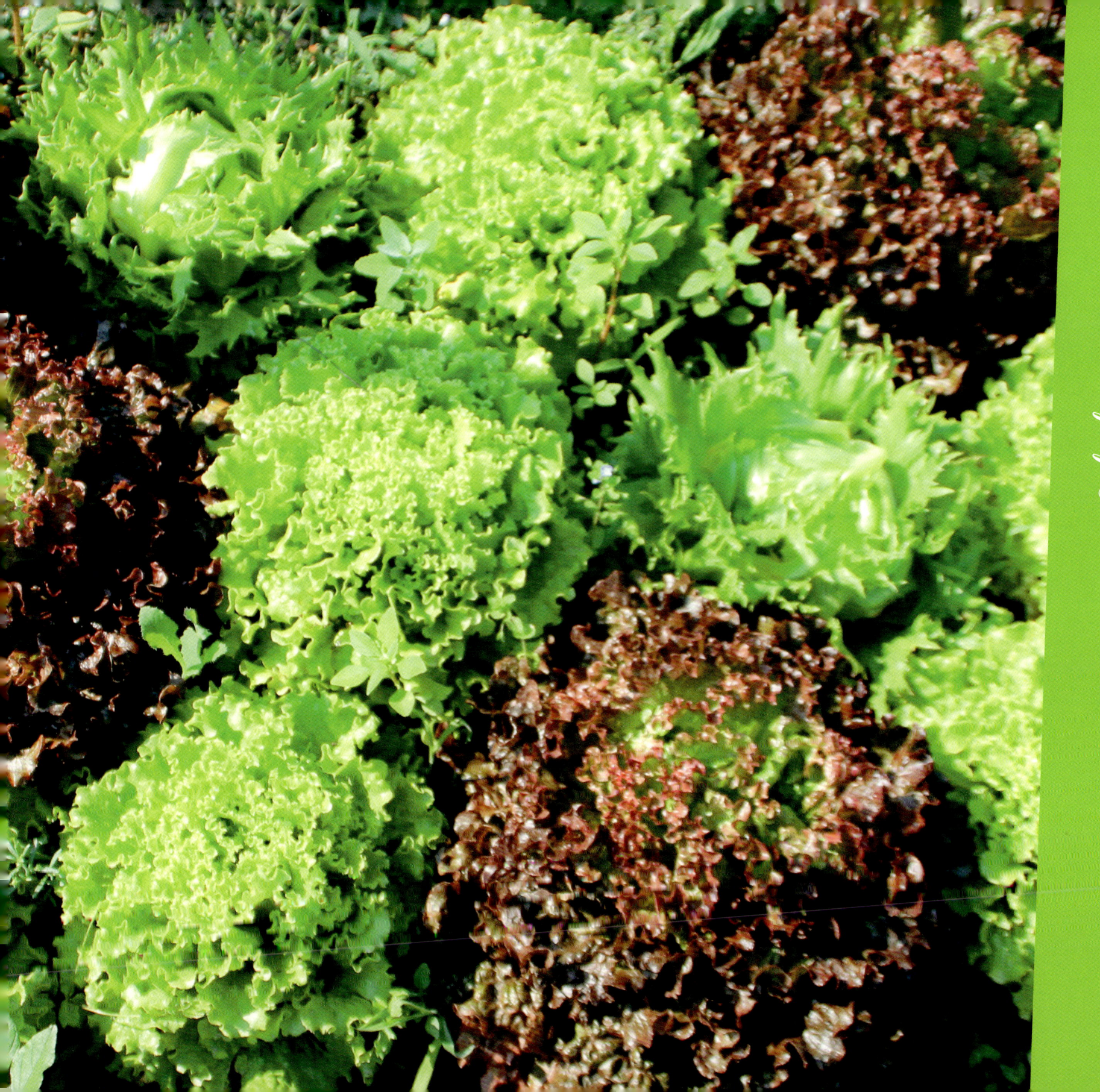

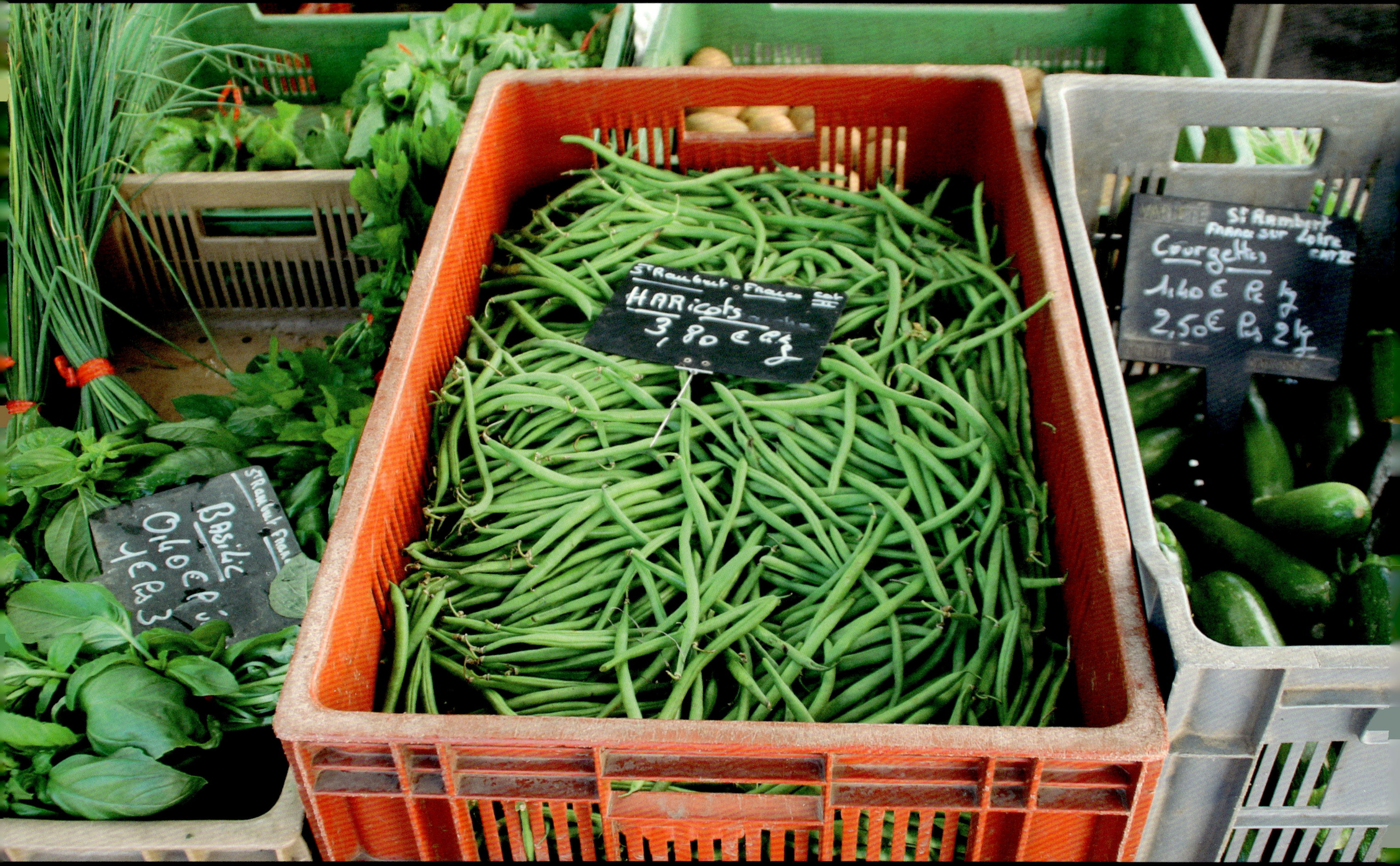
HARicots
3,80 €
Courgettes
1,40 €
2,50 €
Basilic

A healthy choice...

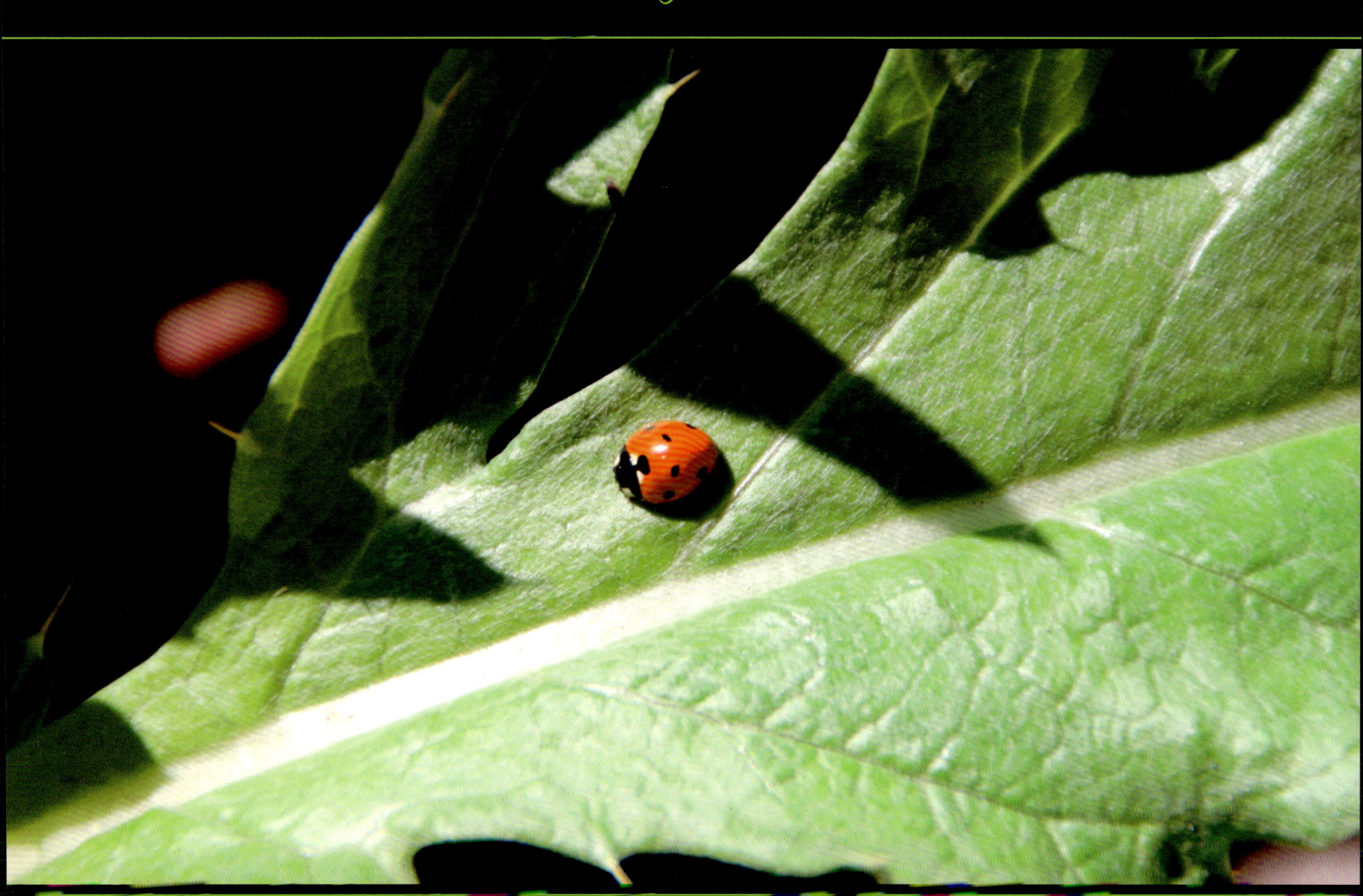

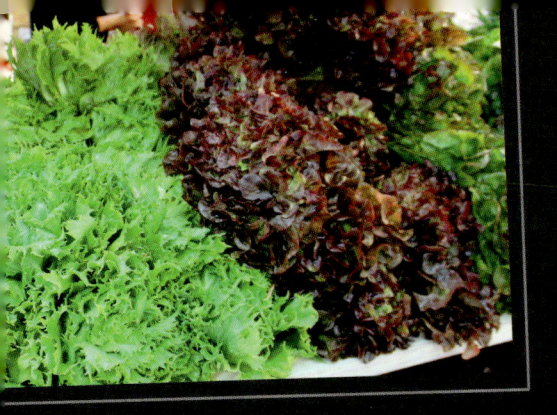

Walnut salad
Salade aux noix

Flavour the bread slices by rubbing with the garlic. Cut into cubes. Heat some oil in a frying pan and fry the bread pieces until golden and crispy. Set aside.

Place the walnuts in a bowl and cover with boiling water. Leave to soak for 1 minute then drain and dry.

Fry the bacon until crispy. Set aside.

Fry the walnuts in the frying pan for several minutes or until they are golden.

Cut the washed salad and place on a serving plate or in a salad bowl.

PREPARE THE VINAIGRETTE according to the recipe (see *recettes de base*), but using the ingredients indicated.

Sprinkle the walnuts and the bacon over the lettuce. Add vinaigrette according to taste and toss well.

Sprinkle with croûtons just before serving.

Serves approx. 12 persons

- 100 g French bread, sliced
- 1 garlic clove, halved
- 70 g walnuts, broken
- 150 g smoked bacon, chopped
- 1 Batavia lettuce (or a mixture of salad leaves)

Vinaigrette:

- 1 tablespoon Dijon mustard
- 3 tablespoons cider vinegar
- 3 tablespoons walnut oil
- 3 tablespoons olive oil
- 3 tablespoons sunflower oil
- Salt and pepper

Salads
Salades

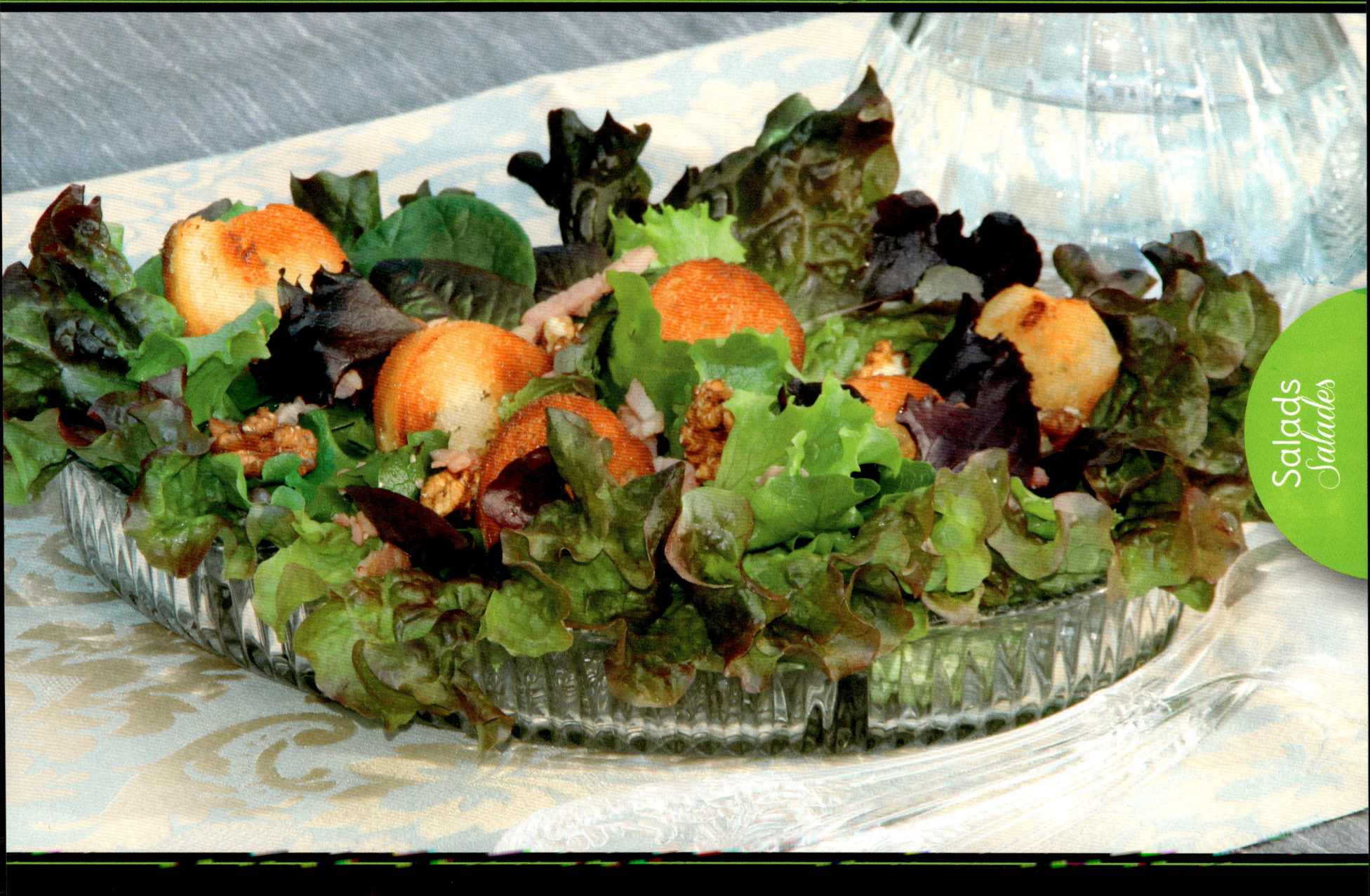

Although more than welcome on any summertime table, salads are always appreciated in any season. The choices and varieties of salads are never-ending.

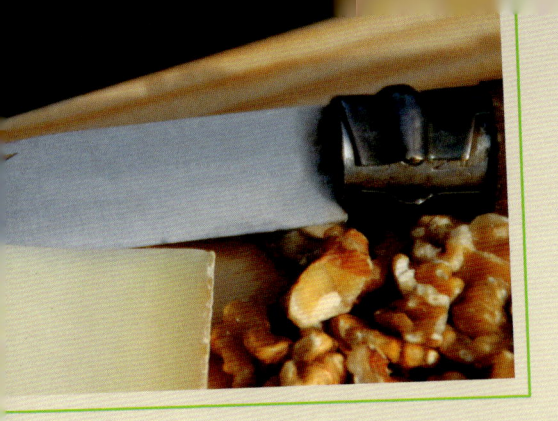

Chicory salad
Salade d'endives

Remove and discard any outer damaged leaves from the chicory. Cut off and discard the hard base. Cut into 1 cm slices.

Peel the hard-boiled egg and mash finely with a fork.

PREPARE THE VINAIGRETTE : Gradually mix in the vinegar, salt, mustard and oils with a fork. Add the mashed egg, chopped shallot and herbs.

Pour the vinaigrette into a salad bowl. Add the chicory, walnuts, cubes of cheese and ham.

Toss the salad in the vinaigrette just before serving. *Do not toss the salad in advance as the chicory quickly turns soggy.*

Serves approx. 3 - 4 persons

- 400 g chicory heads
- 30 g cured ham, cut in pieces
- 30 g *comté* cheese, cubed
- 20 g walnuts
- 1 hard-boiled egg

Vinaigrette:

- 2 teaspoons Dijon mustard
- 1 tablespoon walnut vinegar
- A generous pinch of salt
- 2 tablespoons olive oil
- 2 tablespoons walnut oil
- ½ small shallot, finely chopped
- Fresh herbs (parsley, chives, etc.), washed and finely chopped

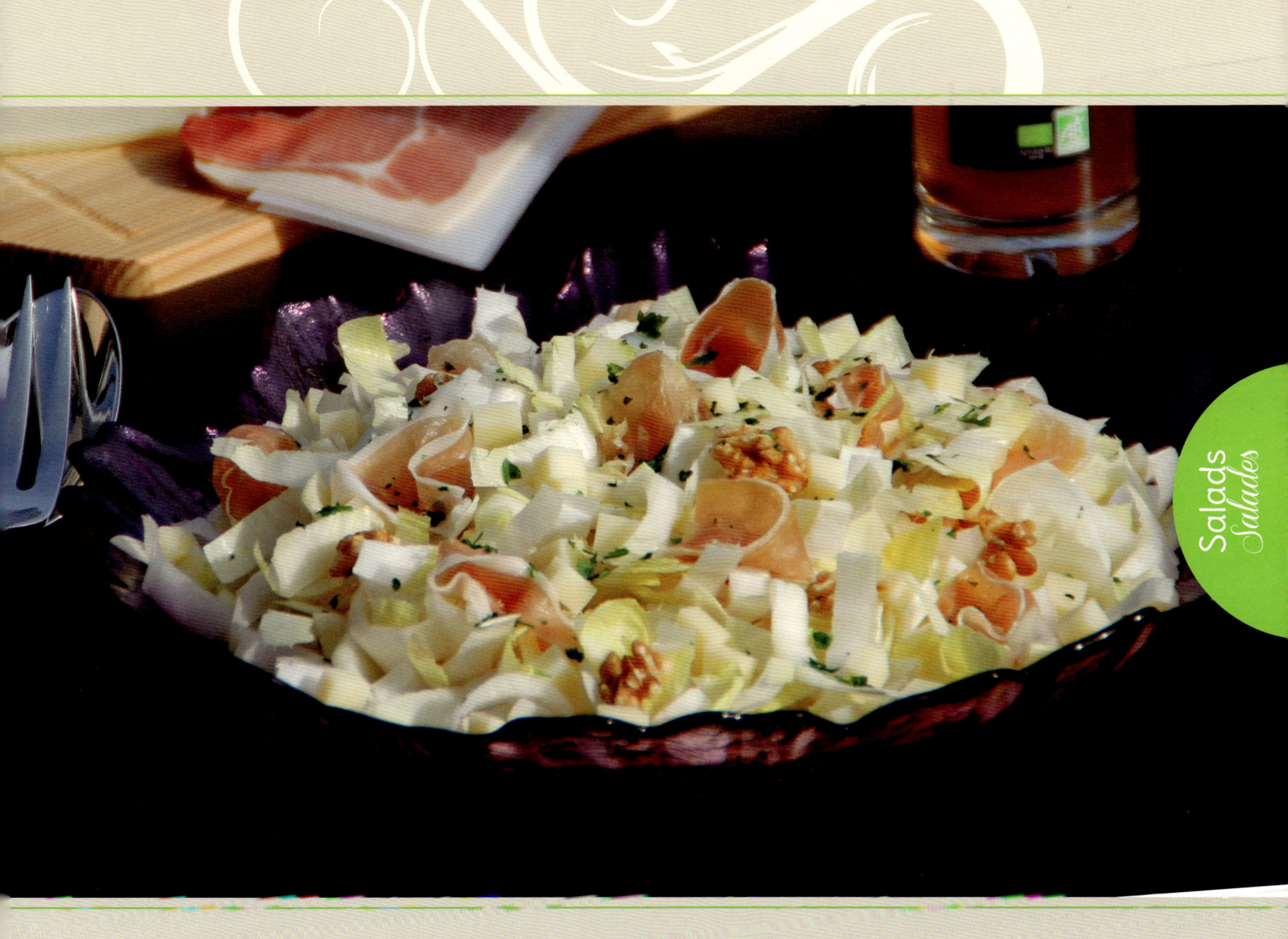

Chicory is the queen of winter salads! Serve it with apples, cubes of *fourme de Montbrison* (a blue cheese), figs, pine nuts, pears, pistachio nuts...

Salads
Salades

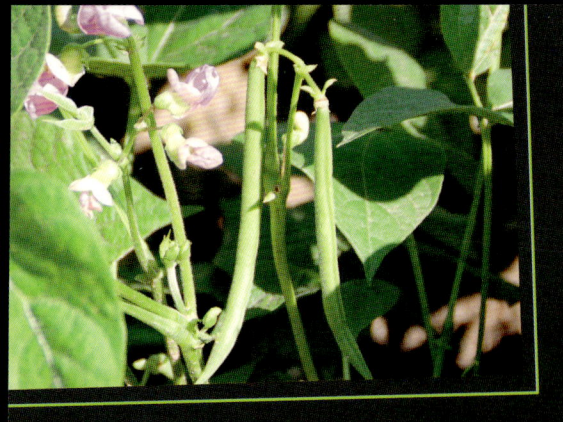

French bean salad
Salade de haricots verts

Boil the potatoes in salted water until soft. Drain them well and cut them in half. Leave aside until cool.

Bring beans to the boil in salted water, cooking for about 10 minutes once the water has begun to boil. Drain well. When cool, place the potatoes, tomatoes, beans, eggs, tuna and anchovies (if using) in a large serving bowl.

PREPARE THE VINAIGRETTE according to the recipe (see *recettes de base*), but using the ingredients as indicated.

Season the salad according to taste with some of the vinaigrette and toss gently.

Sprinkle chopped basil leaves over the top just before serving.

Serves 6 persons

- 350 g small, new potatoes
- 250 g cherry tomatoes
- 500 g fine, French beans, topped and tailed
- 2 hard-boiled eggs
- 200 g tinned tuna in olive oil, drained

Salads
Salades

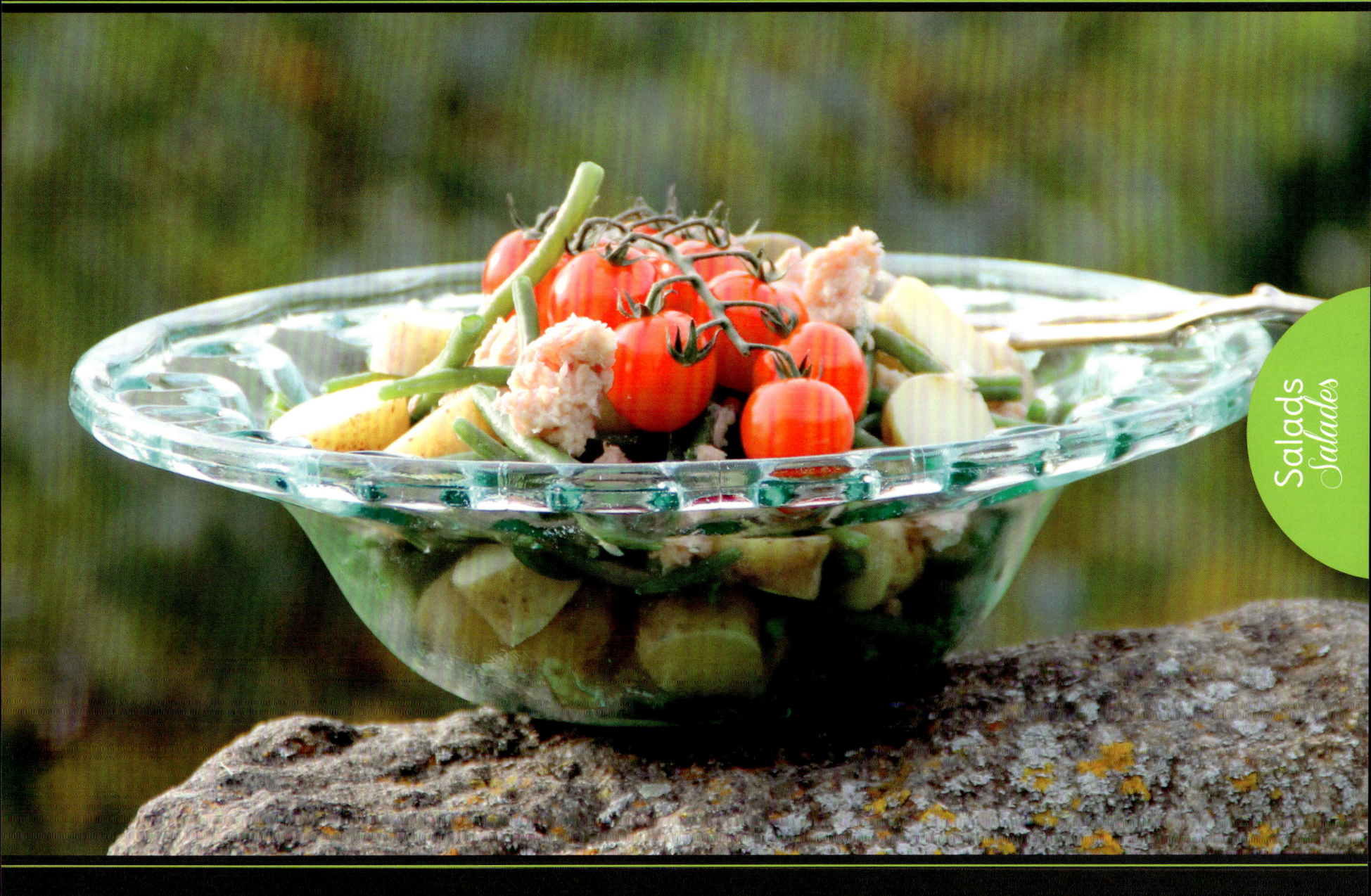

A very tasty, substantial salad which is also ideal for picnics or packed lunches.

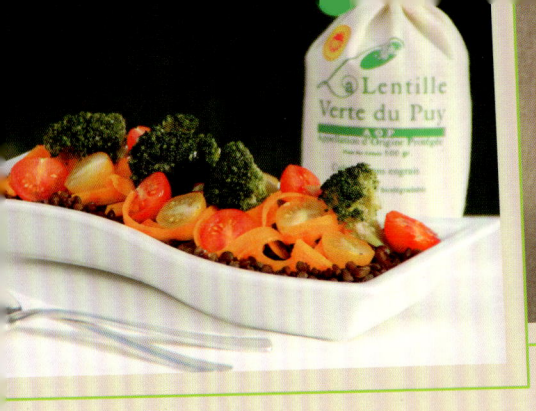

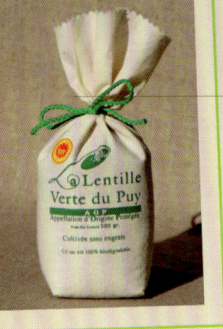

Lentil salad
Salade de lentilles

COOKING LENTILS:

Rinse the lentils quickly with cold water. Prick the onion with the clove. Place all the ingredients in a saucepan with the water. Cover and bring to the boil. Leave to boil steadily for about 20 - 30 minutes depending on preferred hardness. *For softer lentils: add a pinch of bicarbonate of soda to the water at the beginning of cooking.*

Remove the saucepan from the heat and leave to cool. Most of the water will have been absorbed by the lentils. Drain any excess. *This is a healthier way of cooking as it preserves all the valuable nutrients.* Remove and discard the onion.

- 200 g green lentils
- 600 ml cold water, unsalted
- 1 onion, peeled
- 1 whole clove

Lentil salad with bacon and tomatoes
Salade de lentilles aux lardons et tomates

Lightly fry the chopped bacon. Mix with the shallot into the lentils.

MAKE THE VINAIGRETTE according to the recipe and use to season the lentils according to taste. Place in a salad bowl.

Arrange the eggs and tomatoes on top and sprinkle with a few chives.

Serve cold.

- 200 g cooked lentils
- 150 g bacon, chopped
- 2 hard-boiled eggs, sliced
- 2 tomatoes
- 1 shallot, chopped

- 1 quantity of vinaigrette (see *recettes de base*)
- A few chives, chopped for decoration

Lentil salad with broccoli
Salade de lentilles au brocoli

Cut the carrots lengthways into 'ribbons', with a vegetable peeler.

Steam the carrots and broccoli for 20 minutes.

Finely slice the shallot and add to the lentils with the parsley.

MAKE THE VINAIGRETTE according to the recipe.

Place the lentils in a bowl with the carrots, broccoli and cherry tomatoes. Season with the vinaigrette according to taste.

Serve warm or cold.

- 200 g cooked lentils
- 2 carrots, peeled
- 120 g broccoli florets
- 100 g cherry tomatoes
- 4 sprigs fresh parsley, chopped
- 1 shallot

- 1 quantity of vinaigrette (see *recettes de base*)

Add some tuna or finely sliced smoked sausage for a more substantial salad, ideal for a packed lunch.

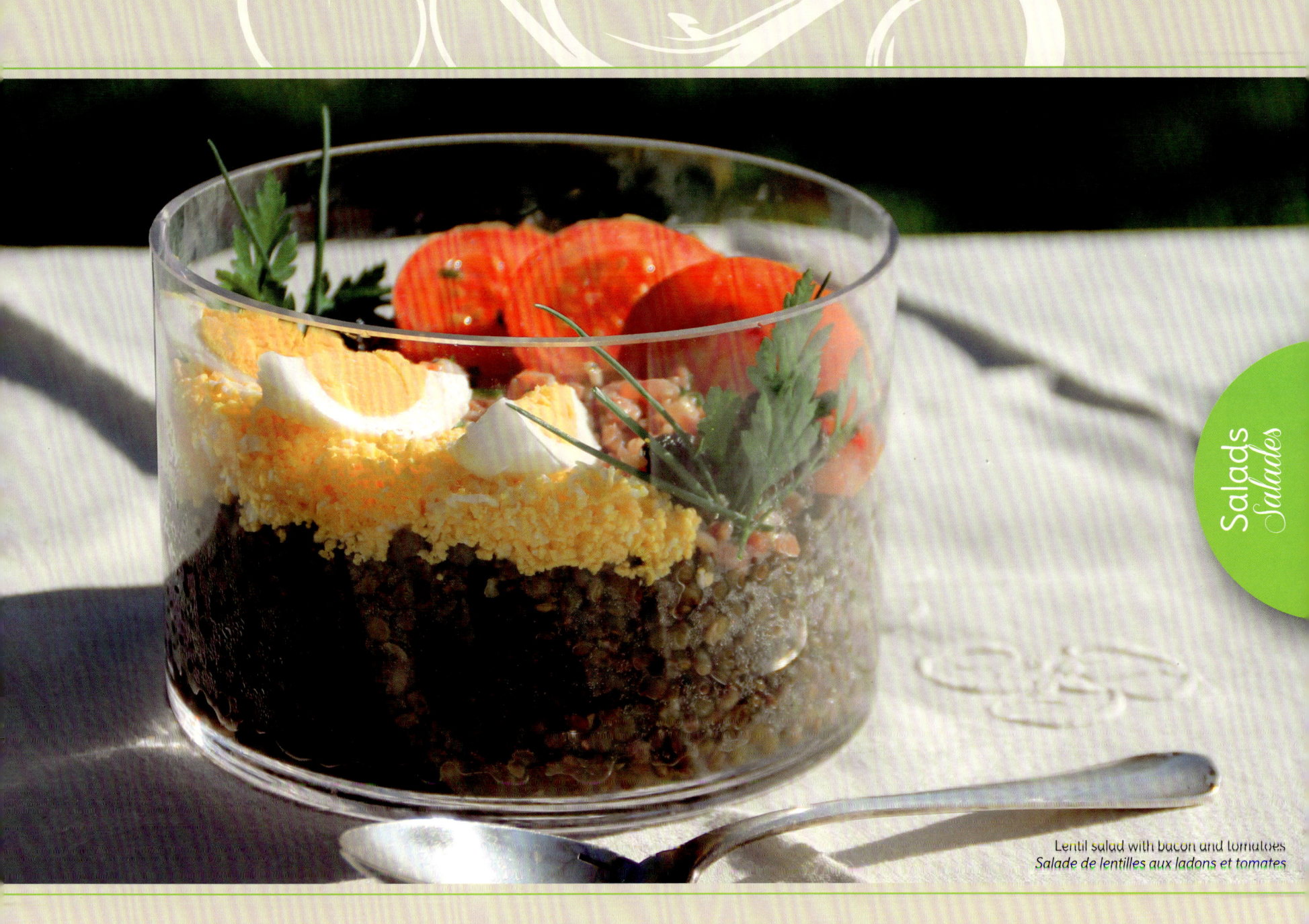

Lentil salad with bacon and tomatoes
Salade de lentilles aux lardons et tomates

Salads
Salades

Lentils are a French speciality and a miraculous pulse containing many unrefined fibres which are nourishing and are easier to digest. They contain four times more fibre than rice, pasta or potatoes, are rich in vitamins (B1, B2, B6), iron and calcium and are known to reduce cholesterol level. A plate of lentils with the same quantity of cereals contains the same amount of protein as one portion of meat.

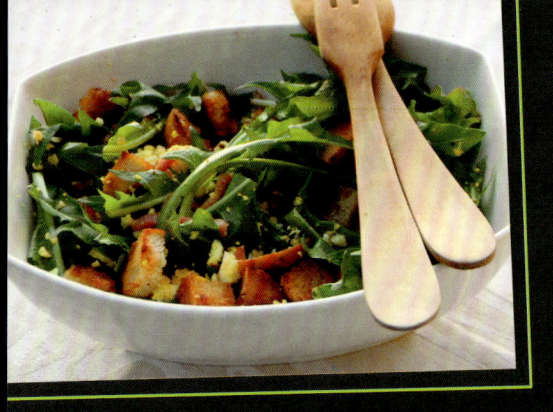

Dandelion and bacon salad
Salade de pissenlits aux lardons

Remove the muddy stalk ends and wash the dandelion leaves thoroughly in water. Cut the smoked bacon and fry until golden. Drain and put aside.

Heat the oil in the same frying pan and fry the pieces of bread until golden. Drain and put aside with the bacon.

Hard boil the egg. Peel and chop it finely.

MAKE THE VINAIGRETTE: Place the mustard, vinegar, salt and pepper, garlic and shallot in a small bowl. Add the oils and mix thoroughly.

Place the dandelion leaves, bacon and bread cubes into a large salad bowl. Drizzle the vinaigrette over the salad then toss together. Sprinkle the hard-boiled egg over the top.

Serve immediately.

Serves approx. 3 - 4 persons

- 100 g dandelion leaves
- 80 g smoked bacon
- 50 g of white bread, cubed
- 2-3 tablespoons oil
- 1 egg

Vinaigrette:

- ½ shallot, finely chopped
- ½ garlic clove, crushed
- 1 ½ tablespoons wine vinegar
- 1 rounded teaspoon strong mustard
- 2 tablespoons olive oil
- 2 tablespoons peanut oil
- 1 tablespoon walnut oil
- Salt and pepper

Choose dandelions which have not yet come into flower. Once they flower the leaves become too bitter.

When washing dandelion or lettuce leaves—especially if grown wild or in the garden—they should be rinsed in five changes of water.

Salads
Salades

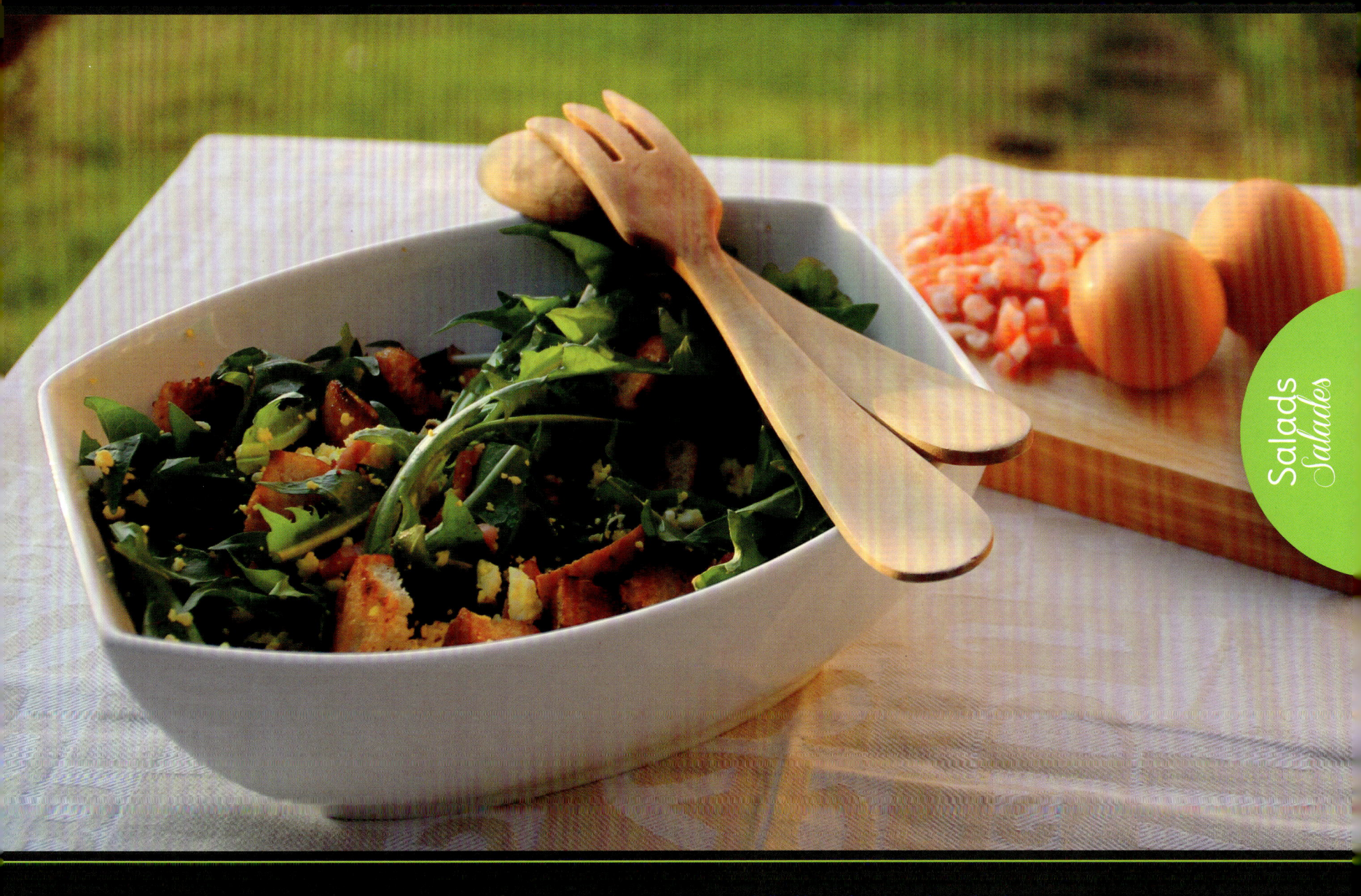

Dandelions are not just a garden weed—they are full of beneficial medicinal values.
The young leaves contain vitamin C and beta-carotene and are regarded as a laxative and a tonic as well as being dietetic

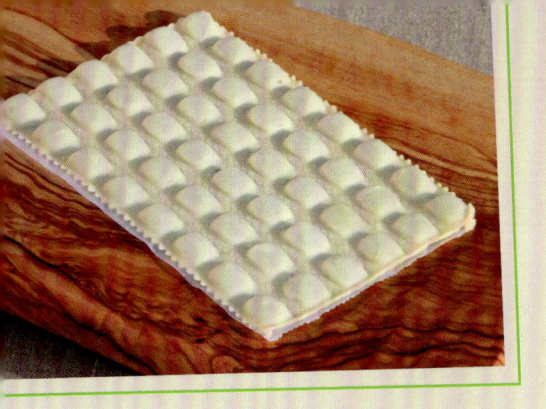

Lamb's lettuce with *ravioles* and walnuts
Salade de mâche aux ravioles et noix

Plunge the *ravioles* in 1 litre of boiling, salted water and cook for 1 minute.

Carefully remove them using a slotted spoon and plunge them in cold water. Separate them one by one. Drain.

Arrange the lamb's lettuce onto 4 separate plates, topping with the *ravioles*, walnuts and parsley.

PREPARE THE VINAIGRETTE by mixing all the ingredients together, and drizzle over the salad according to taste, just before serving. *You may not need all the vinaigrette.*

Serves approx. 4 persons

- 1 sheet of *ravioles*
- 1 handful walnuts
- 3 - 4 handfuls lamb's lettuce
- Parsley, chopped

Vinaigrette:

- 1 tablespoon walnut vinegar
- 2 tablespoons walnut oil
- 1 tablespoon oil
- Salt and pepper

Salads
Salades

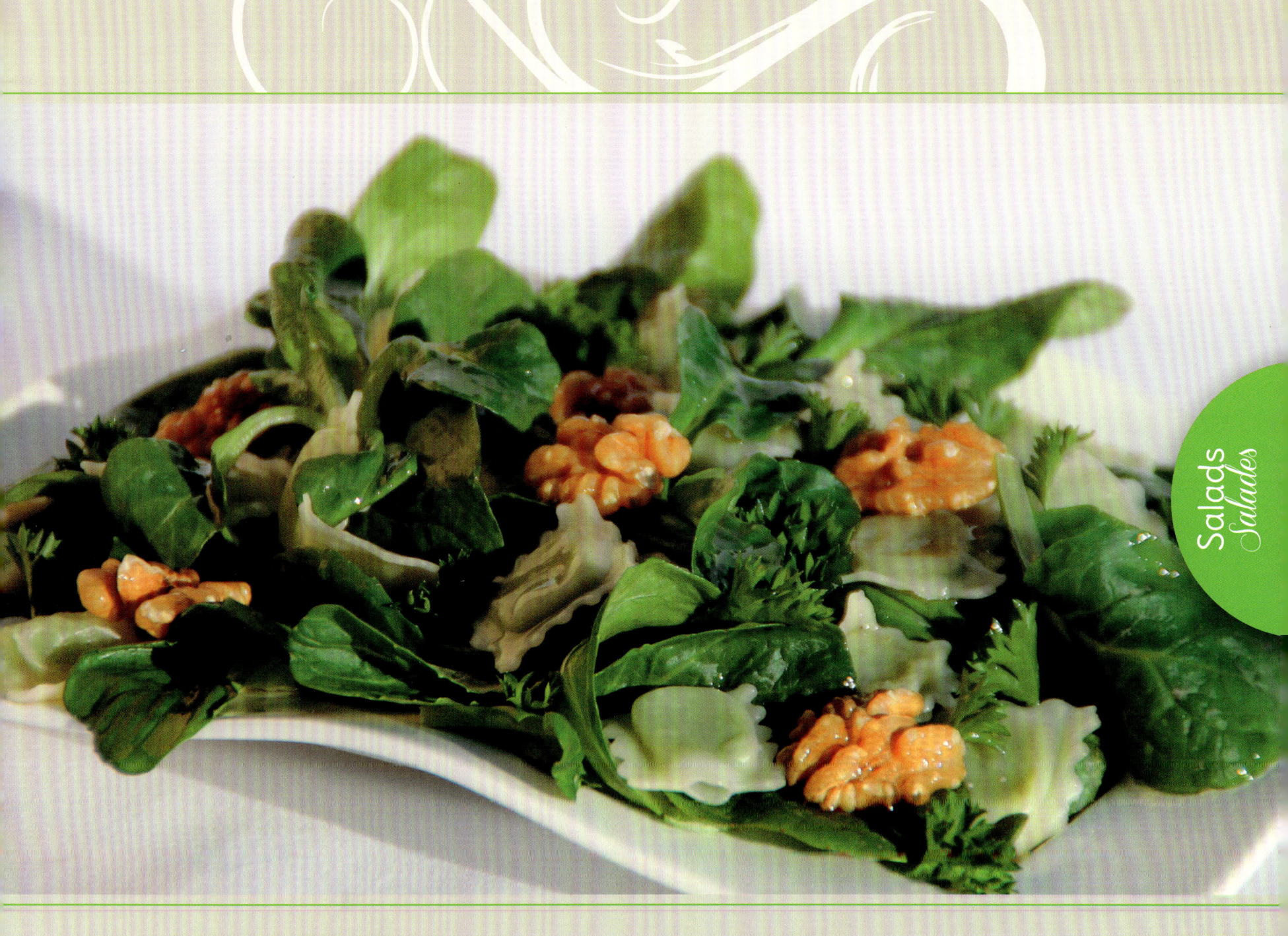

Lamb's lettuce contains three times more vitamin C, beta-carotene and antioxidants than other lettuces.
Ravioles are small pasta shapes filled with a mixture of *fromage frais*, *emmental* or *comté* cheese, fresh eggs and parsley.
They are made in Romans (near Valence) and were for a long time mistakenly thought to be a copy of the Italian ravioli.

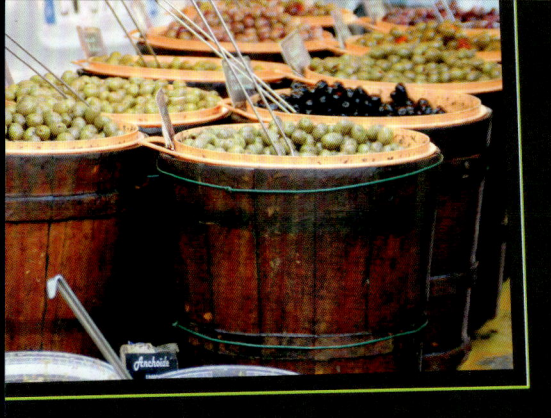

Niçoise salad
Salade niçoise

Wash the lettuce, tomatoes, pepper and cucumber.

Rub a serving plate with the garlic clove and arrange the lettuce.

Flake the tuna on top.

Cut the pepper into strips and place on the lettuce with the olives and onions.

Cut the hard-boiled eggs into quarters, slice the tomatoes and cucumber and scatter through the salad.

Sprinkle over some parsley or basil.

Arrange the anchovy fillets on top.

MAKE THE VINAIGRETTE sauce by mixing all the ingredients together.

Drizzle a little vinaigrette over the salad as desired. *It may not be necessary to use all the vinaigrette.*

- 200 g mixed green lettuce
- 1 garlic clove, peeled and halved
- 2 tomatoes
- 1 pepper
- ½ cucumber
- 150 g tuna
- 70 g small, black olives
- 2 or 3 small, white or red onions, sliced
- 2 hard-boiled eggs
- Parsley or basil, chopped
- 8 anchovy fillets

Vinaigrette:
- 2 tablespoons cider vinegar

Salads
Salades

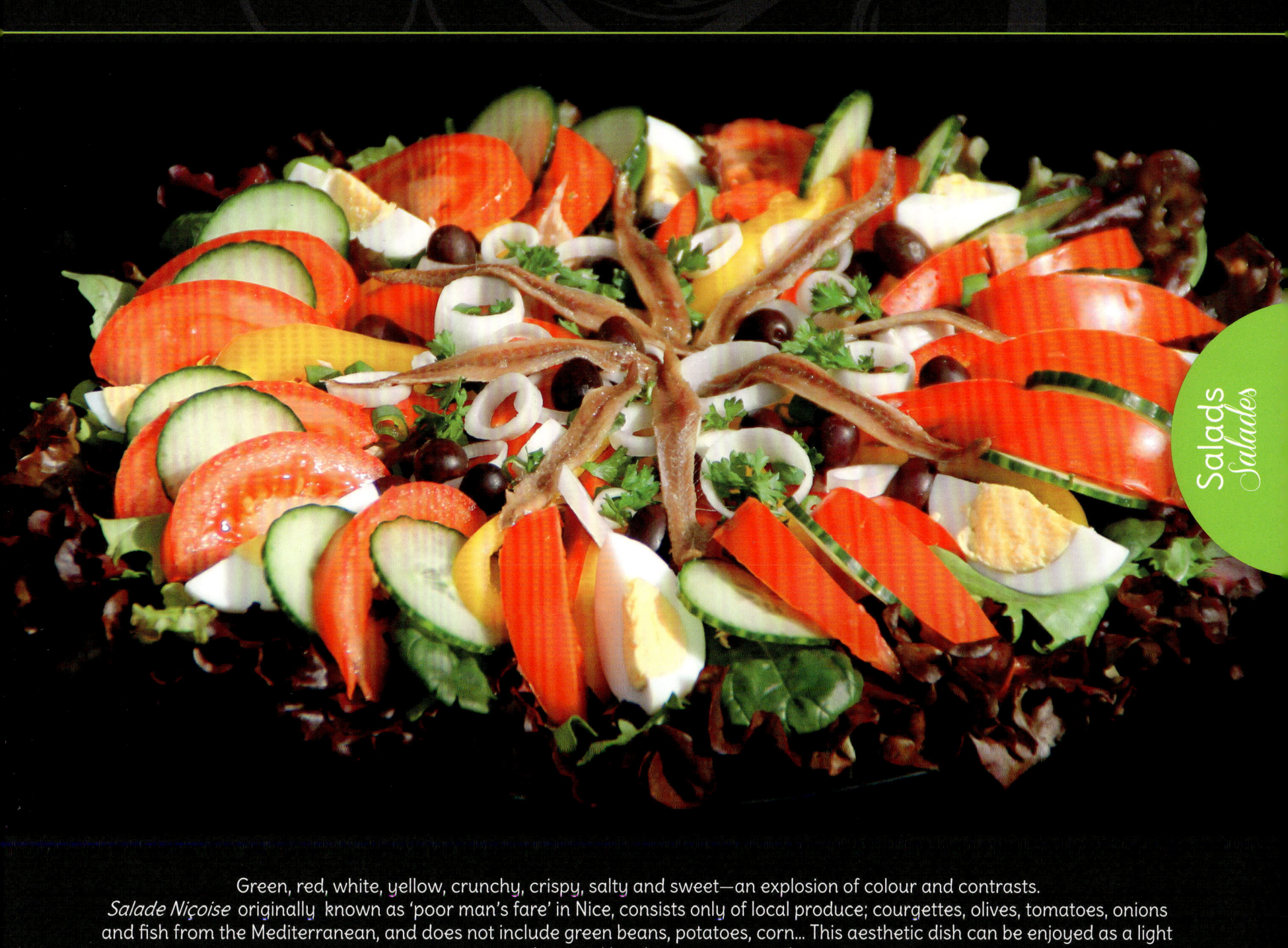

Green, red, white, yellow, crunchy, crispy, salty and sweet—an explosion of colour and contrasts. *Salade Niçoise* originally known as 'poor man's fare' in Nice, consists only of local produce; courgettes, olives, tomatoes, onions and fish from the Mediterranean, and does not include green beans, potatoes, corn... This aesthetic dish can be enjoyed as a light yet substantial lunch or evening meal.

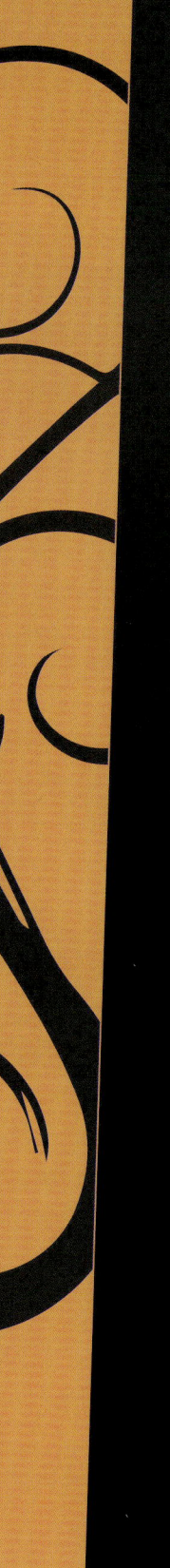

Starters
Entrées

80   Asparagus with *vinaigrette* sauce
Asperges à la vinaigrette

80   Asparagus with hollandaise sauce
Asperges avec sauce hollandaise

82   Artichokes with *vinaigrette* sauce
Artichauts à la vinaigrette

84   Ham and mushroom filled crêpes
Aumônières au jambon et champignons

86   Rolled crêpes with ham
Crêpes roulées au jambon

88   Crab-filled avocados
Avocats garnis

90   Ham and olive cakes
Cakes au jambon et olives

92   Courgette and goat's cheese cakes
Cakes aux courgettes et au fromage de chèvre

94   Creamy pizza
Crémière

96   Assortment of crudités
Assortiment de crudités

98   Grated carrots
Carottes râpées

98   Baked camembert served with crudités
Camembert au four accompagné de crudités

100   Leek pie
Flamiche aux poireaux

102   *Fougasse*
Fougasse

104   Bacon *fougasse*
Fougasse aux lardons

106   *Gougères*
Gougères

108   Melon with cured ham
Melon au jambon cru

110   Melon with port
Melon au porto

112   Mimosa eggs
Oeufs mimosa

114	Provençale-style pizza *Pissaladière*
116	Quiche Lorraine *Quiche Lorraine*
118	Cheese soufflé *Soufflé au fromage*
120	Onion tart *Tarte à l'oignon*
120	Onion tart with bacon *Tarte à l'oignon aux lardons*
122	Provençale-style tart *Tarte à la provençale*
124	Cheese soufflé tartlets *Tartelettes soufflées au fromage*
126	*Foie gras* with spiced honey loaf *Toasts au foie gras*
126	Red onion chutney *Confit d'oignons rouges*
128	Avocado-filled tomatoes *Tomates garnies*

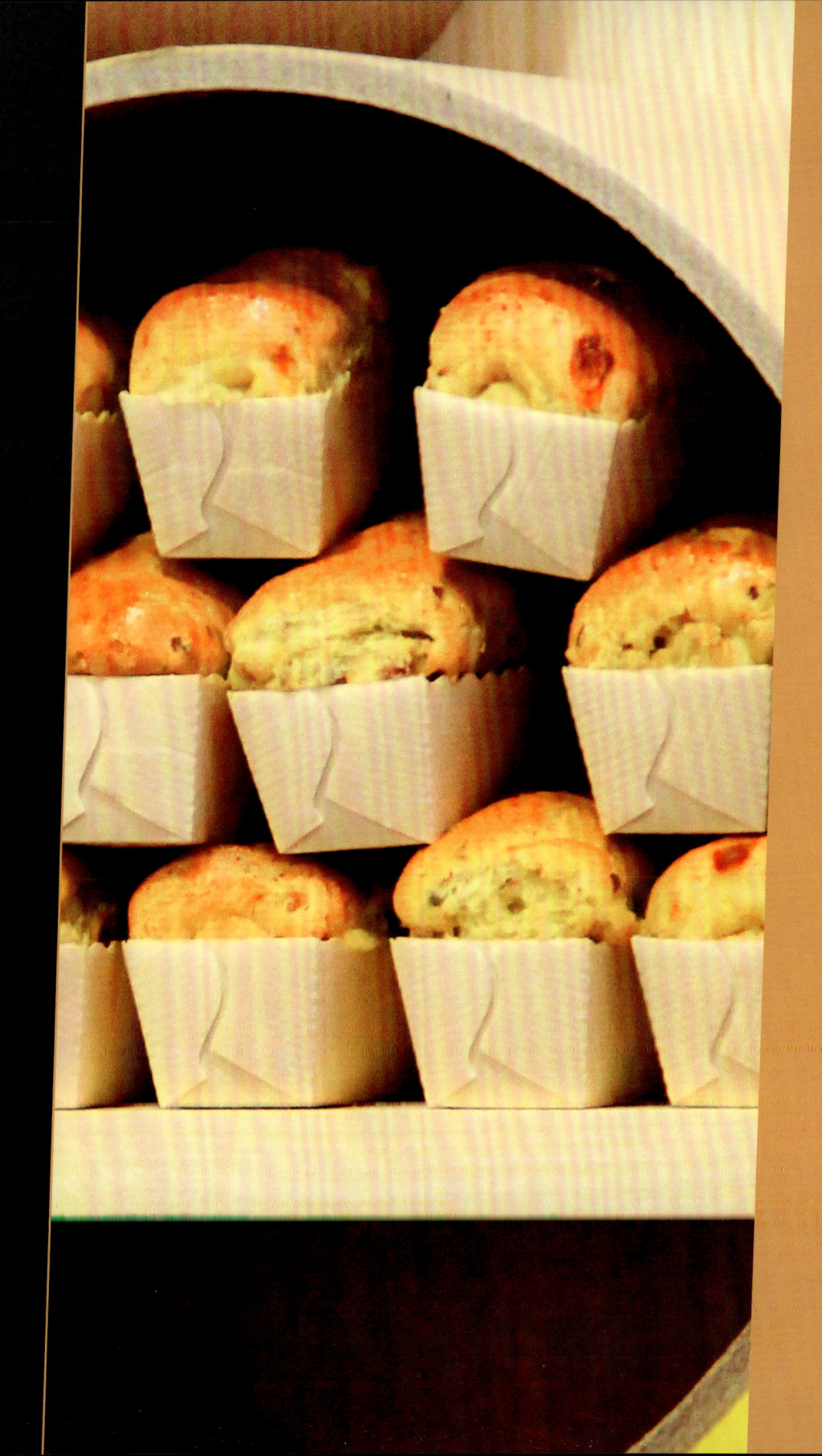

Warning !
Some recipes contain alcohol.

Starters *Entrées*

77

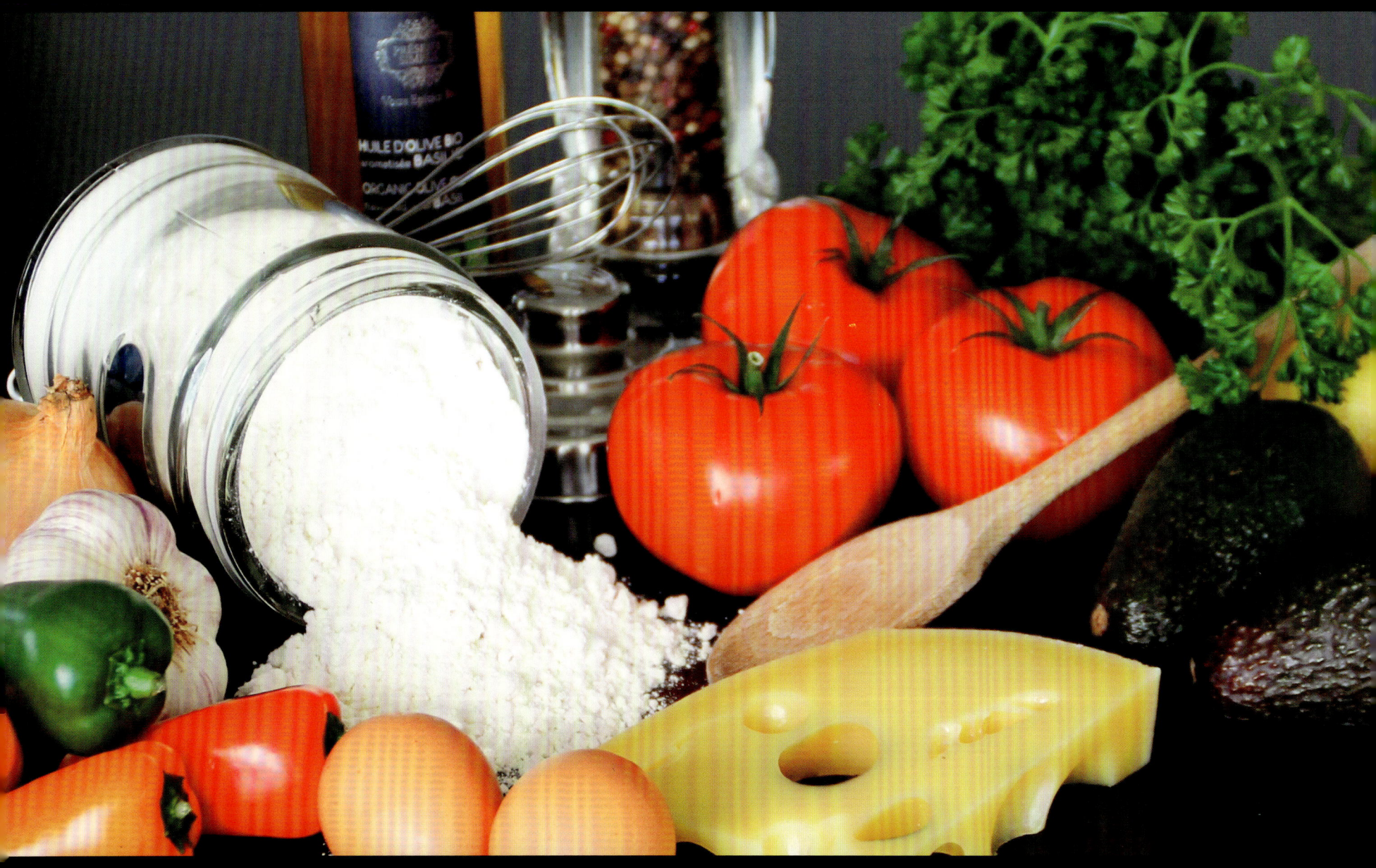

To whet the appetite...

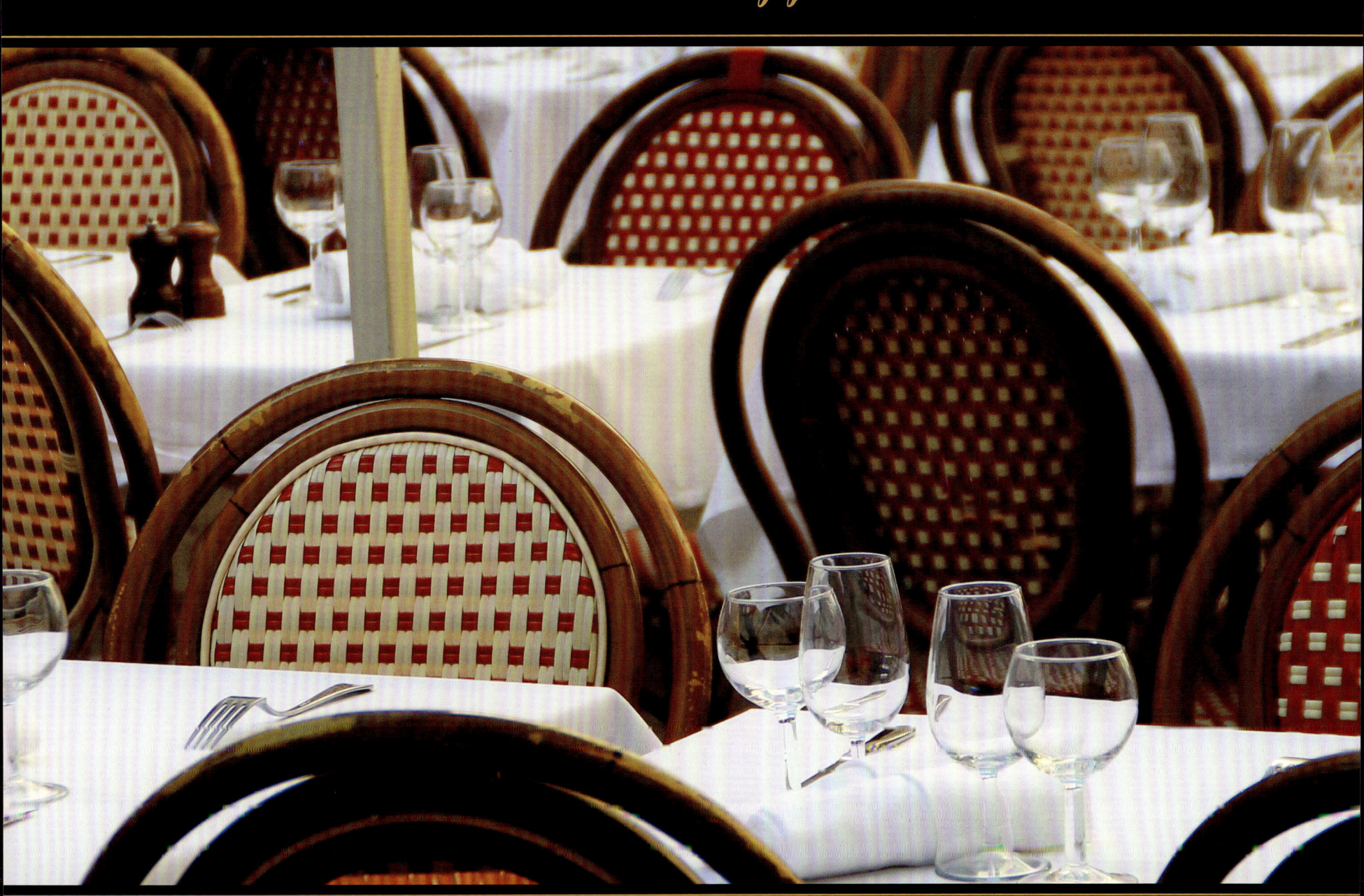

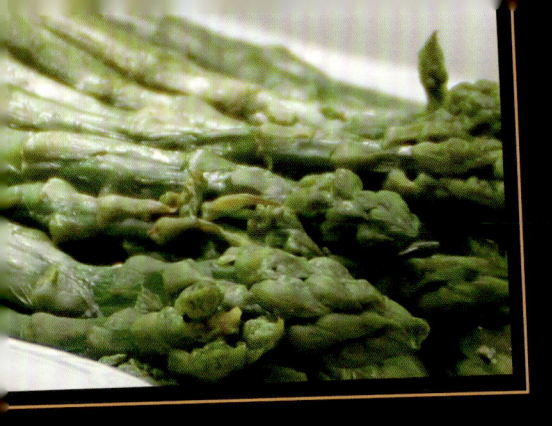

Asparagus with *vinaigrette* sauce
Asperges à la vinaigrette

Carefully peel the asparagus, taking off the hard stalk ends. *If using small asparagus, it won't be necessary to peel them.* Quickly rinse them under fresh running water and divide them into 2 bunches, tied round with string. This will stop them from breaking up while cooking.

Bring 2½ litres of water to the boil in a large saucepan and add the salt. Add the asparagus and bring the water back to the boil. Reduce the heat if necessary, leaving the water just simmering. Cook for about 15 - 25 minutes depending on the type and size of asparagus. If you can easily prick the stalk with a sharp knife, they are cooked. Drain into a colander. Remove the string.

PREPARE THE *VINAIGRETTE* according to the recipe (see *recettes de base*).

Serve the asparagus warm with the *vinaigrette*.

Asperges à la vinaigrette is also delicious served with mayonnaise (see *recettes de base*)

Serves approx. 4 persons

- 1 kg asparagus
- 1 tablespoon coarse ground salt
- 2 quantities of *vinaigrette* (see *recettes de base*)

Asparagus with hollandaise sauce
Asperges avec sauce hollandaise

For a richer, creamy alternative, prepare one quantity of *sauce hollandaise* (see *recettes de base*). Pour over the warm asparagus and serve immediately.

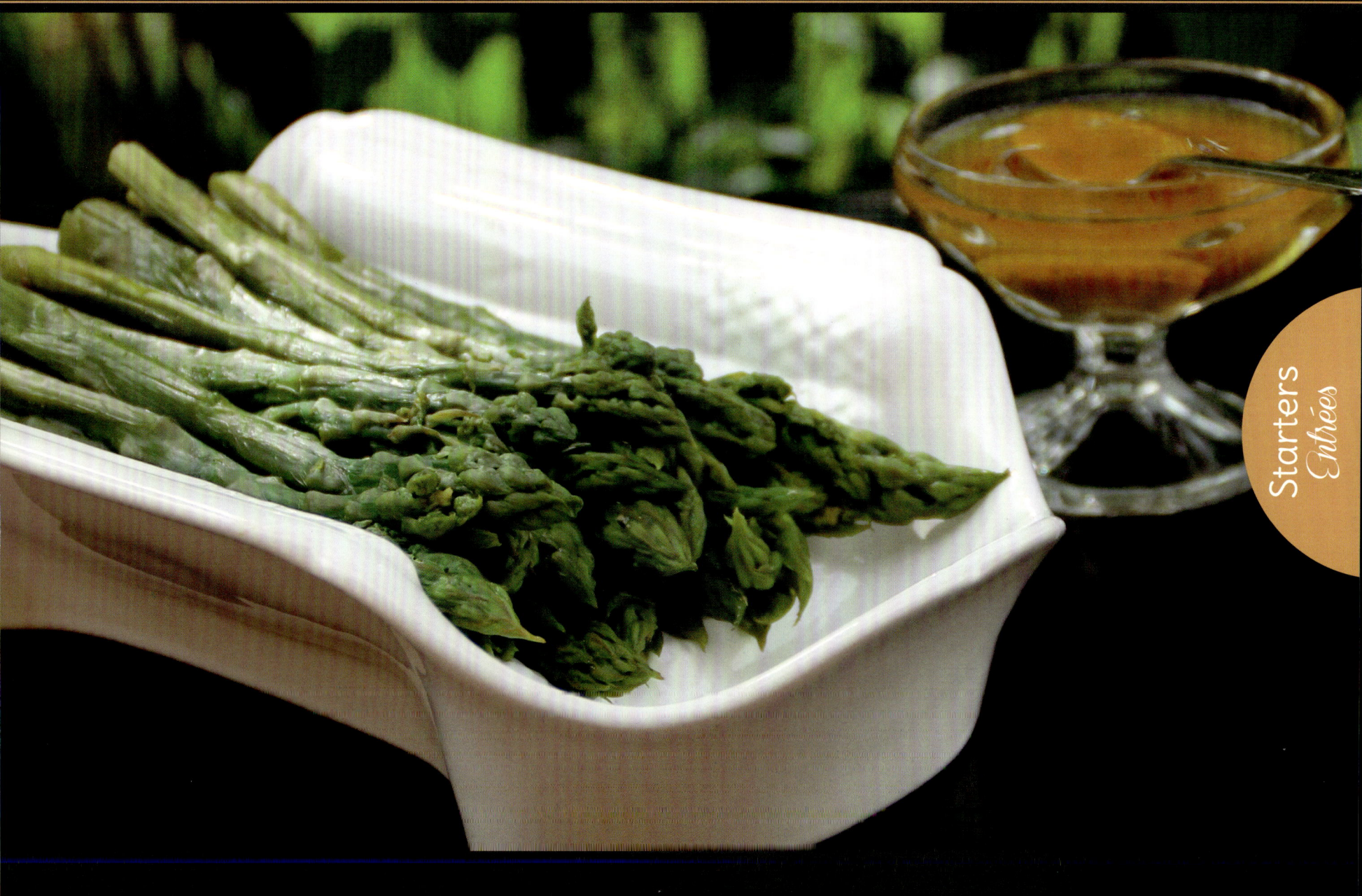

Asparagus are at their best in the spring, when they are tender and green.
They are a good source of fibre, potassium and antioxidants such as vitamins A and C.

Starters *Entrées*

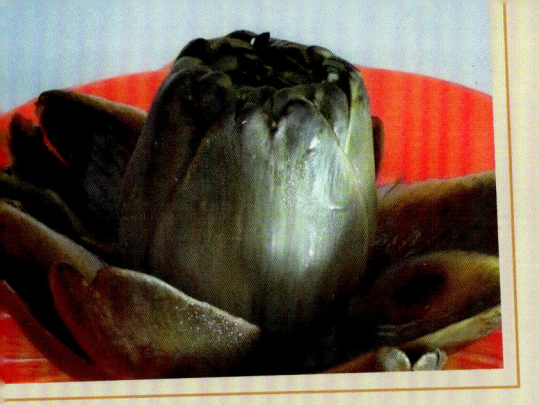

Artichokes with *vinaigrette* sauce
Artichauts à la vinaigrette

Bring a large saucepan of salted water to the boil and add the lemon juice. *Adding the lemon juice preserves the colour of the artichoke.*

Trim the stalks from the artichokes and remove the damaged and outer leaves.

Place the artichokes into the boiling water and cover. Cook for approximately 20 minutes then turn them upside-down and cook for another 20 – 30 minutes or until a leaf can be pulled out easily (or they are tender when pierced with a knife). *The cooking time will depend on the size and type of the artichokes.*

Drain them upside down.

PREPARE THE *VINAIGRETTE* according to the recipe.

Place the artichokes on individual serving plates and carefully open out the leaves. Pour over some *vinaigrette* and sprinkle with parsley. Serve the rest of the *vinaigrette* in a small bowl.

The correct way to eat an artichoke is to pull off an outer leaf, dip it in the *vinaigrette* and nibble the fleshy inside. The cup-shaped base can be eaten after removing the choke with a teaspoon.

Serves 4 persons

- 4 artichokes, small purple variety
- Juice of 1 lemon

- 1 quantity of *vinaigrette* (see *recettes de base*)
- A few sprigs of parsley, chopped

Starters *Entrées*

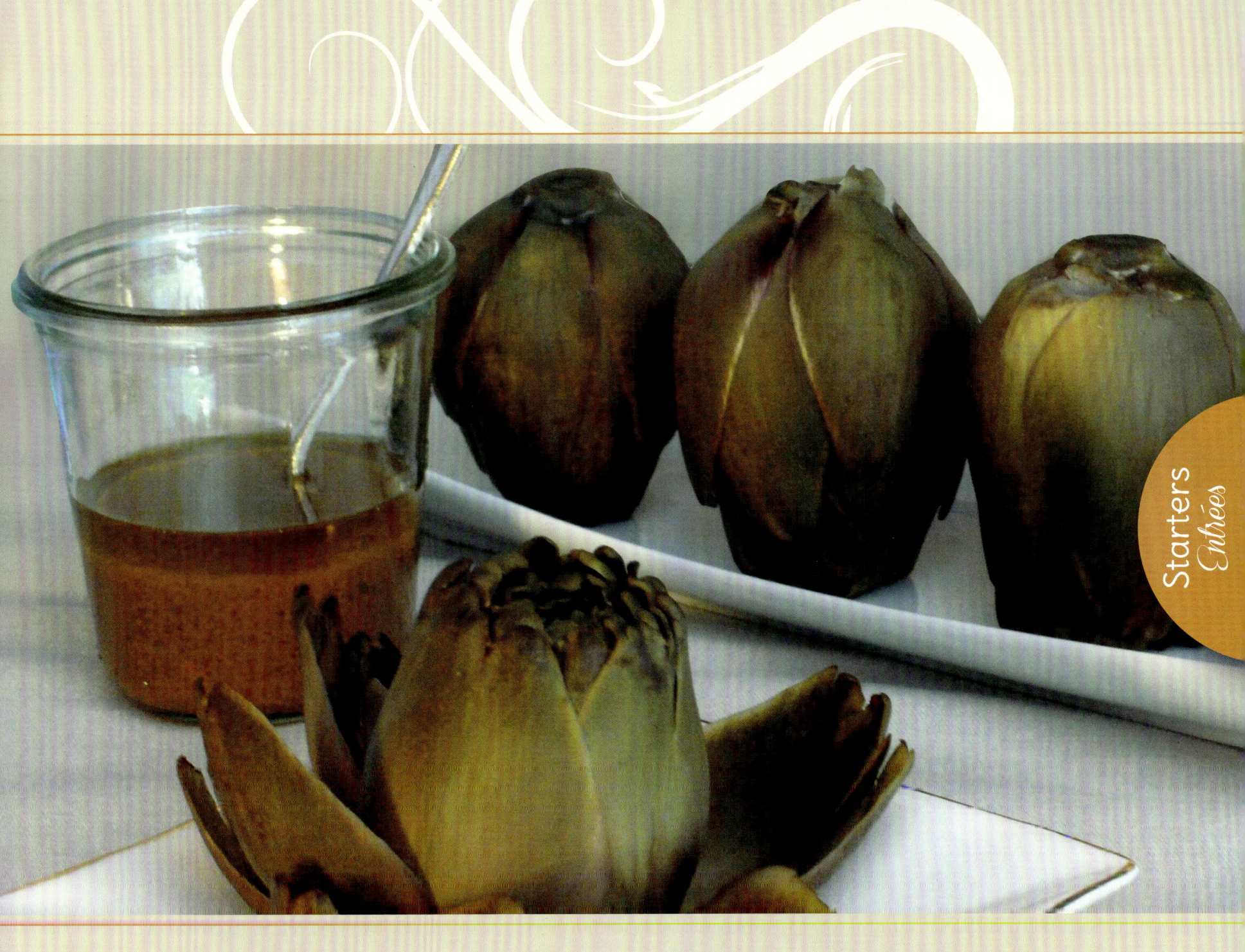

Artichokes are a classic familiar starter and are served more often with a *vinaigrette* than anything else.
They are rich in vitamins B1, B2, B3, B5, B6, C and K, antioxidants, calcium and magnesium.

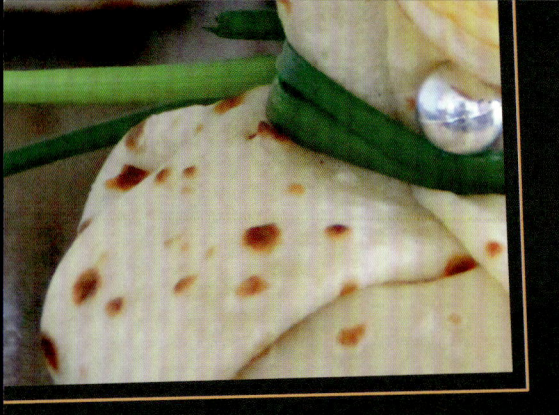

Ham and mushroom filled crêpes
Aumonières au jambon et champignons

MAKE THE CRÊPES: Mix the flour and salt together in a large bowl and make a well in the centre. In another bowl mix together the eggs and the milk. Slowly pour the liquid into the well mixing continuously until a smooth batter is formed. Add the oil. Cover and leave to rest in the fridge for about 20 minutes.

Melt some butter or oil in a shallow frying pan. Pour in enough crêpe mixture to cover the base of the pan. Cook on a medium heat for about 1½ minutes or until it is starting to come away from the pan. Flip it over and leave to cook again for about 1½ minutes or until beginning to turn golden.

Place the cooked crêpe onto a plate and repeat this process until all the mixture is used up, piling the crêpes one on top of the other.

PREPARE THE FILLING: Make the *sauce béchamel* according to the recipe adding 20 g more flour than is shown in the recipe (50 g instead of 30 g).

Heat the oil in a frying pan and add the onion. Cook until beginning to turn transparent.

Place a spoonful of *sauce béchamel* on each crêpe, sprinkle with the bacon, mushroom, onion and grated cheese. Close the crêpe round the filling, tying the top with either a toothpick or a whole chive.

Place in a warm oven for a few minutes before serving.

VARIATION
Rolled crêpes with ham .... P. 86

Makes approx. 10 crêpes of 22 cm diameter

Crêpe:
- 250 g plain flour
- A pinch of salt
- 2 eggs, beaten
- 600 ml milk
- 1 tablespoon oil

Filling:
- 1 quantity *sauce béchamel* (see *recettes de base*)
- 2 tablespoons olive oil
- 1 onion, finely chopped
- 250 g mushrooms, sliced and fried
- 150 g cooked bacon or ham, finely chopped
- 200 g grated cheese

Starters
Entrées

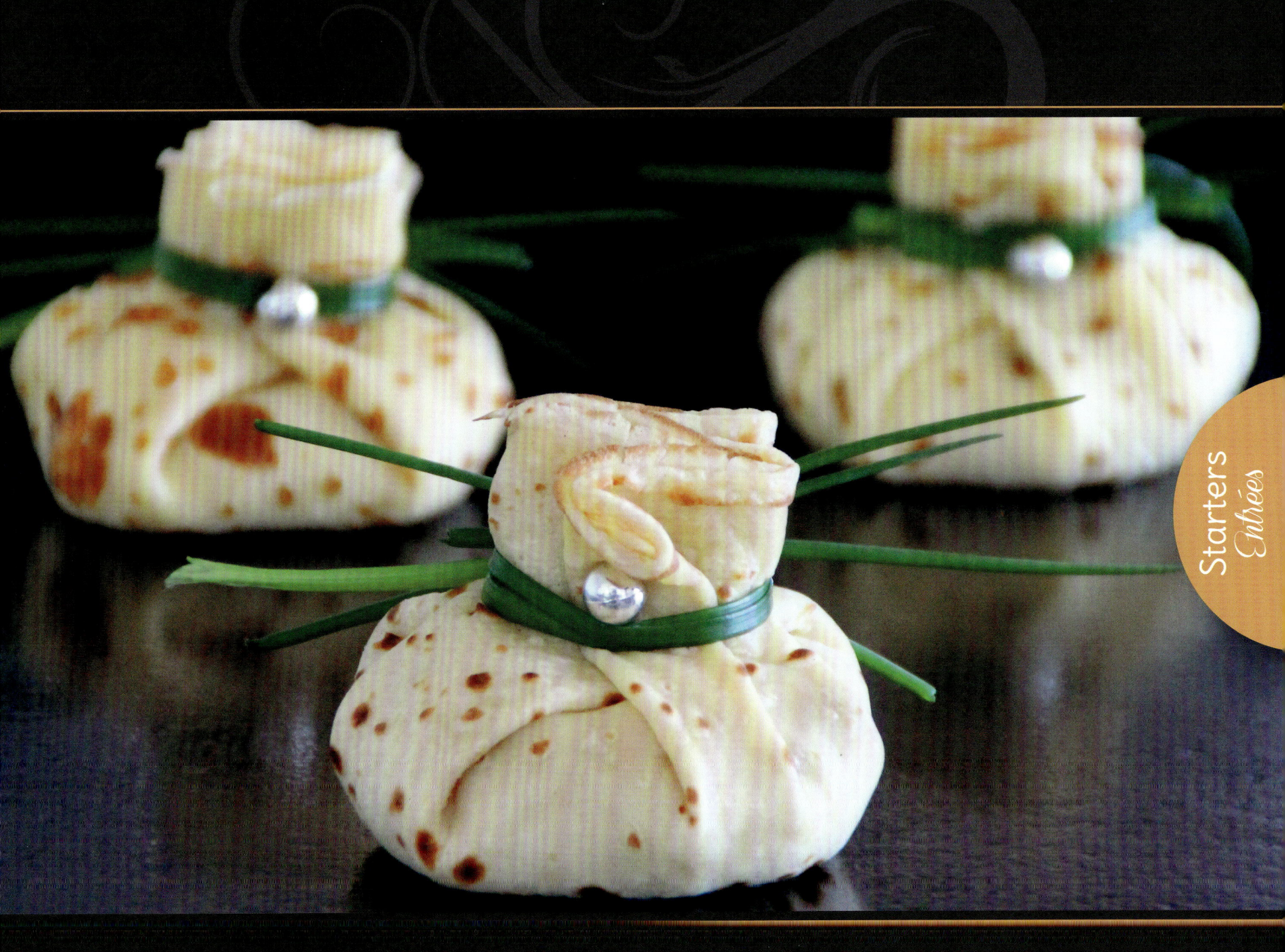

This attractive starter is simple to prepare and can also be enjoyed as a main meal, served with a fresh green salad.

85

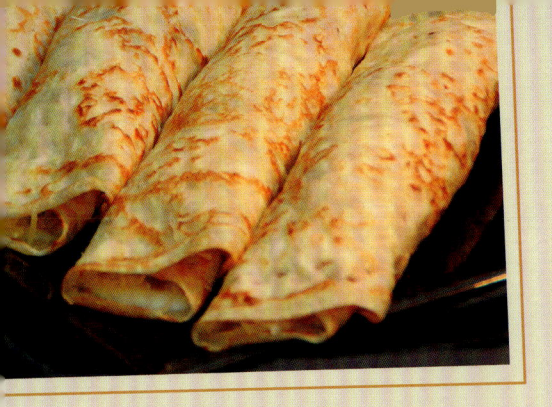

Rolled crêpes with ham
Crêpes roulées au jambon

MAKE THE CREPES as indicated previously.

PREPARE THE FILLING: Make the *sauce béchamel* according to the recipe, but add 20 g more flour than is shown in the recipe (50 g instead of 30 g).

Heat the oil in a frying pan and add the chopped onions. Cook until they are beginning to turn transparent.

ASSEMBLE THE CREPES: Spread a tablespoon of *sauce béchamel* on each crêpe, cover with a slice of ham and sprinkle the onions and grated cheese over the top.

Roll up like a swiss roll.

Place in a warm oven for a few minutes before serving.

Makes approx. 10 crêpes of 22 cm diameter

- 1 quantity of crêpe mixture (see previous recipe)

Filling:
- 1 quantity *sauce béchamel* (see *recettes de base*)
- 4 tablespoons olive oil
- 2 onions
- 300 g sliced ham
- 300 g grated cheese

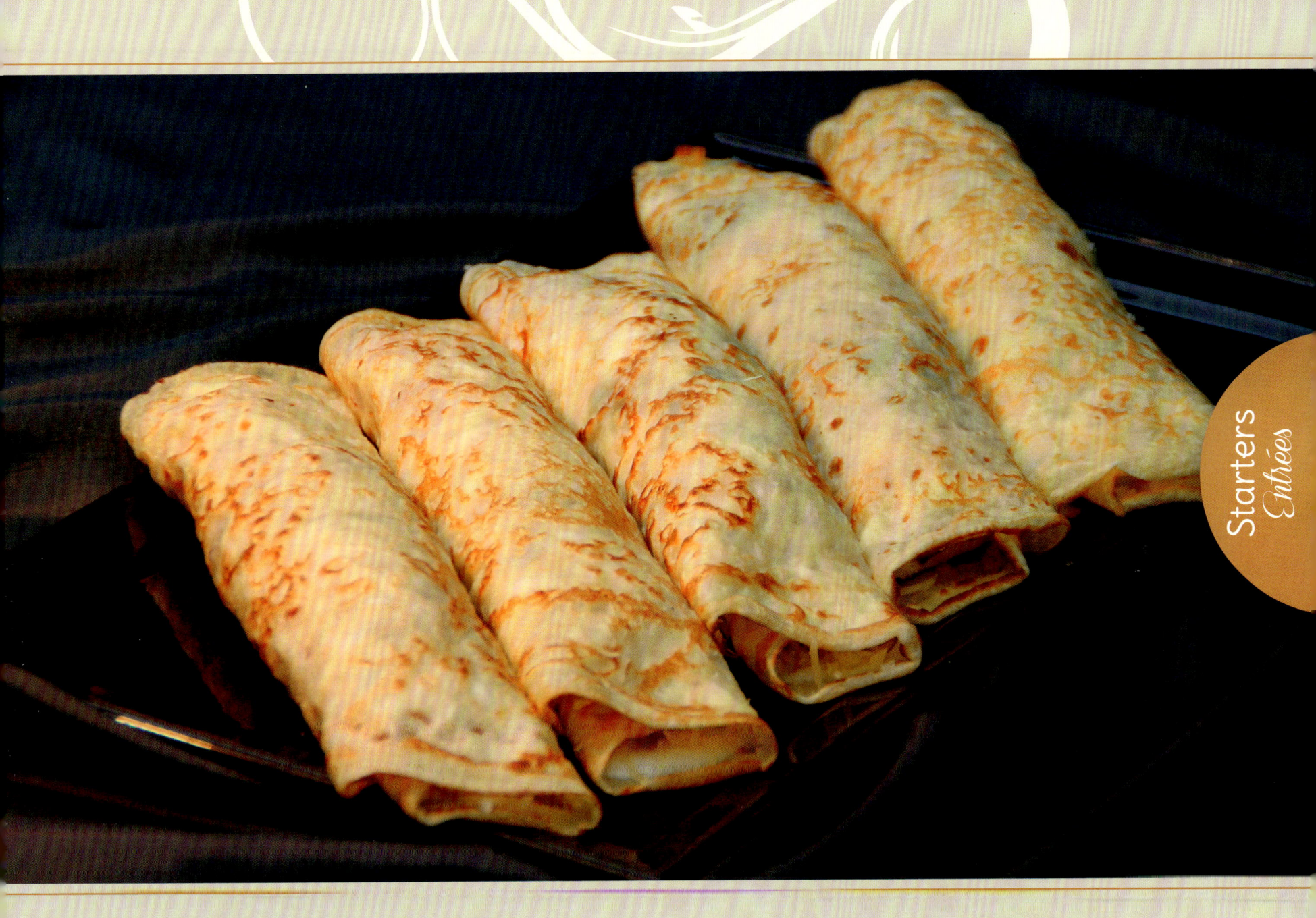

Delicious as well as simple to prepare and are an ideal stand-by snack or supper when everything else fails!
Visitors, young and old, will enjoy them!

Starters *Entrées*

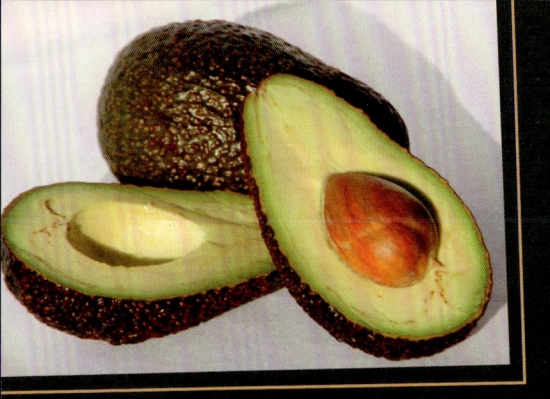

Crab-filled avocados
Avocats garnis

Cut the avocado in half. Remove the stone.

Drain the crab meat well. Mix with the mayonnaise and *sauce cocktail* and use to fill the inside of the avocado.

Decorate each with a prawn, parsley, half a slice of lemon and a slice of smoked salmon (optional).

As a variation use the filling to stuff tomato halves or use to garnish sliced tomatoes.

When choosing an avocado, press it gently to check how ripe it is, remembering also that they turn slightly brown as they ripen. Avoid those that are bruised or that have brown or black marks on them. If any avocados are not ripe, place them in a brown paper bag for a couple of days at room temperature.

Starters
Entrées

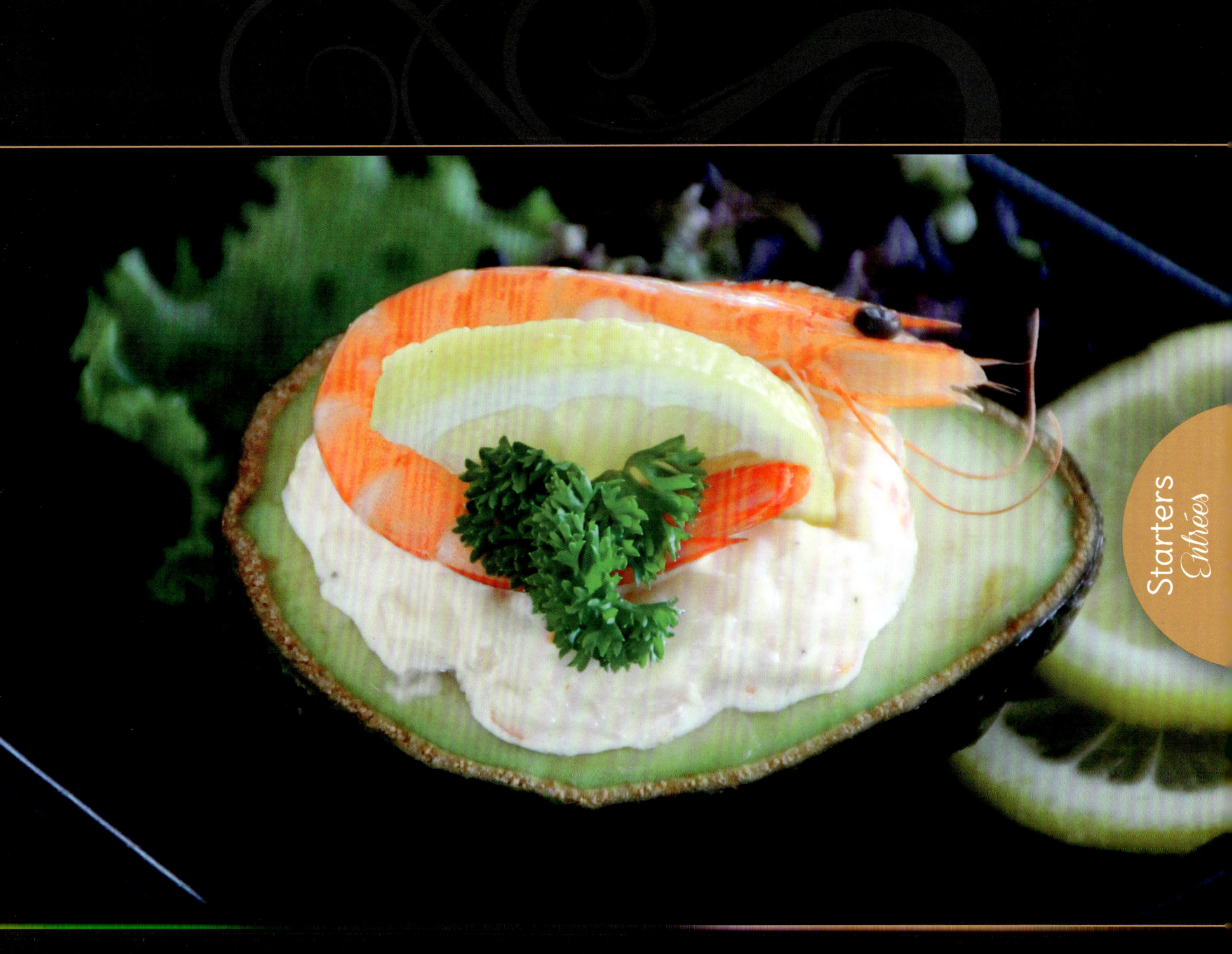

Avocados are a very healthy choice as they contain no sodium or cholesterol and are full of minerals such as magnesium and potassium as well as being rich in fibres and vitamins (B6, K and E).

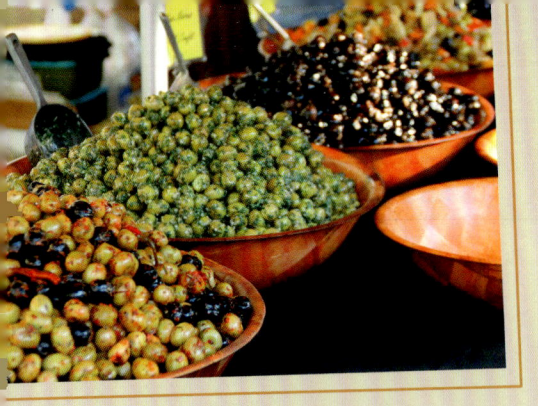

Ham and olive cakes
Cakes au jambon et olives

Beat the eggs with the melted butter. Add the cream, salt and pepper.

Add the flour and baking powder, wine, ham and olives. Mix together.

Divide into well-greased muffin tins.

Cook for about 20 minutes or until risen and golden.

Makes approx. 18 individual cakes

Oven: 200°C

- 4 eggs
- 100 g butter, melted
- 150 ml double cream
- Salt and pepper
- 250 g plain flour
- 2 teaspoons baking powder
- 100 ml dry white wine
- 200 g chopped ham or bacon, cooked
- 70 g green olives, stoned and halved

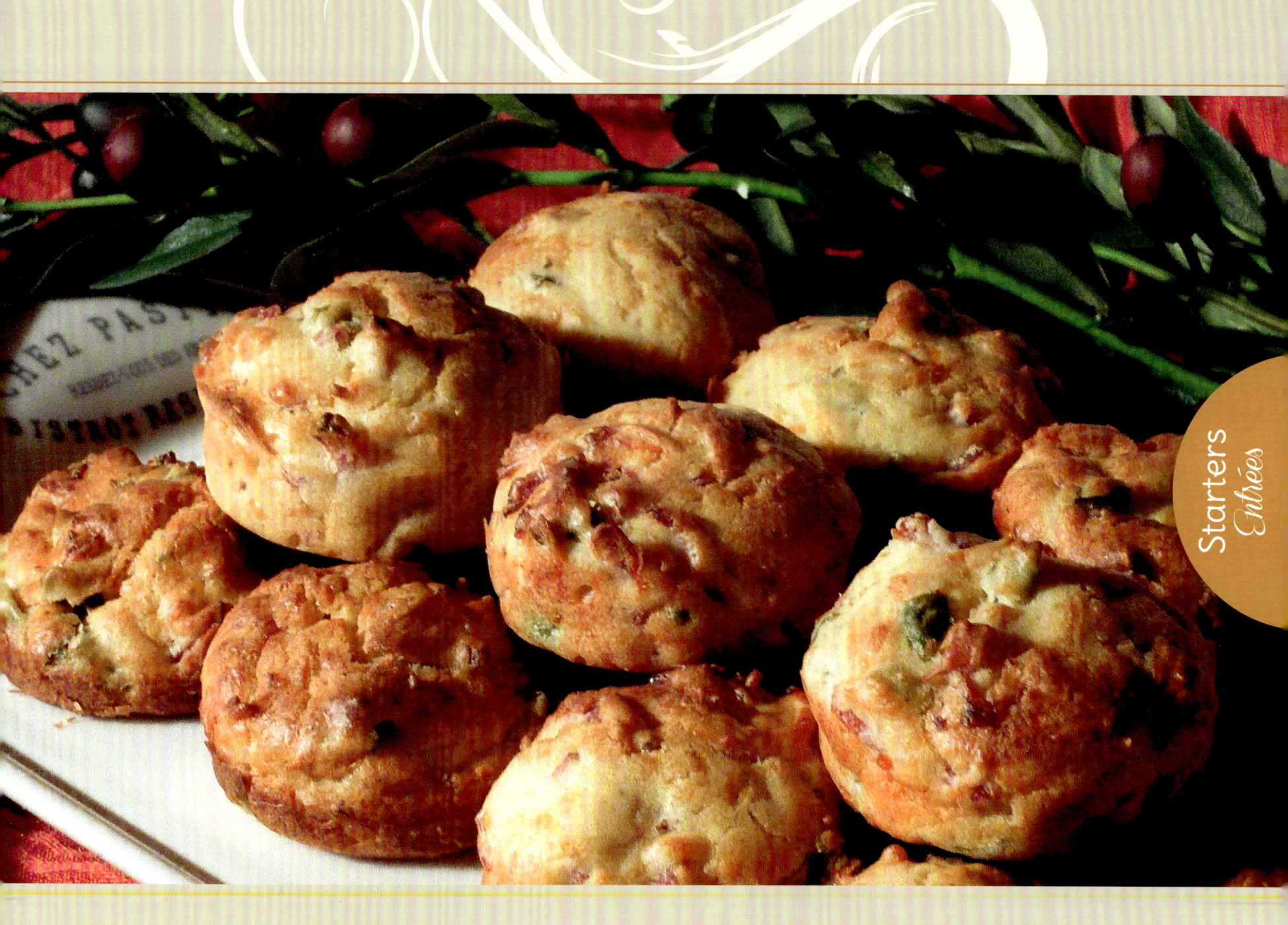

These small savoury cakes are ideal as a starter. Serve warm with a fresh, green salad tossed with *vinaigrette*.

Starters
Entrées

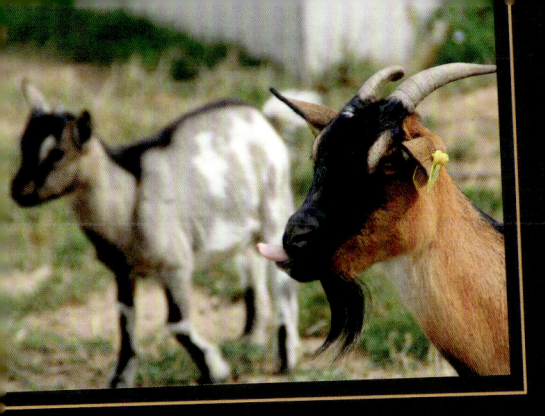

Courgette and goat's cheese cakes
Cakes aux courgettes et au fromage de chèvre

Heat 2 tablespoons of the oil in a frying pan. Chop the courgettes into small pieces, leaving on the skins. Fry the courgettes in the hot oil for about 15 minutes or until soft. Season with salt.

Beat the eggs with the milk, 80 ml of olive oil and a pinch of salt and pepper for seasoning.

Mix the baking powder into the flour and add to the egg mixture. Mix until smooth.

Add the courgettes, cheese and herbs. Mix all together and divide between the individual well-greased cake moulds.

Cook for about 20 minutes or until risen and golden.

Serve warm with a green salad.

Makes 6 - 8 individual cakes

Oven: 180°C

- 200 g courgettes *(zucchini)*
- 80 ml olive oil plus 2 tablespoons for frying
- 3 eggs
- 100 ml milk
- Salt and pepper
- 170 g plain flour
- 10 g baking powder
- 100 g goat's cheese, cubed
- 1 teaspoon *herbes de Provence*

If preferred, change the goat's cheese for another type of cheese such as raclette cheese.

Starters *Entrées*

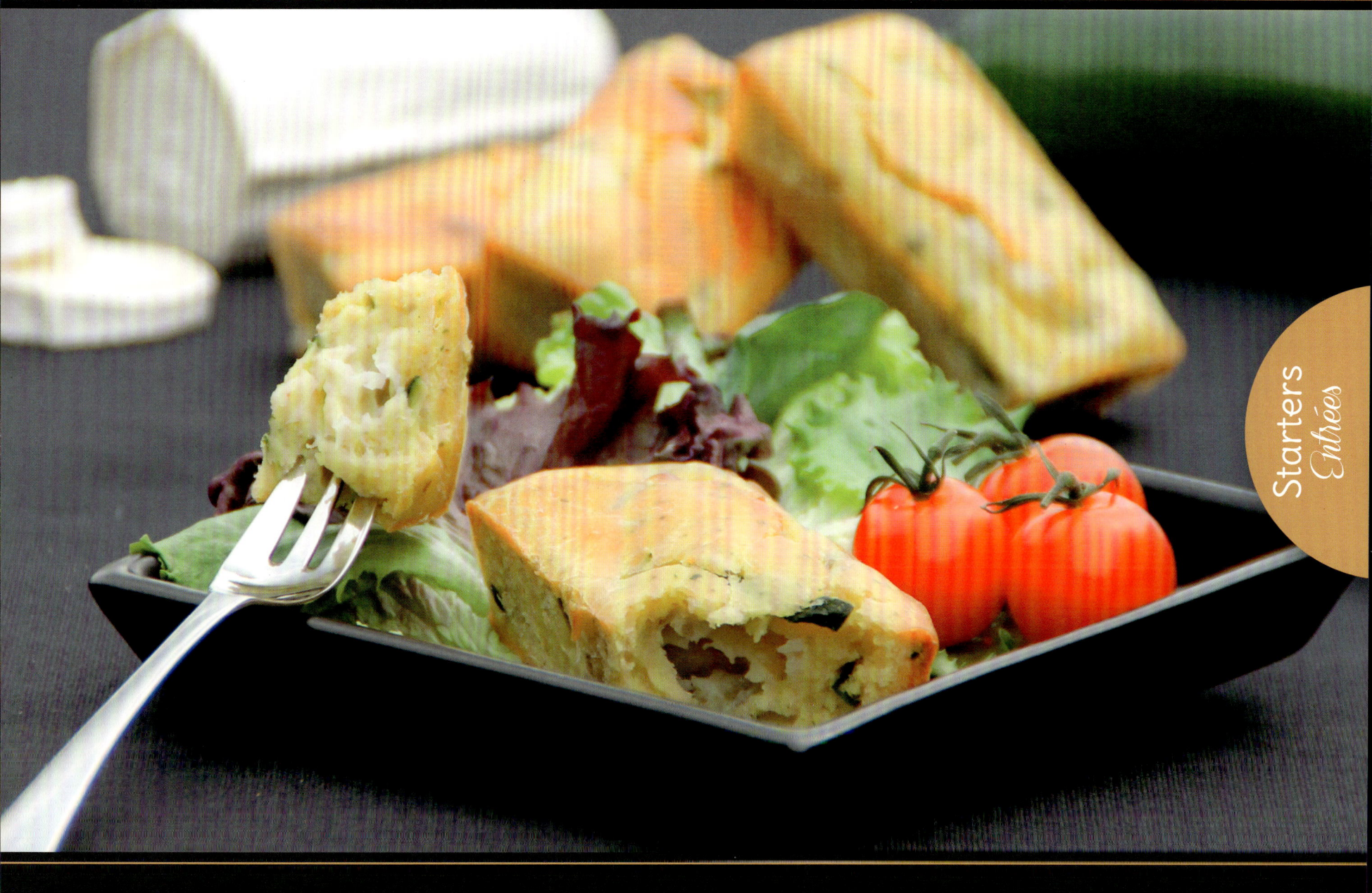

Goat's cheese is lower in fat, calories and cholesterol than cheese derived from cow's milk.

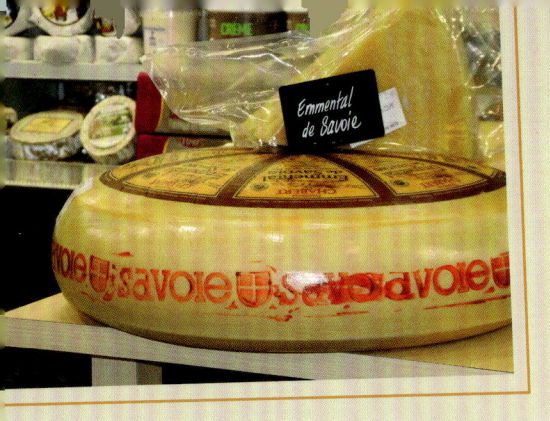

Creamy pizza
Crémière

MAKE THE PIZZA BASE: Dissolve the yeast in the water with the sugar. Mix together all the other ingredients. Add the yeast mixture. Knead the dough until smooth. Roll out on a lightly-floured surface and use to line a well-greased baking tray (40 x 30 cm).

MAKE THE TOPPING: Chop the onion finely and fry with the bacon. Sprinkle over the dough.

In a mixing bowl, mix together the cream and milk with the herbs and salt. Pour the bacon and onions over and sprinkle over the cheese.

Leave to rise then cook for about 15 - 20 minutes or until beginning to turn golden.

Serves approx. 12 persons

Oven: 175°C

Pizza base:
- 250 g strong white flour
- 150 g warm water
- 10 g fresh yeast
- ½ teaspoon sugar
- 2 tablespoons olive oil
- ½ teaspoon salt
- 1 teaspoon *herbes de Provence*

Topping:
- 1 large onion
- 200 g smoked bacon, chopped
- 250 ml thick double cream
- 3 tablespoons milk
- 1 teaspoon *herbes de Provence*
- 150 g grated cheese
- Pinch of salt

Starters *Entrées*

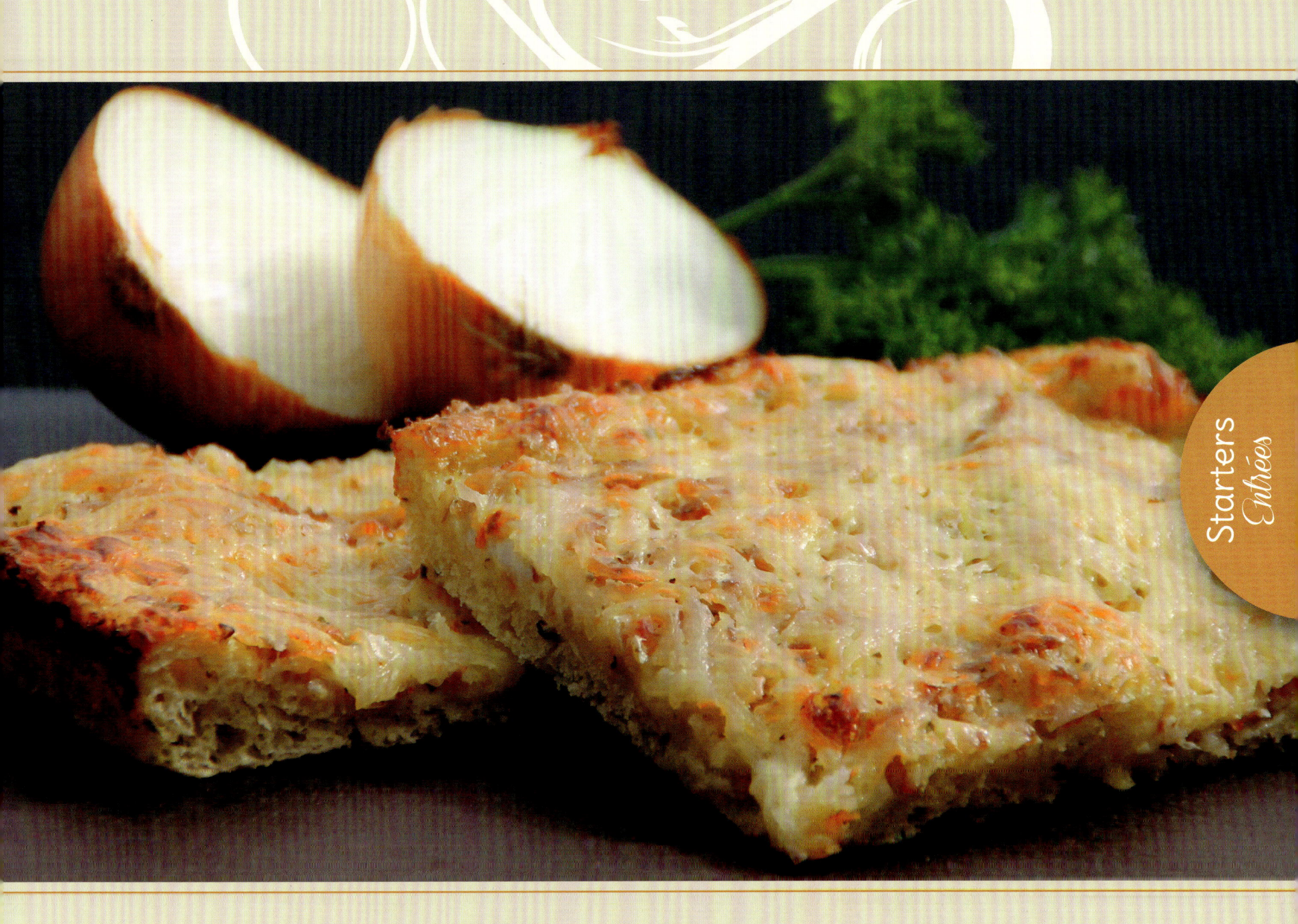

A delicious creamy change to a pizza!
This recipe is easy to make and tastes lovely served warm with a fresh green salad.

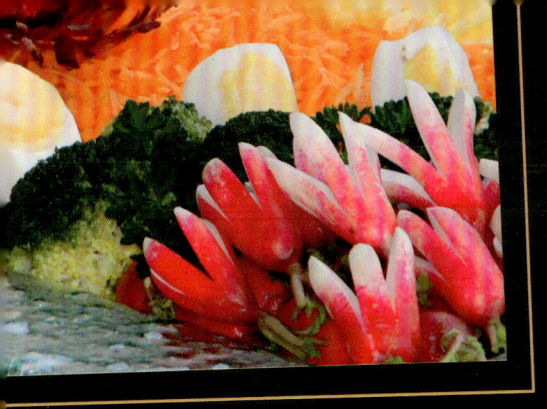

Assortment of crudités
Assortiment de crudités

Cook the broccoli in boiling salted water for 10 - 15 minutes. Drain and leave aside to cool.

Top and tail the radishes and wash thoroughly in cold water.

Peel the carrots and grate them finely.

Arrange the broccoli, carrots and radishes on a serving plate and decorate with the hard-boiled eggs.

Make the mayonnaise and *vinaigrette* according to the recipe and serve separately.

- 400 g broccoli florets
- A bunch of radishes
- 600 g carrots
- 4 hard-boiled eggs
- 1 quantity of mayonnaise (see *recettes de base*)
- 1 quantity of *vinaigrette* (see *recettes de base*)

Grated carrots..P. 98
Carottes rapées

Baked camembert served with crudités........................P. 98
Camembert au four accompagné de crudités

Starters
Entrées

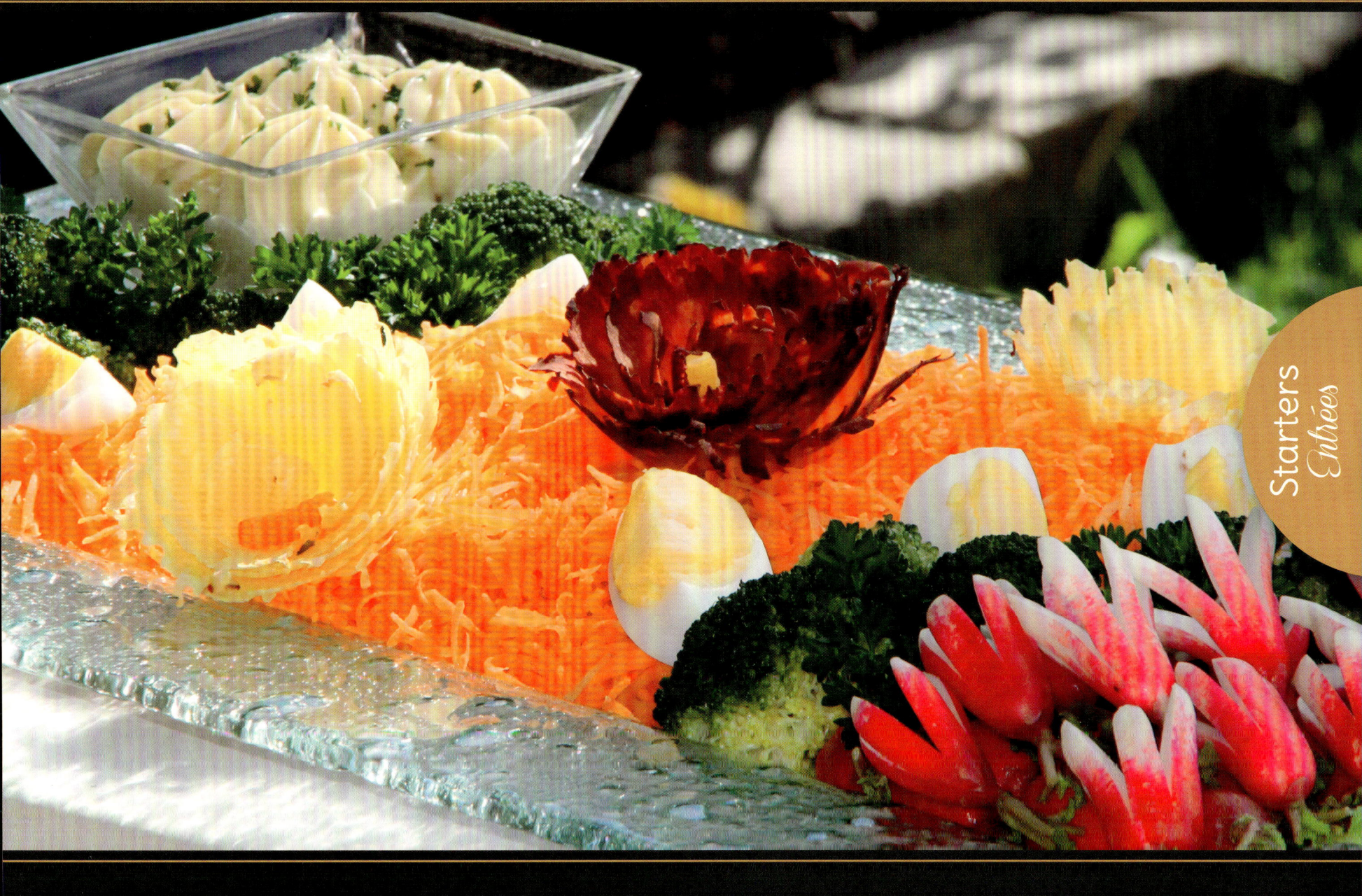

For a healthy starter packed full of vitamins, all you need is fresh, grated vegetables and a light dressing. Dare to mix colours and tastes to create a stunning centrepiece!

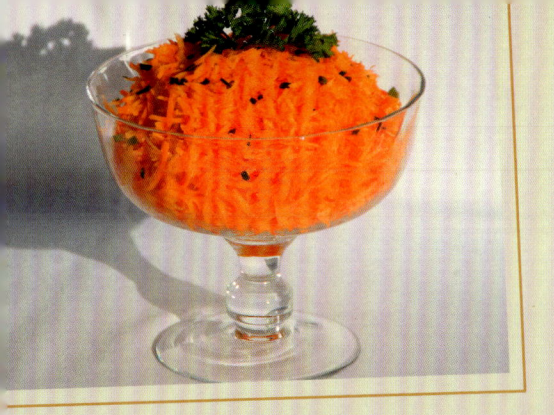

Grated carrots
Carottes rapées

Peel the carrots and grate them finely. Place in a serving dish.

MAKE THE *VINAIGRETTE* according to the recipe. Season with the *vinaigrette* according to taste and decorate with the fresh herbs.

Serve immediately.

- 500 g carrots
- A few sprigs fresh herbs

- 1 quantity of *vinaigrette* (see *recettes de base*)

Baked camembert served with crudités
Camembert au four accompagné de crudités

Prepare the crudités.

Remove the camembert from its paper and replace it in the box. Score a circle on the white surface of the camembert, 1 cm in from the edges. *Do not replace the lid on the box.* Wrap the box in foil.

Cook for about 20 minutes. Remove the foil and discard the scored top and serve with the crudités.

Oven: 180°C

- A selection of different crudités cut into sticks (carrots, celery, peppers, cucumber...)
- 1 whole round camembert cheese

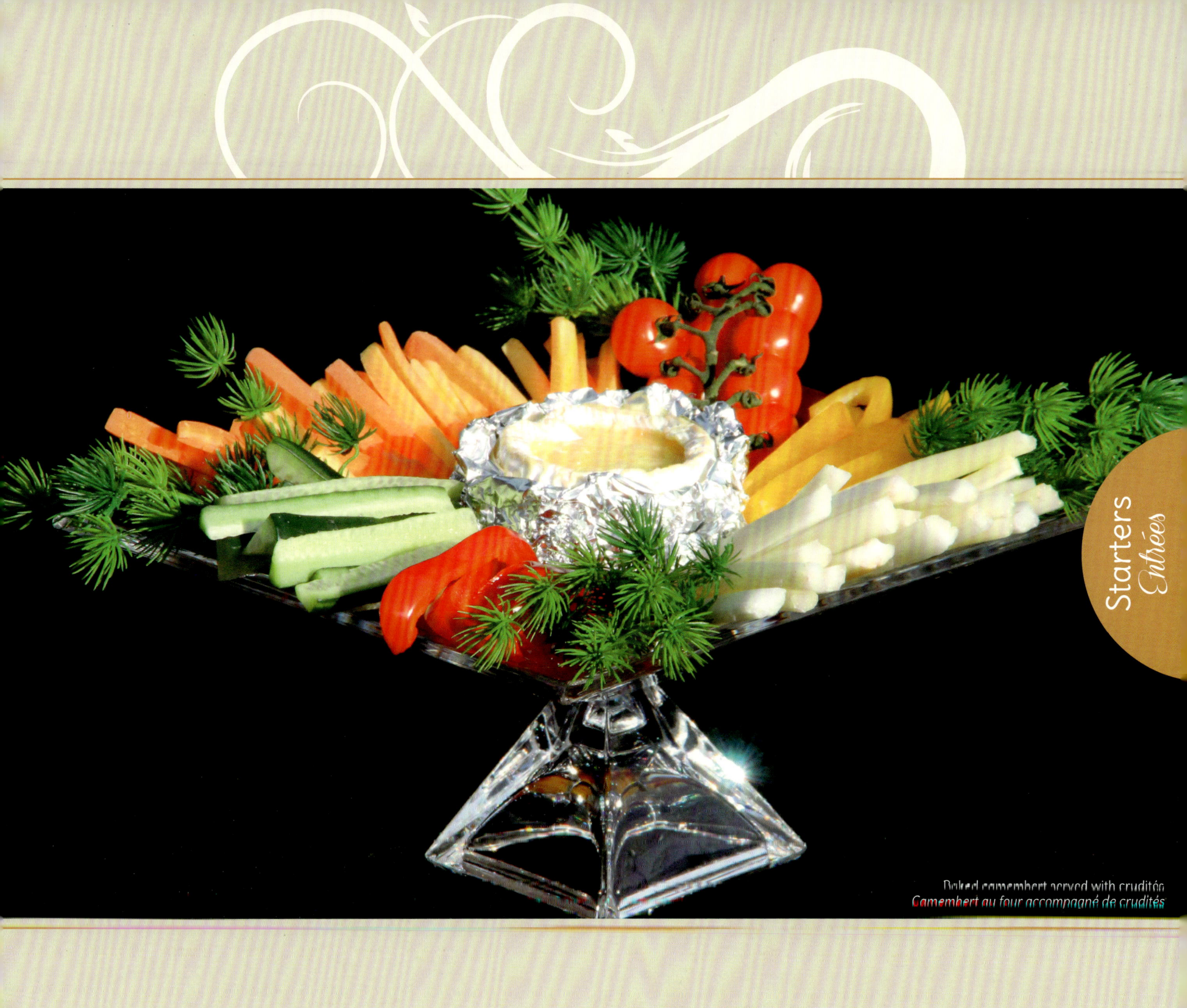

Baked camembert served with crudités
Camembert au four accompagné de crudités

Starters
Entrées

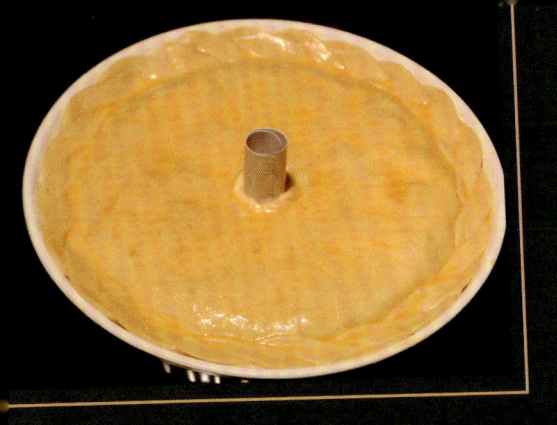

Leek pie
Flamiche aux poireaux

Wash the leeks and cut them into 2 - 3 cm chunks. Heat the oil in a saucepan and lightly fry the onion. Add the leeks and continue cooking on a low heat for about 30 minutes.

MAKE THE *PÂTE BRISÉE*: according to the recipe.

Divide the pastry into 2 separate parts, one slightly bigger than the other. Roll out the larger piece to fit the base and sides of a 28 cm well-greased and floured ovenproof pie dish.

PREPARE THE FILLING: Mix together the cream with the egg and egg yolk. Add the onion and leek mixture with the grated cheese. Mix well. Season with salt, pepper and nutmeg.

Pour the leek mixture into the pastry case.

ASSEMBLE THE PIE: Roll out the other half of the pastry and use to cover the pie. Dampen the edges and seal. Cut the edges neatly and use the leftover pastry to decorate the pie. Trace a lattice pattern with a sharp knife and cut out a small round of pastry in the centre for the chimney.

GLAZE THE PIE: Beat the egg yolk with the milk in a bowl and brush over the pie.

Make the chimney with a rectangle of card, and place in the hole. Cook for about 1 hour then cover with foil and cook for a further 15 minutes. *Take care not to allow the chimney to become blocked with the cream during cooking.*

Remove the chimney and serve hot.

Serves 8 - 12 persons

Oven: 175°C

2 quantities *pâte brisée* (see *recettes de base*)

Filling:
- 800 g leeks (approx. 5 leeks)
- 80 ml olive oil
- 1 onion, finely chopped
- 250 ml double cream
- 1 egg
- 1 egg yolk
- 100 g grated cheese
- Salt and pepper
- Pinch of ground nutmeg

Glaze:
- 1 egg yolk
- 1 tablespoon milk

Starters *Entrées*

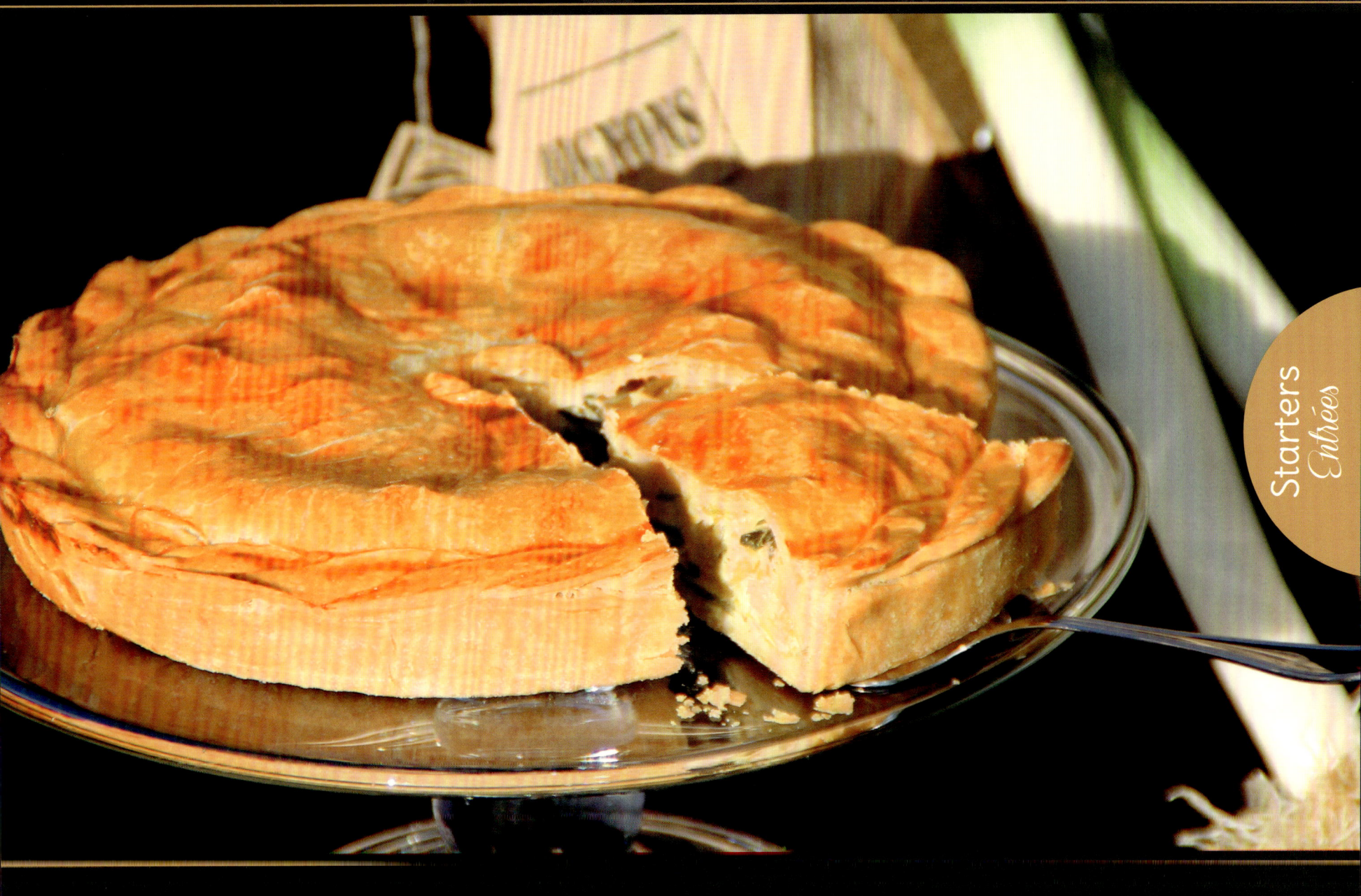

Flamiche aux poireaux is believed to be the *Picardie* equivalent of the Quiche Lorraine and the first recipe was said to have dated back to the 18th century where it was found in a French soldier's notebook. Some *Picardie* locals like to add other additional vegetables such as broccoli or carrots.

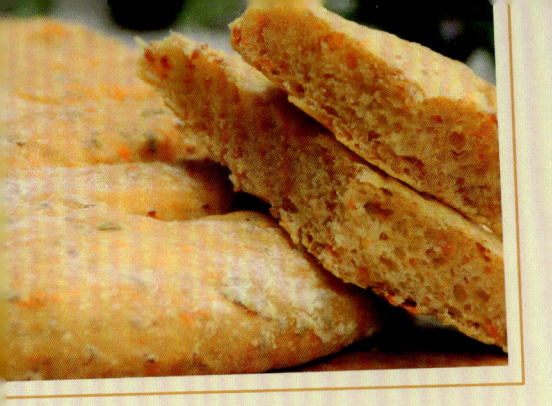

Fougasse
Fougasse

MAKE THE *PÂTE À PIZZA* according to the recipe and knead until smooth. Knead in the ham and olives (or dried tomatoes). *If necessary, add a little more flour (15 – 20 g) if the dough becomes too sticky after adding the olives or tomatoes.*

Leave covered in a warm place until doubled in size. Knock back the dough, knead again then divide in half. Roll out to an oval shape (15 x 25 cm). Repeat with the other half. Make cuts down the length (a little like buttonholes slightly slanted) and stretch the dough lengthways to allow the cuts to open out.

Leave covered in a warm place again until doubled in size.

Cook for about 20 minutes.

As a variation, sprinkle with grated cheese before cooking.

Makes 2 *fougasses*

Oven: 200°C

- 2 quantities *pâte à pizza* (see *recettes de base*)

- 150 g grated smoked ham
- 80 g olives or dried tomatoes, chopped

VARIATION
Bacon *fougasse* ....P. 104
Fougasse aux lardons

Starters
Entrées

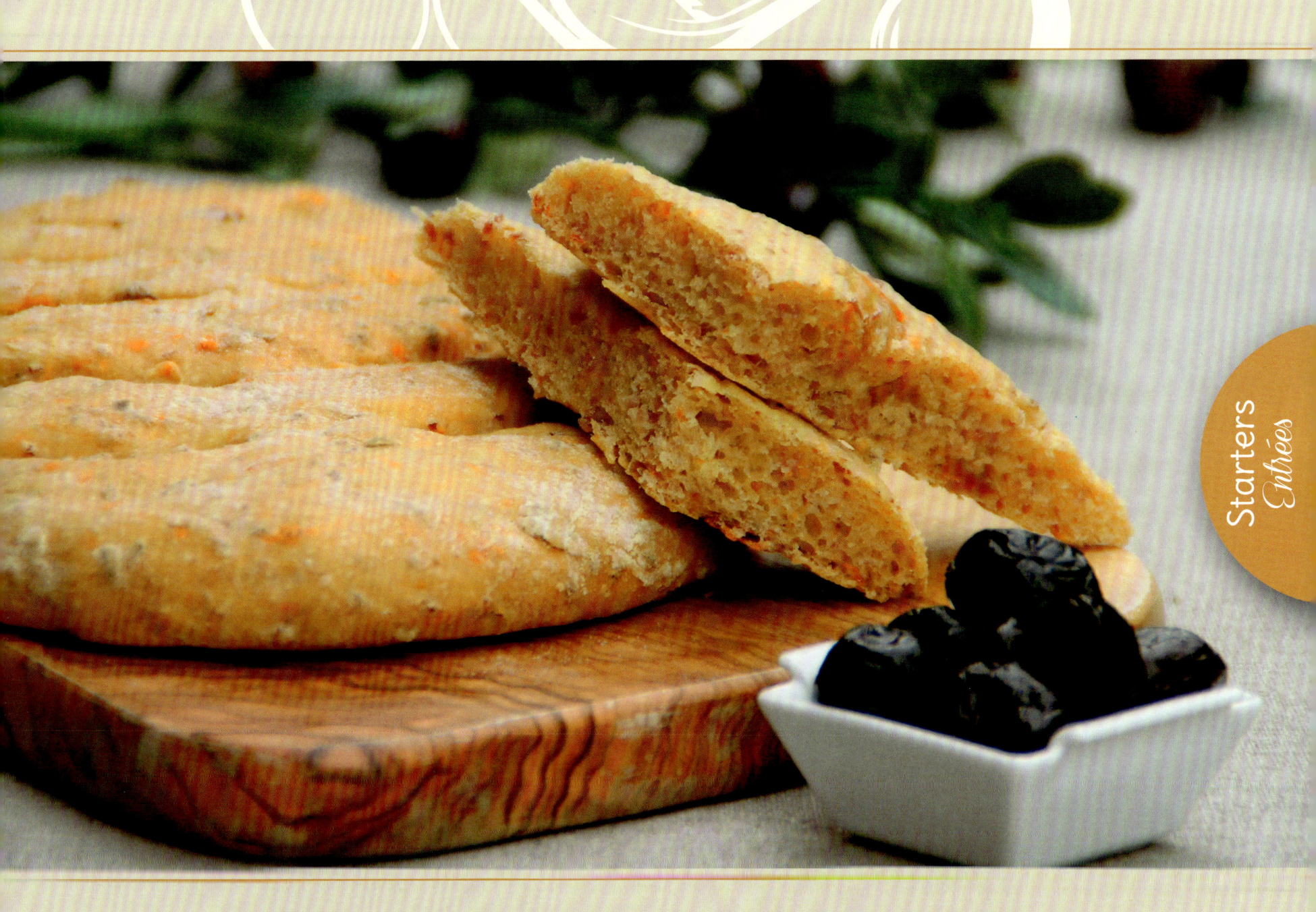

Fougasse comes from the latin word *focacius* meaning baked on the hearth or fireplace. Originally *fougasse* was a bread designed to test the temperature of the bread oven. To avoid waste, bakers invented different fillings and created the first *fougasses*!

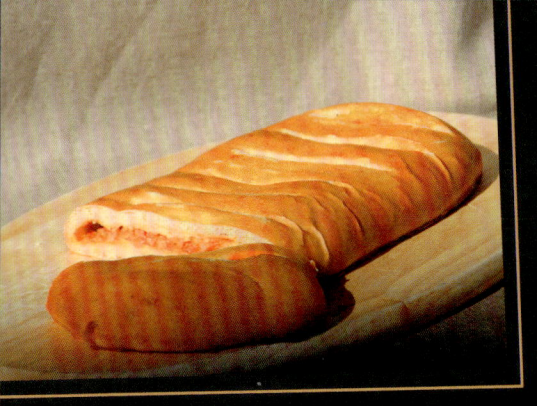

Bacon fougasse
Fougasse aux lardons

MAKE THE DOUGH: Crumble the yeast with the sugar into the warm water. Leave aside in a warm place until the yeast froths.

Put the flour in a large bowl and make a well in the centre. Add the salt, olive oil and egg. Pour in the yeast liquid and knead together until smooth and the sides of the bowl clean. Leave covered in a warm place until double in size.

MAKE THE FILLING: Fry the bacon until just cooked. Mix together all the rest of the ingredients for the filling. Add the bacon.

Divide the dough in half. Roll out one half into a rectangle approximately 5 mm thick. For a plaited effect, cut strips on one third of the longer side and do the same on the opposite side. The strips should be slanted slightly and not horizontal.

Place half of the filling in the centre of the rectangle then plait the *fougasse* enclosing the filling.

Repeat with the other half of the dough and filling.

Leave to rise, covered, in a warm place for at least 1½ hours.

Glaze with the egg then cook for about 20 - 25 minutes. *If the top is beginning to brown before it is completely cooked, cover with foil.*

Turn out onto a cooling rack and cover with a tea towel.

Serve warm with a green salad.

The variations for *fougasse* are endless: olives, dried tomatoes, thyme, bacon, blue cheese, onion...

For a different style *fougasse*: roll into an oval shape and place the filling over one half and cut incisions into the dough like buttonholes, on the other half, stretching the edges to enlarge the holes. Fold over on top of the filling, pressing the edges together to seal the filling. Brush with olive oil before cooking.

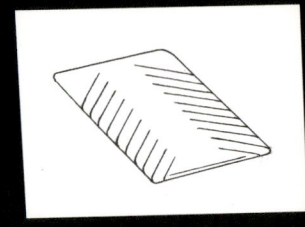

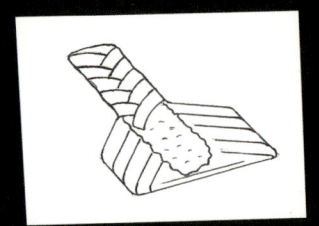

Makes 2 *fougasses*

Oven: 180°C

Dough:
- 20 g fresh yeast
- 1 tablespoon sugar
- 300 ml warm water
- 560 g plain flour
- 2 teaspoons salt
- 70 ml olive oil
- 1 egg

Filling:
- 300 g smoked bacon, chopped
- 200 g grated cheese
- 200 g seasoned *coulis de tomates* (see *recettes de base*)
- 100 g thick double cream

Glaze:
- 1 beaten egg

Starters *Entrées*

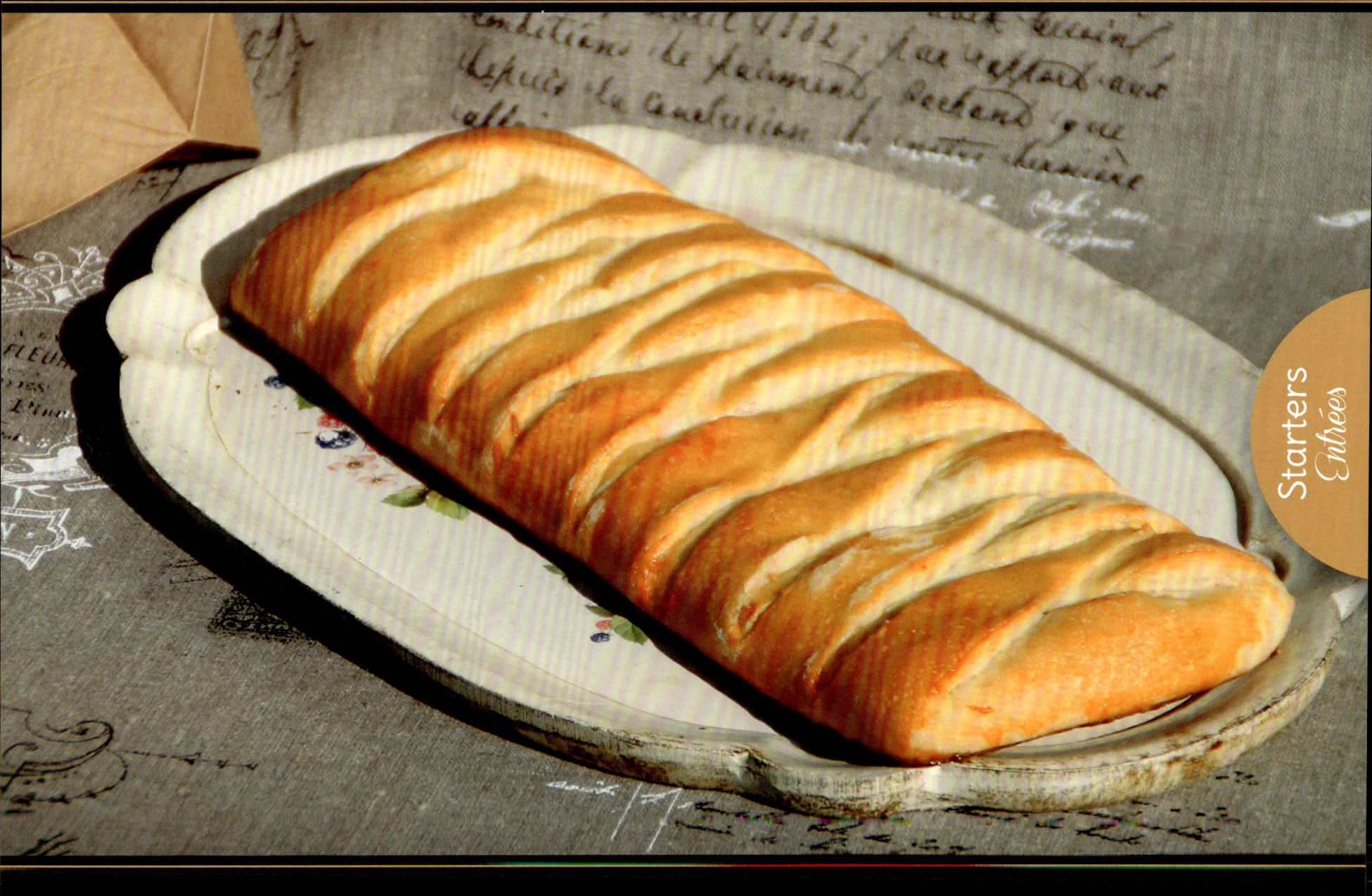

France is the biggest manufacturer of *fougasse* with every region having its own speciality, but it is particularly popular in *Provence*, *Côte d'Azur* and the Alps. They normally include lardons, olives and anchovies in their ingredients.

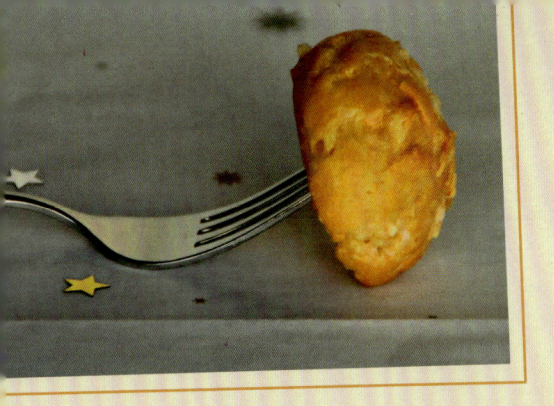

Gougères
Gougères

Put the water and the butter into a saucepan. Heat until the butter is melted and the water boiling.

Take off the heat and add the flour and salt. Stir with a wooden spoon until well combined. Put back on the heat and cook for about 2 - 3 minutes until the sides of the saucepan are clean. Leave to cool slightly.

Add the eggs one at a time, beating between each addition. The mixture should be smooth and glossy. Stir in the grated cheese.

Pipe small rounds of the pastry onto a baking sheet. *They will rise to about double this size.*

Sprinkle a little extra grated cheese over each *gougère*.

Cook in a hot oven for about 20 minutes. *Do not open the oven during cooking.* After 20 minutes, open the oven door and without removing them, make a small slit, with a sharp, pointed knife, in the side of each *gougère* to help them dry out and prevent them from being soggy inside. Cook for a further 3-4 minutes or until golden and crispy.

Serve warm as a starter with a green salad.

Makes 40 - 50 *gougères*

Oven: 190°C

- 450 ml water
- 150 g butter
- 200 g plain flour
- Pinch of salt
- 5 medium or 6 small eggs
- 150 g grated cheese plus extra for sprinkling over the top.

Variation: add some cooked bacon or ham with the cheese.

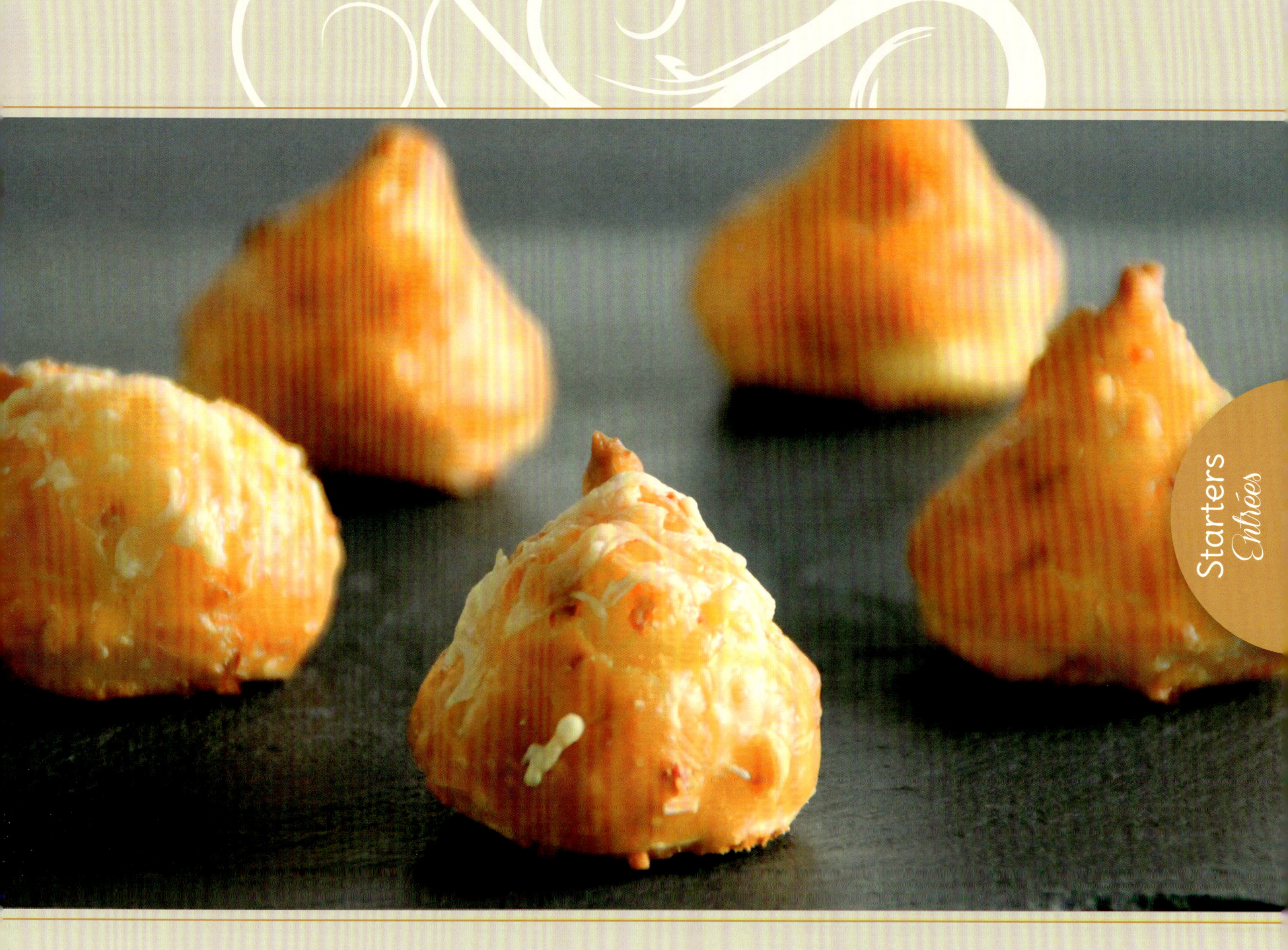

Gougères are little choux pastries enriched with cheese and originated from *Bourgogne* and *Franche-Comté*.
Serve as a starter or make smaller ones for an *apéritif*.

Starters *Entrées*

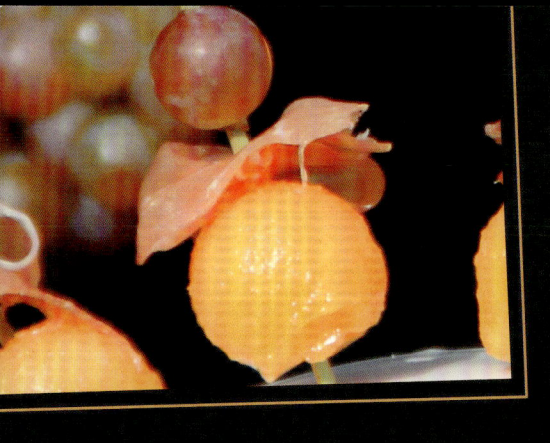

Melon with cured ham
Melon au jambon cru

Cut the melon in half and remove the seeds. Remove the flesh and cut into big cubes or scoop out into balls with a melon baller.

Cut the slices of ham into thin strips.

Fix the pieces of melon onto a cocktail stick with a slice of ham and a grape to finish. *If desired, wrap the ham around the melon before fixing it onto the cocktail stick and adding half a cherry tomato.*

Sprinkle with pepper and serve chilled.

- 1 melon
- 4 thin slices cured ham
- Bunch of grapes
- Freshly ground pepper

Starters *Entrées*

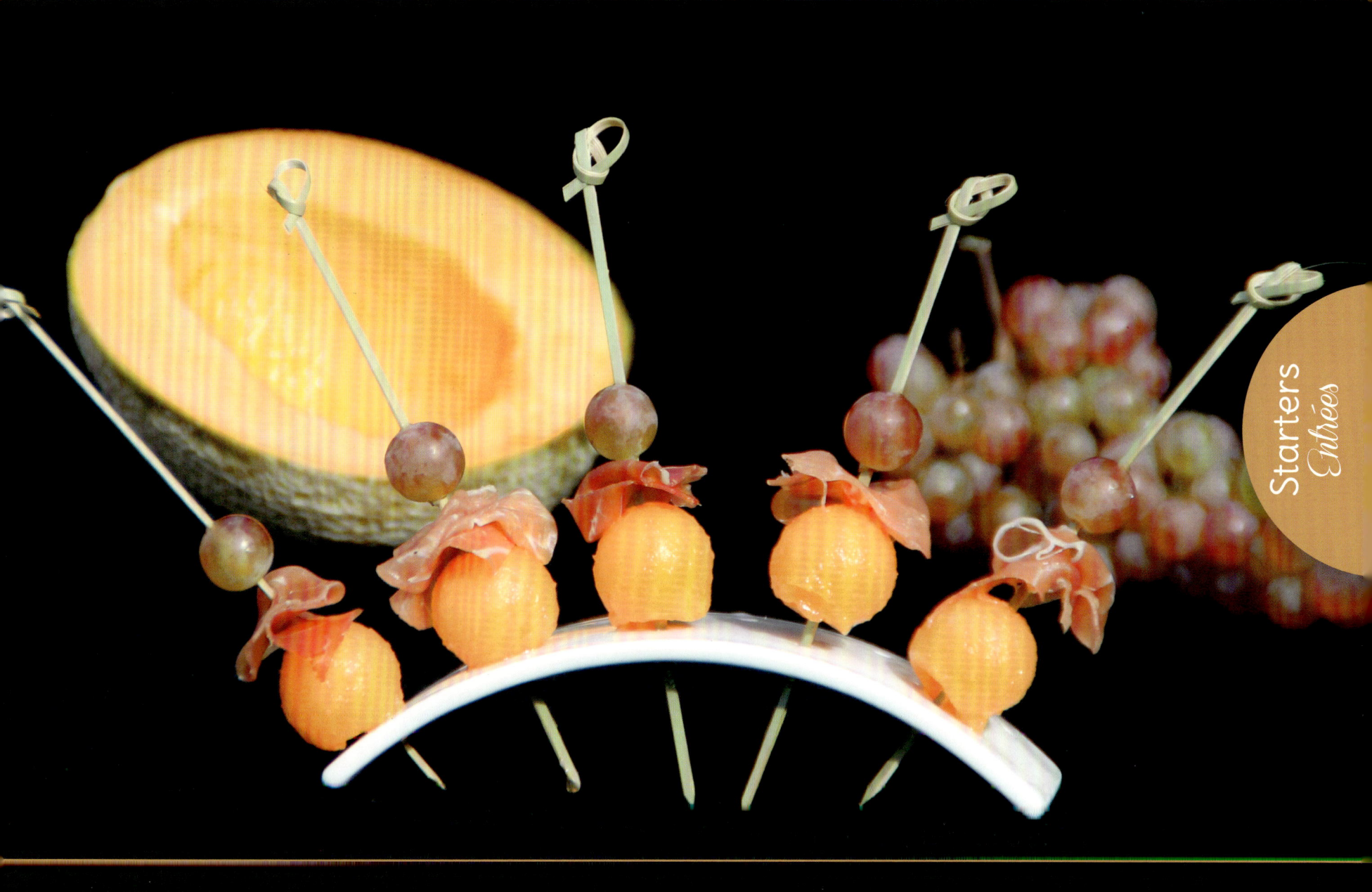

A sure sign of summer is when melons begin to appear on the market stalls!
Whether it's *melon au porto* or *melon au jambon cru*, there are many ways to enjoy this delicious sweet, juicy fruit with its unique flavour.
The salty flavour of cured ham with the sweetness of melon makes it a perfect combination.

109

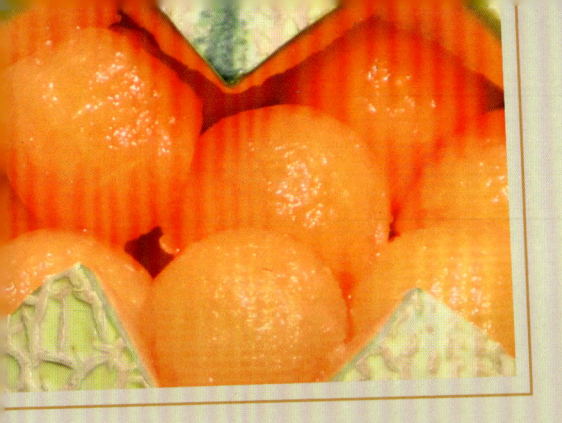

Melon with port
Melon au porto

Cut a lid off the melon by making zigzag patterns, like the teeth of a saw.

Carefully remove the lid. Remove the seeds with a tablespoon.

Scoop out the flesh using a melon baller. Replace them inside the melon.

Pour over the port.

Serve chilled.

Serves approx. 6 persons

- 2 melons
- 4 tablespoons port

As a variation, use small melons and cut in half. Scoop out the seeds and pour the port inside the hole. Serve individual half melons per person.

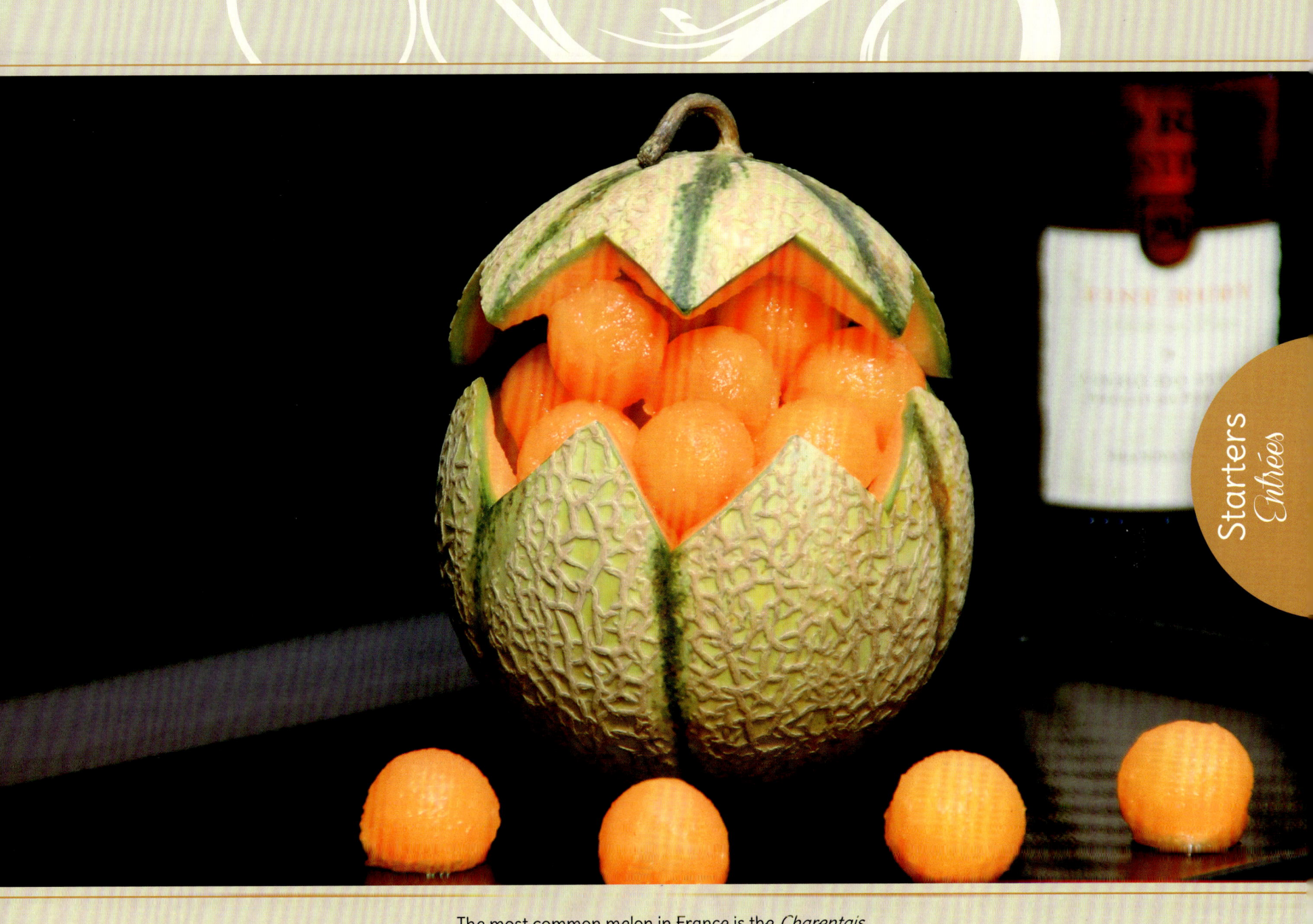

The most common melon in France is the *Charentais*.
The skin of this type of melon is slightly patterned and turns yellow as it matures.

There are 4 points to keep in mind when choosing a melon:
1. It must feel heavy to hold.
2. Its light-green skin is turning yellow and should show well-marked grooves.
3. There is a crack around the peduncle and the stalk is removed easily.
4. It should be delicately fragrant.

Starters *Entrées*

111

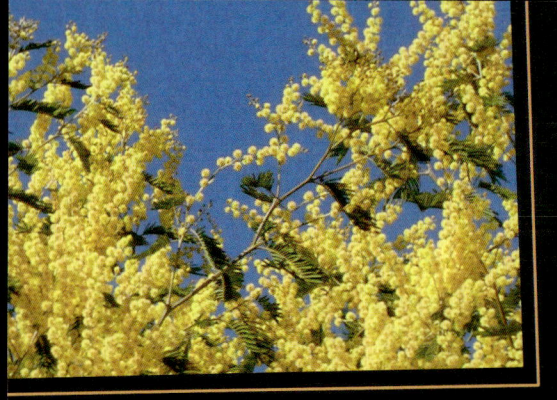

Mimosa eggs
Oeufs mimosa

Boil the eggs for 10 minutes. *For perfect rounded eggs (without an air pocket), pierce 2 or 3 holes at the base (the rounded end) with a pin or a needle before cooking, to allow any air to escape. Immersing them in cold water after cooking makes shelling easier.*

PREPARE THE MAYONNAISE according to the recipe.

Peel the eggs and cut in half lengthways, separating the yolks from the white.

Place 6 half yolks into a shallow bowl and mash them with a fork. Add the mayonnaise and mix together. Season with salt and pepper according to taste.

Fill each half egg white with the mixture.

Finely grate the remaining yolks and sprinkle over the eggs.

Decorate with black olives.

Serve chilled.

Serves 4 persons

- 4 eggs
- 60 g mayonnaise (see *recettes de base*)
- Black olives, for decoration

Can be served with a green salad or as an accompaniment to crudités.

As a variation, add herbs (such as chives or tarragon), mustard or tomato ketchup, crab meat or tuna to the filling.

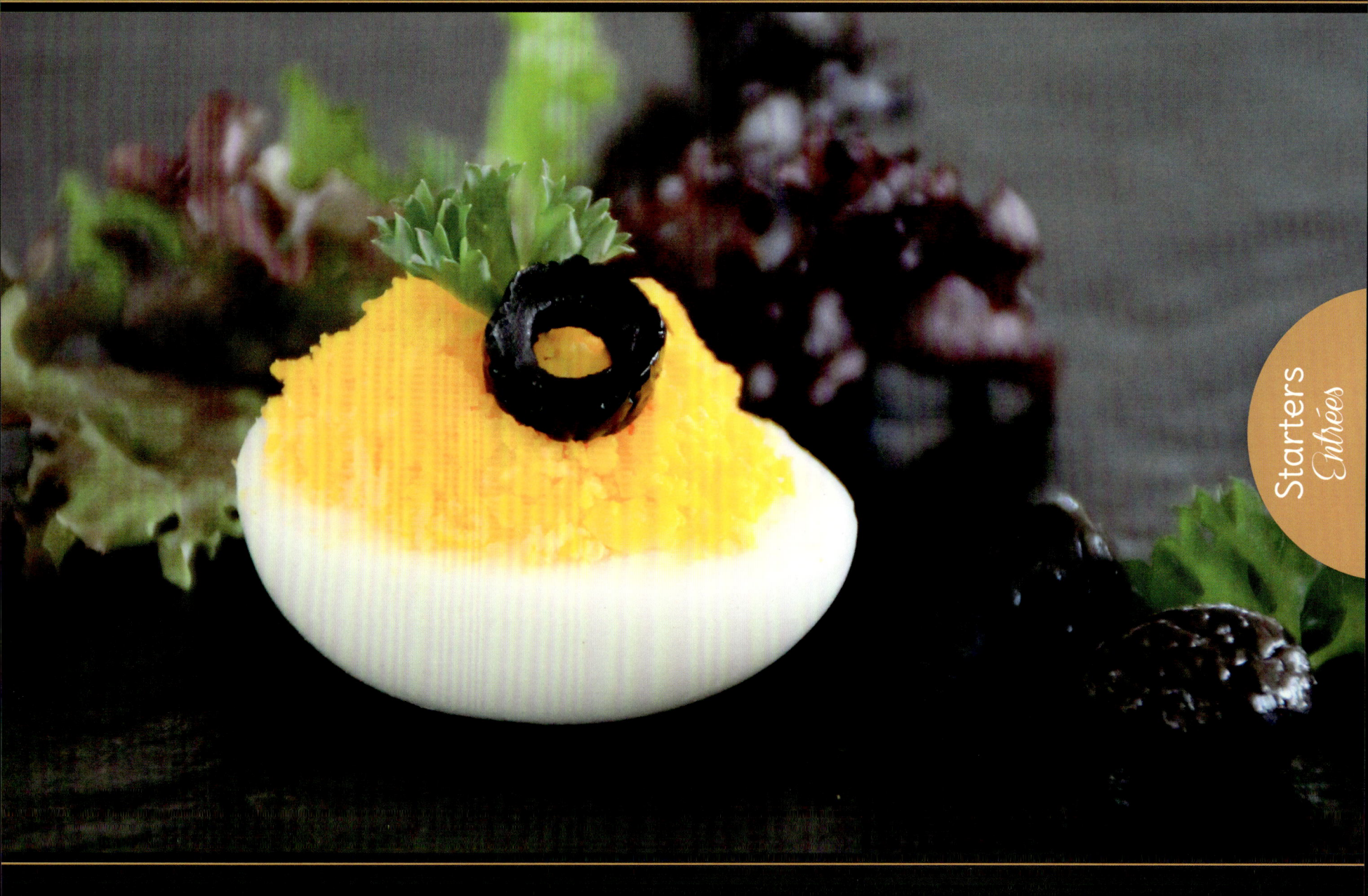

Oeufs mimosa are a typical starter of *grand-mère's époque*, yet enjoyed just as much today.
This recipe gets its name from the mimosa tree, which is very common in the South of France, as the grated yolks look just like the tiny, yellow flowers which bloom from late winter to early spring.

Starters
Entrées

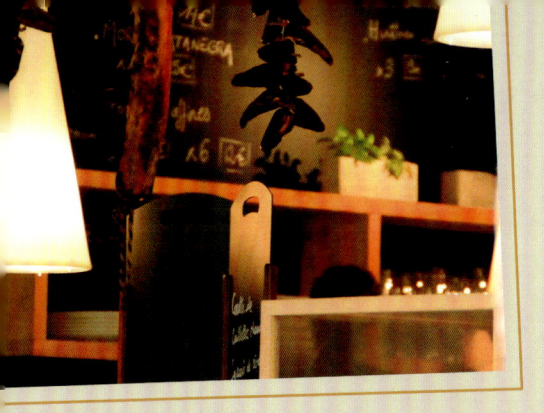

Provençale-style pizza
Pissaladière

MAKE THE *PATE À PIZZA* according to the recipe and leave in a warm place to rise until doubled in size.

MAKE THE TOPPING: Peel and finely slice the onions. *Use a mandolin cutter to make it easier.*

Heat 4 tablespoons of olive oil in a frying pan. Add the chopped onions, garlic, thyme, salt, pepper and sugar and cook on a gentle heat for about 45 minutes until the onions are soft, but not coloured.

Roll out the *pâte à pizza* and use to cover a rectangular greased baking tray (approx. 30 x 25 cm).

Brush the surface of the dough with 2 tablespoons of olive oil.

Cover with the cooked onions and then place the anchovies in a lattice pattern on top.

Place a black olive between the anchovies and sprinkle with a little more chopped thyme.

Leave to rise again in a warm place and cook for about 20 - 25 minutes.

Serve warm or hot.

Best served with a green salad as a starter.

Serves approx. 10 persons

Oven: 200°C

1 quantity *pâte à pizza* (see *recettes de base*)

Topping :
- 6 tablespoons olive oil
- 1 kg onions
- Salt
- Freshly ground pepper
- 2 garlic cloves, crushed
- A teaspoon of thyme
- 1 teaspoon sugar
- 12 - 18 anchovies, rinsed (cut in 2 or 4 lengthways)
- Black olives

Starters *Entrées*

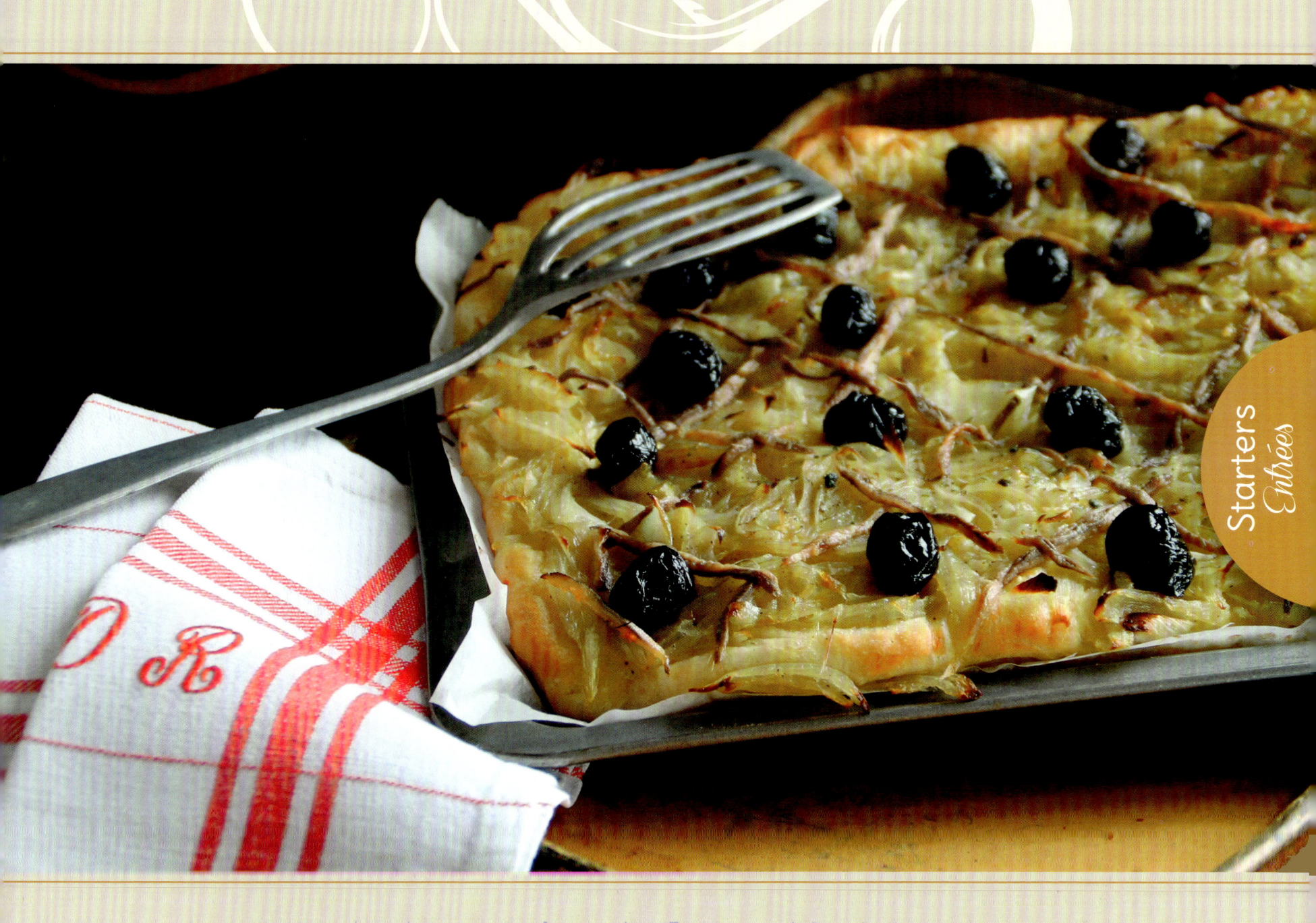

Pissaladière is a traditional *niçoise* recipe, from southern France, named after *pissalat* meaning anchovy paste, and is easily recognised by the lattice pattern of the anchovies.
There are many versions of this recipe: just add anchovy paste with garlic or add tomatoes to the anchovies and onions.

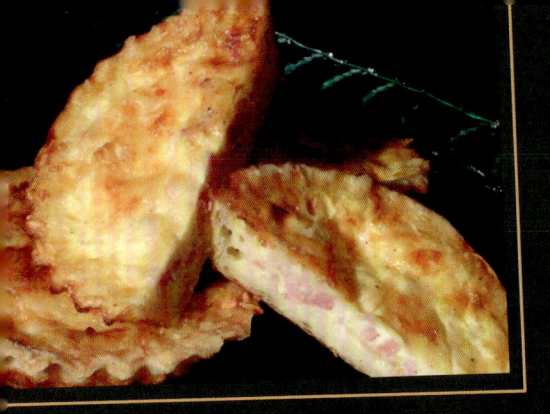

Quiche Lorraine

Quiche Lorraine

MAKE THE *PÂTE BRISÉE* according to the recipe.

Roll out the pastry to fit the base and sides of a well-greased and floured ovenproof pie dish (28 cm diameter). Cover with greaseproof paper, fill with baking beans and bake blind for about 30 minutes. Remove the baking beans and spread with the mustard. Cook uncovered for a further 5 minutes. *It is important that the pastry is completely cooked or it will become soggy when filled.*

MAKE THE FILLING: Lightly fry the bacon and leave aside to cool slightly.

Mix together the eggs, cream and milk. Season with the salt, freshly ground pepper and nutmeg. *Take care not to add too much salt as the bacon is already salted!*

Sprinkle the bacon over the pastry case and pour over the egg and cream mixture. Cook for about 40 - 45 minutes or until set and golden.

Serves approx. 6 persons

Oven: 180°C

- 1 quantity of *pâte brisée* (see *recettes de base*)
- 1 tablespoon Dijon mustard

Filling:
- 200 g smoked bacon, finely chopped
- 3 eggs
- 200 ml double cream
- 200 ml milk
- Salt
- Freshly ground pepper
- Nutmeg

Starters *Entrées*

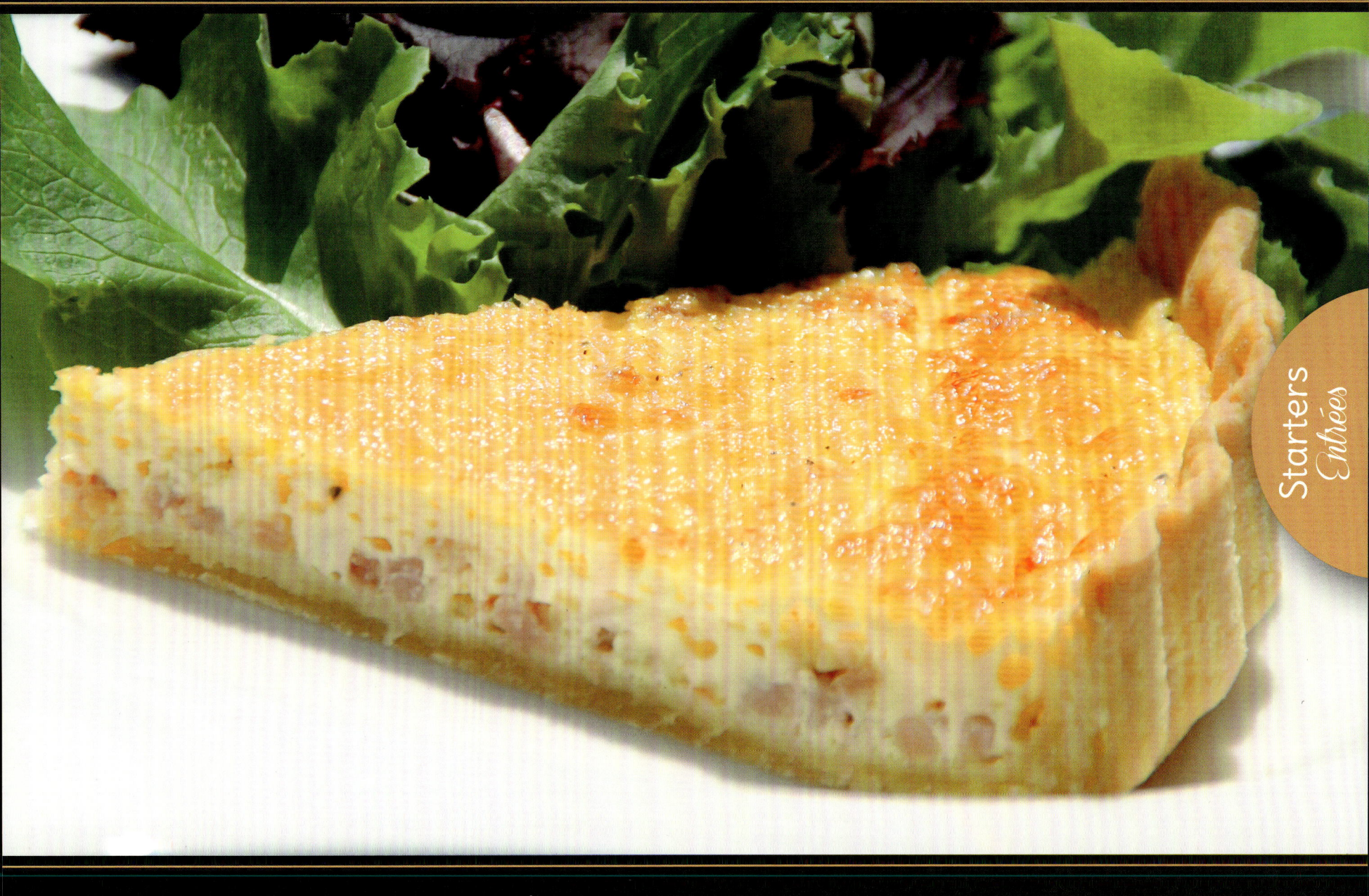

This is the original quiche recipe, from *Lorraine*, which does not have any cheese in it.
For a richer version, grated cheese can be added with the bacon.

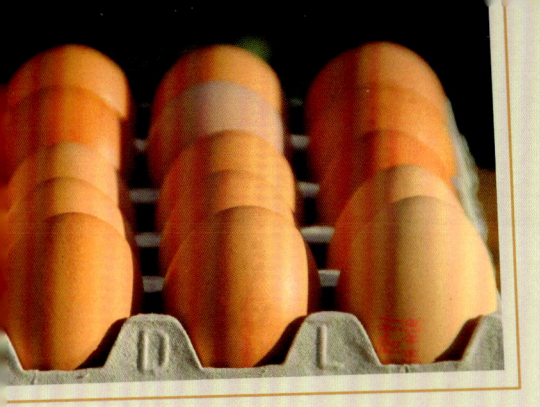

Cheese soufflé
Soufflé au fromage

Place the cornflour in a saucepan, and gradually blend with the cold milk. Bring to the boil, stirring all the time. Remove from the heat. Add the butter, grated cheese, nutmeg, and salt and pepper.

Leave to cool.

Add the yolks one by one, mixing well.

Whisk the egg whites with a pinch of salt until firm and glossy. Carefully fold the egg whites into the cheese mixture. Pour it into a well-greased soufflé dish filling it about 2/3 full. Chill for about 2 hours.

Heat the oven to 200°C.

Place in the oven once it has reached temperature, then immediately reduce the temperature to 150°C and bake for about 20 minutes. Increase the temperature to 200°C and cook for another 20 minutes.

Serve immediately (as it starts to sink very quickly).

Serves 4 - 6 persons

Oven: 200°C / 150°C

- 50 g cornflour
- 580 ml milk
- 100 g butter, cut into cubes
- Pinch of nutmeg
- 210 g grated cheese
- Salt and pepper
- 4 eggs, separated

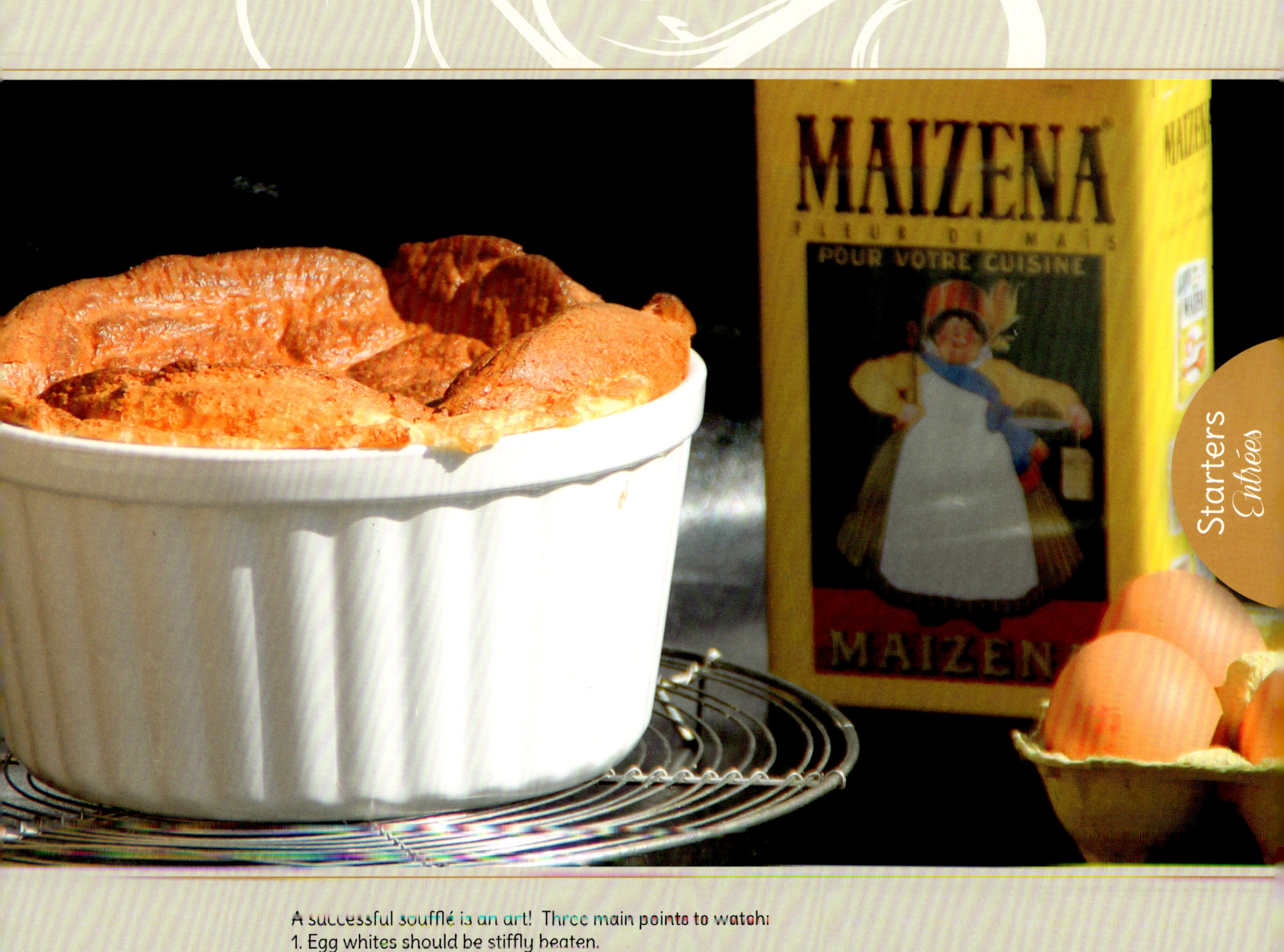

A successful soufflé is an art! Three main points to watch:
1. Egg whites should be stiffly beaten.
2. The soufflé base is the right consistency (not too liquid, nor too heavy).
3. Careful folding of the egg whites into the soufflé base.
Season the soufflé base well as it will become bland once the egg whites have been added.

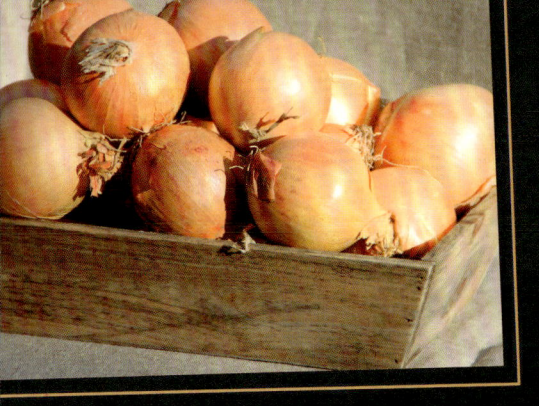

Onion tart
Tarte à l'oignon

Heat the olive oil in a large frying pan. Add the onions and cook on a medium heat for about 10 - 15 minutes until transparent but not coloured, stirring from time to time to avoid them burning. Add the thyme and mix well. Leave aside to cool.

MAKE THE *PÂTE BRISÉE* according to the recipe. Roll out to line a 28 cm diameter well-greased and floured ovenproof pie dish. Cover with greaseproof paper, fill with baking beans and bake blind for 10 - 15 minutes. Remove the baking beans and cook for a further 5 minutes.

MAKE THE FILLING: In a large bowl, mix together the cream and eggs. Season with salt, pepper and nutmeg according to taste.

Fill the pastry case with the onions. Sprinkle with the cheese and pour over the egg and cream mixture.

Cook for 35 - 40 minutes or until golden. Leave to stand in the dish for 5 minutes before serving.

VARIATION:

Onion tart with bacon
Tarte à l'oignon aux lardons

Add 100 g cooked smoked bacon, chopped, with the onions. Continue as above

Starters *Entrées*

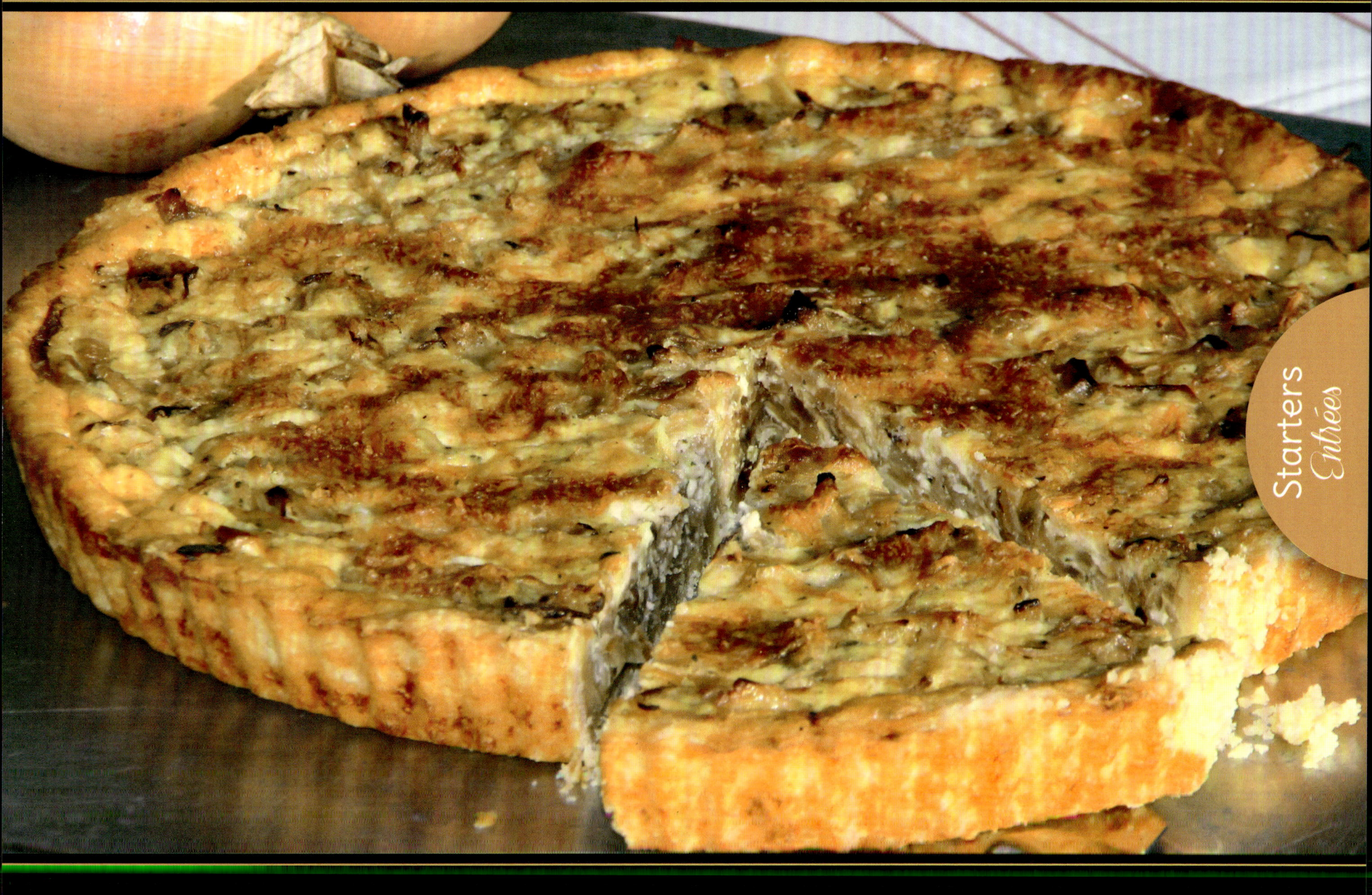

A crispy and melt in the mouth tart, this speciality from Alsace is delicious served with a fresh salad.

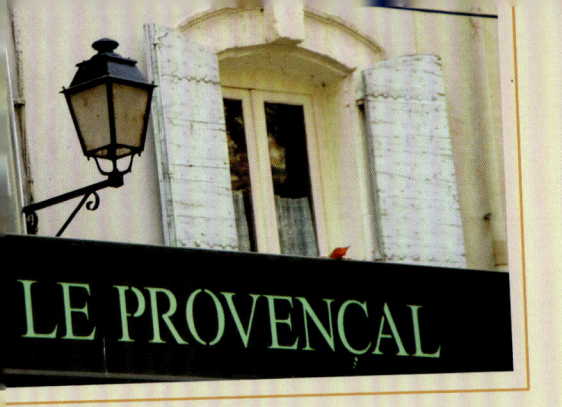

Provençale-style tart
Tarte à la provençale

MAKE THE PASTRY: Rub the butter into the flour until it becomes like fine breadcrumbs. Add the egg yolk and the water to make a pliable pastry dough. Leave covered in the fridge for about half an hour.

PREPARE THE TOPPING: Heat the oil in a frying pan and fry the onion until soft and transparent. Add the garlic, tomatoes and tomato paste. Stir in the bicarbonate of soda and dried oregano. Simmer on a low heat until it thickens.

Roll out the pastry to either fit one large 30 x 30 cm greased and floured baking tray or two smaller 30 x 18 cm baking trays. Prick the surface but do not pierce the pastry right through. Leave to rest in the fridge for another 30 minutes.

Cut the peppers into quarters lengthways and remove the seeds. Place skin side up under a grill and heat until the skins are black and blistering. Leave to cool. Peel off the skin and slice finely into strips.

Cover the pastry with greaseproof paper and fill with baking beans. Cook blind for about 10 - 15 minutes. Remove the baking beans and cook for another 5 minutes. *Continue cooking a little longer if the pastry appears uncooked.*

Spread the tomato mixture over the cooked pastry base. Arrange the peppers, anchovy fillets and olives on top. Cook for about 20 minutes.

Decorate with fresh oregano leaves before serving.

Serves approx. 10 persons

Oven: 180°C

Pastry:
- 250 g plain flour
- 150 g butter, diced
- 1 egg yolk, beaten
- 40 ml water

Topping:
- 2 tablespoons olive oil
- 1 large onion, chopped
- 2 garlic cloves, crushed
- 2 tins (400 g) chopped tomatoes (or 10 fresh tomatoes, skinned)
- 1 tablespoon concentrated tomato paste
- A pinch of bicarbonate of soda
- 1 teaspoon dried oregano
- 1 red pepper
- 1 yellow pepper
- 12 anchovy fillets
- Approx. 12 black olives, stoned
- Oregano leaves for decoration

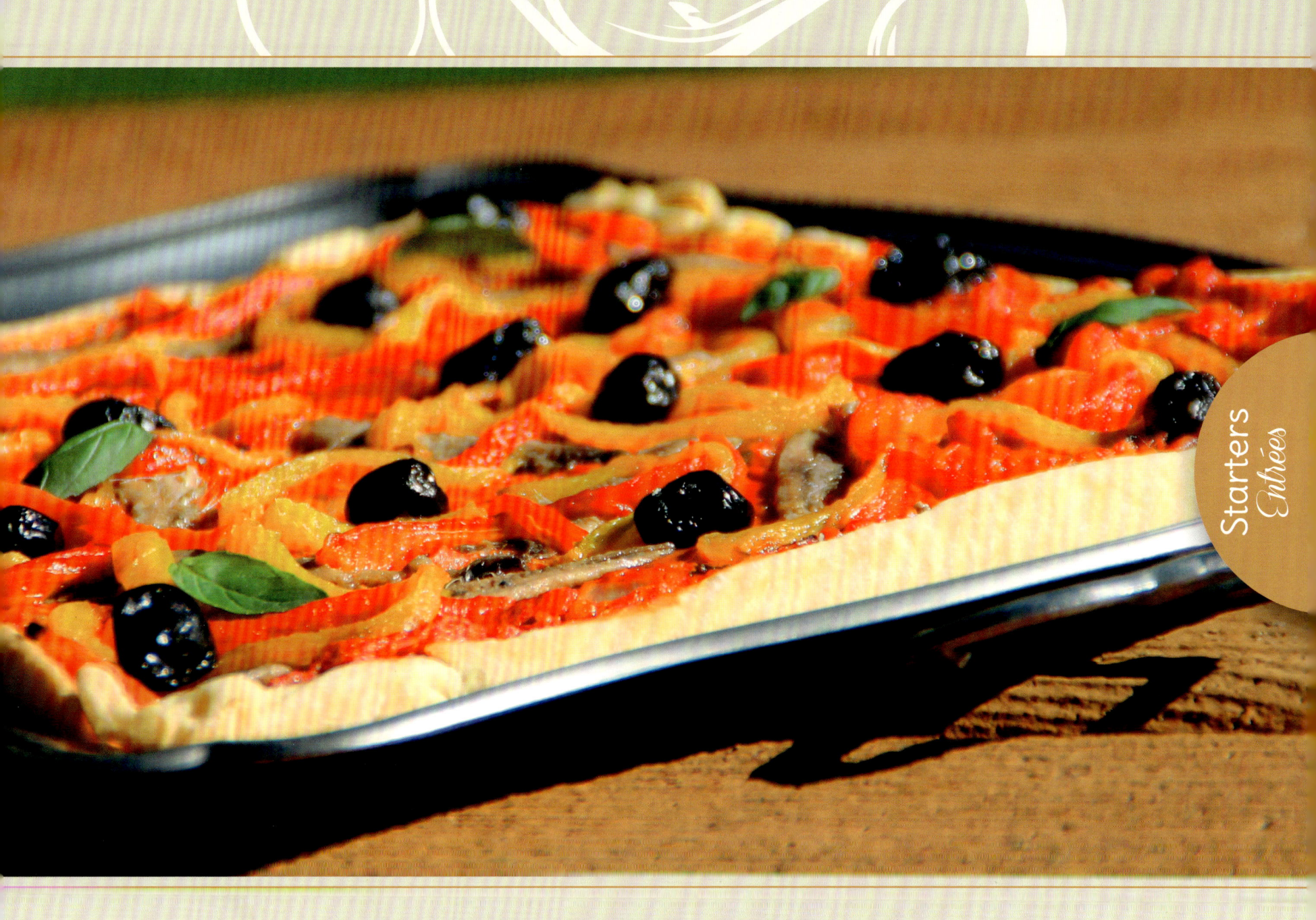

Tarte à la Provençale instantly spells tastes and colours of summer.
Grilling the peppers removes the bitter taste which is found in the skins.

Starters *Entrées*

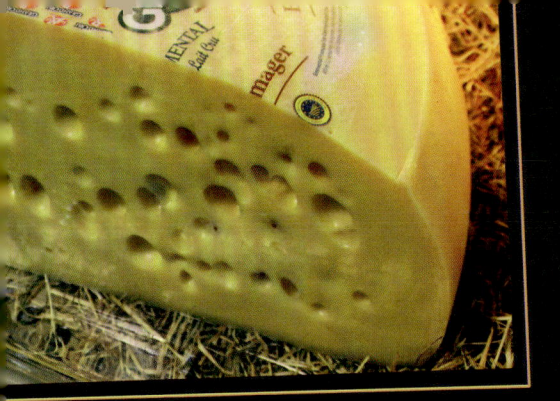

Cheese soufflé tartlets
Tartelettes soufflées au fromage

Roll out the pastry and cut into individual rounds. Press into well-greased 7 cm diameter moulds.

Slice the cheese using a vegetable peeler to make long, thin strips and place in the pastry bases.

Mix together the egg yolks with the flour, milk, cream, salt, pepper and nutmeg.

Whisk the egg whites until stiff then carefully fold into the egg and cream mixture.

Spoon the mixture into the pastry moulds.

Cook for about 20 minutes or until risen and set.

Serve warm

Makes approx. 28 mini tartlets

Oven: 200°C

- 2 ready-to-roll puff pastry (each of 230 g)
- 250 g *comté* cheese (or 150 g *comté* cheese plus 100 g *emmental* cheese)
- 4 eggs, separated
- 2 tablespoons plain flour
- 200 ml milk
- 250 ml double cream
- Salt and pepper
- 1 teaspoon nutmeg

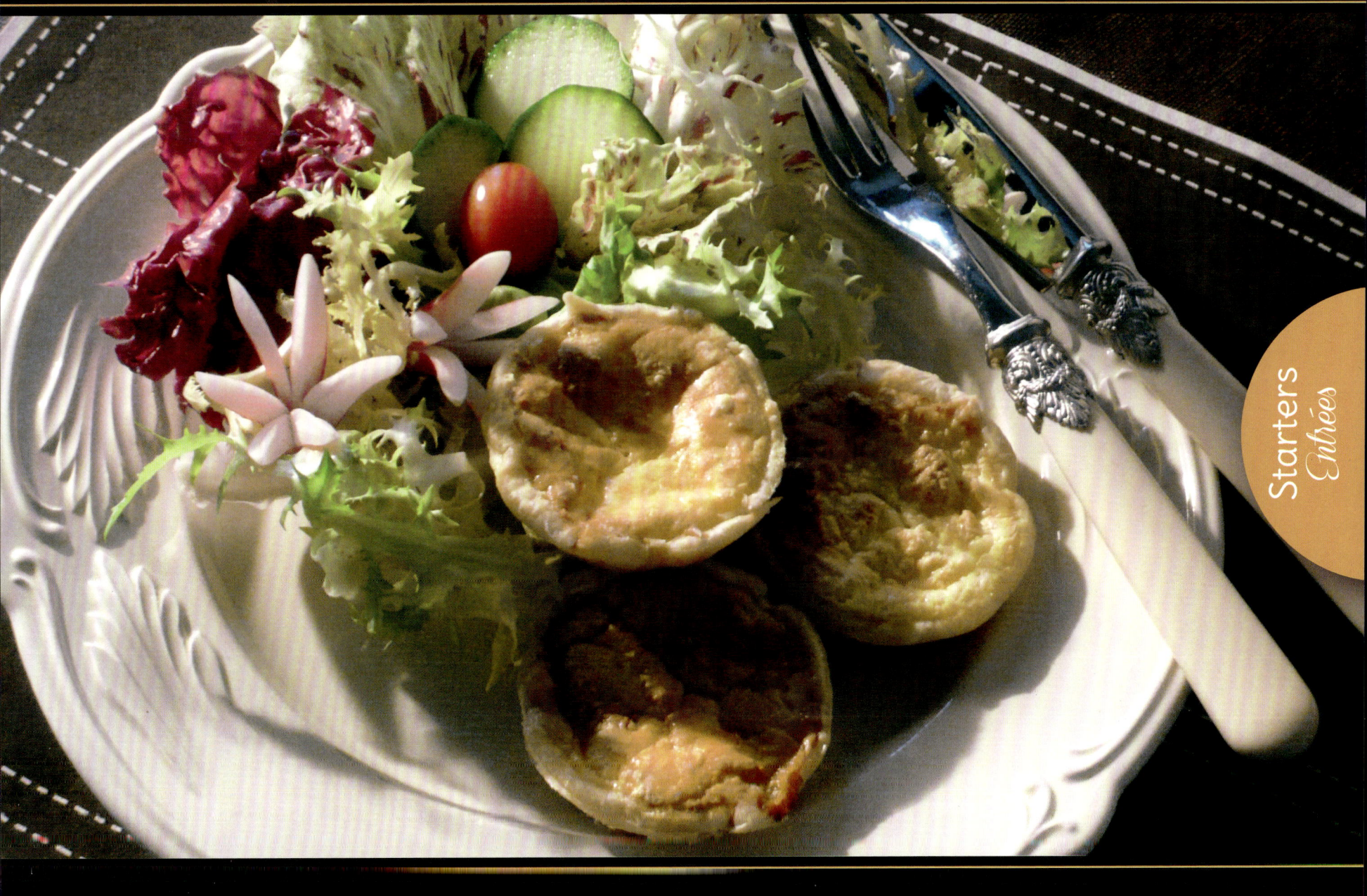

Lighter than a quiche, *tartelettes soufflées au fromage* are a delicate starter served with a fresh green salad.

Starters *Entrées*

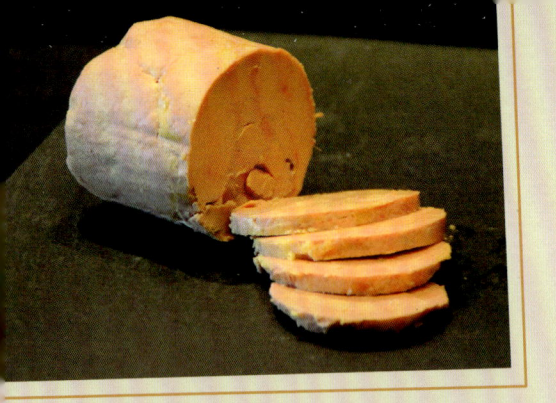

Foie gras with spiced honey loaf
Toasts au foie gras

Slice the *pain d'épices*.

Cut into square 'toasts' (approx. 3 x 3 cm).

Slice the *foie gras* the same thickness as the little 'toasts'.

Cut into squares and place on top of the *pain d'épices*.

Serve with *confit d'oignons rouges* (see recipe below).

Serves 4 persons

- 100 g *foie gras* (at room temperature)
- 100 g *pain d'épices* (see recipe page 44 volume 2—made with only 250 g of honey)

Red onion chutney
Confit d'oignons rouges

Finely slice the onions and place in a saucepan with the wine and vinegar. Cook on a low heat until all the liquid has evaporated (about 1 hour).

Add the water and honey and continue cooking for about 35 - 40 minutes. Stir from time to time to prevent it sticking to the base of the saucepan.

Add the butter, salt and pepper and stir well.

Place in warm, sterile jars and close the lids.

Serve with *toasts au foie gras*.

Red onion chutney:
- 600 g red onions
- 500 ml red wine
- 100 ml red wine vinegar
- 500 ml water
- 70 g honey
- 40 g butter
- Salt and pepper

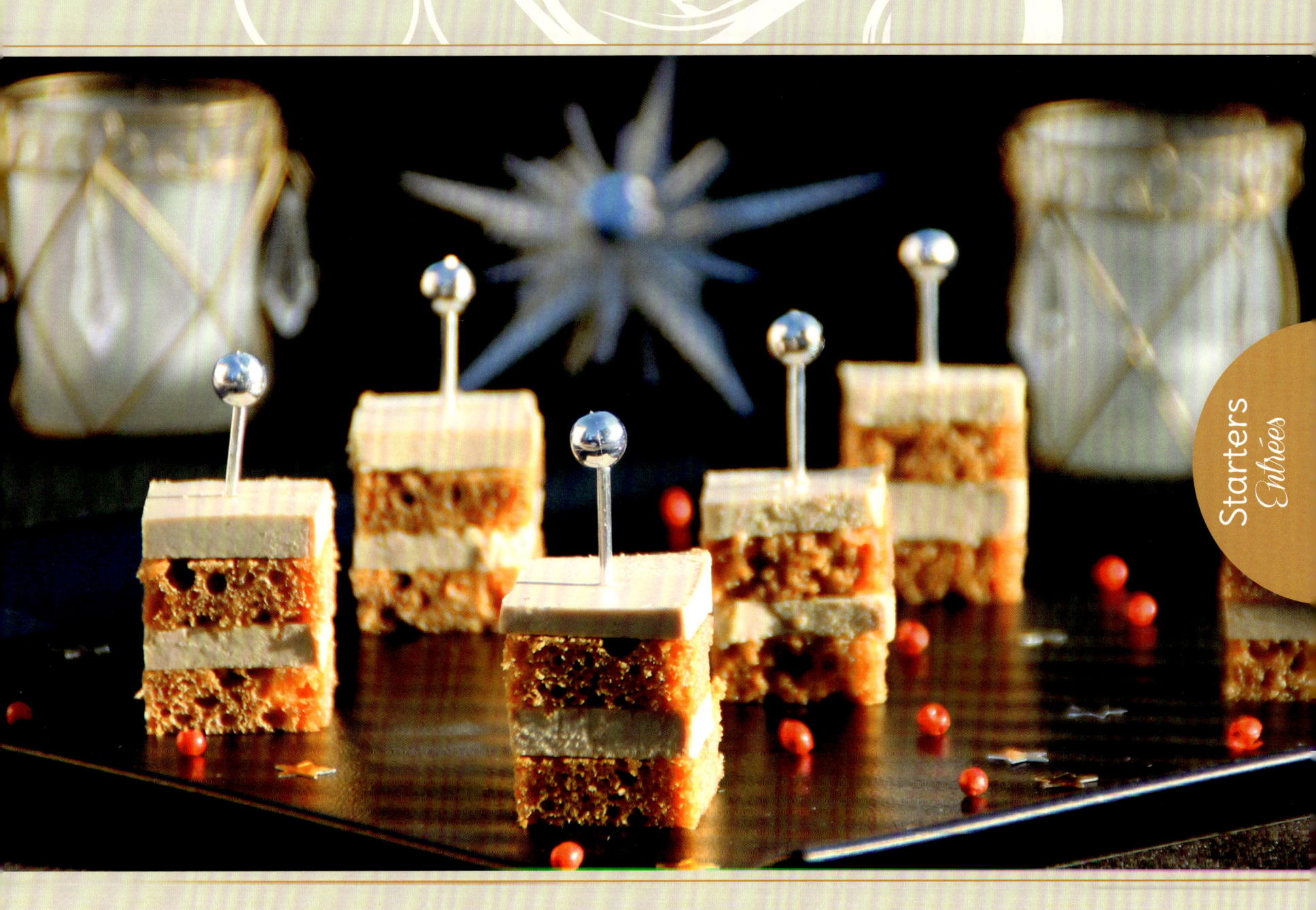

Subtle contrasts between sweet and savoury accentuates the delicate flavour of *foie gras*.

Starters *Entrées*

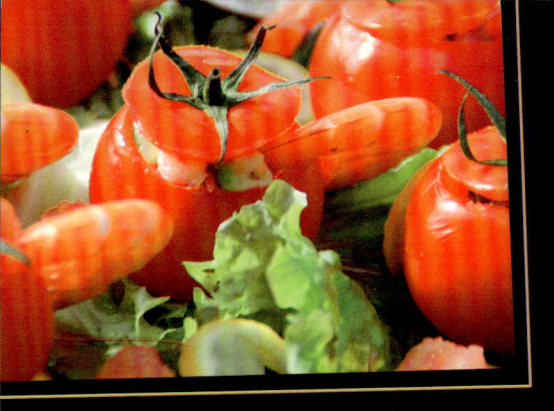

Avocado-filled tom[atoes]

Tomates garnies

Wash the tomatoes well and cut off the top of each one. Reserve. Scoop out the insides of each tomato and discard. Season the interior with salt and freshly ground pepper.

Peel the avocado and chop into cubes. Sprinkle them with the lemon juice to avoid them browning. Rinse the shrimps well and dry thoroughly.

Peel the grapefruit and separate the segments. Cut each segment into small pieces, keeping aside a few whole segments for decoration.

Mix together the pieces of avocado, shrimps and grapefruit. Season with salt and pepper and fill the tomatoes with this mixture. Replace the tops.

Place the stuffed tomatoes on a serving plate lined with salad leaves. Decorate with the reserved segments of grapefruit and the prawns.

Serve with a *vinaigrette* (see *recettes de base*) or *sauce cocktail* (see *recettes de base*)

Starters
Entrées

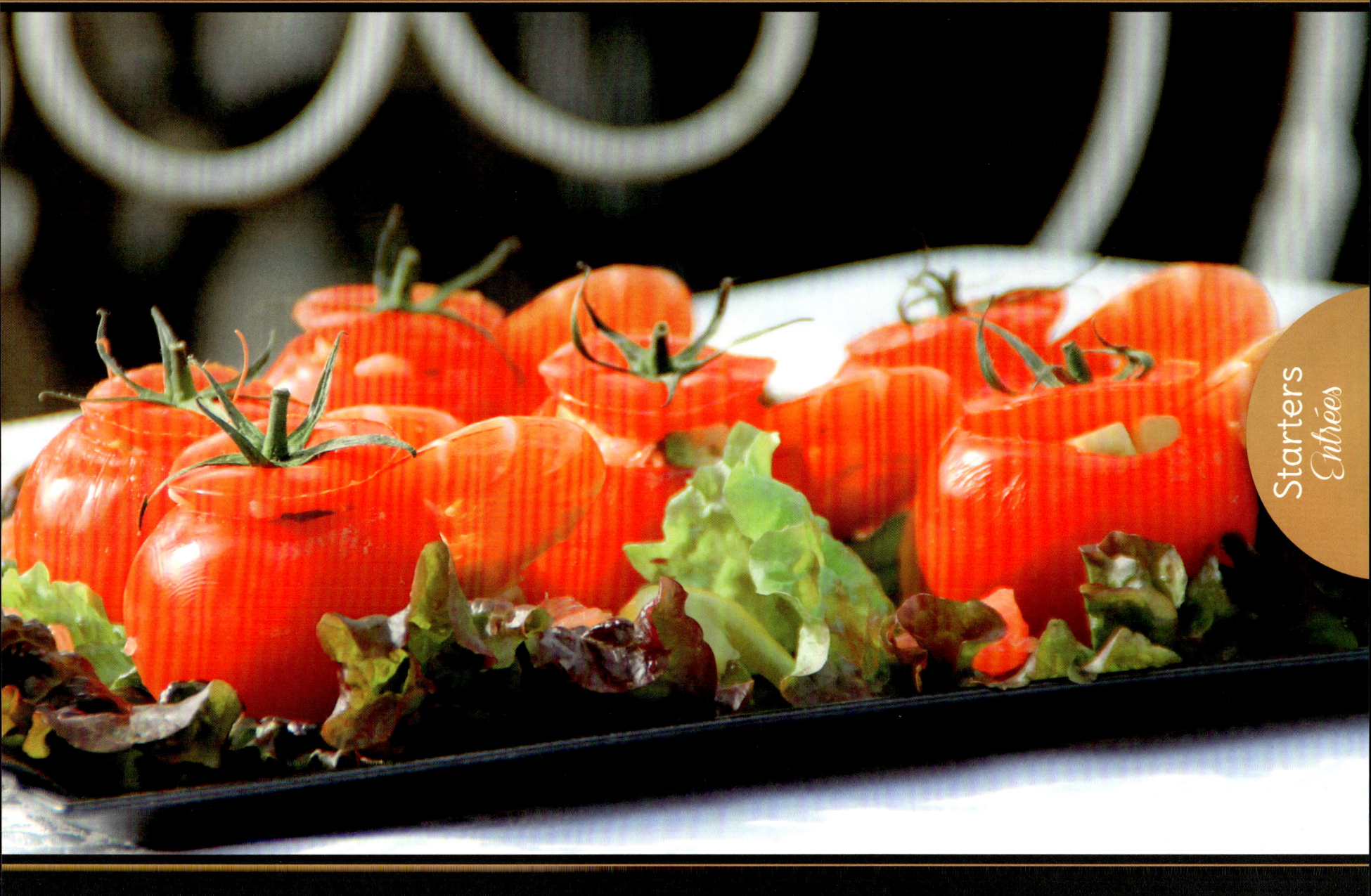

For a colourful and healthy summery starter.
Just 100 g of tomatoes covers an adult's daily requirement of vitamins A, B and C.

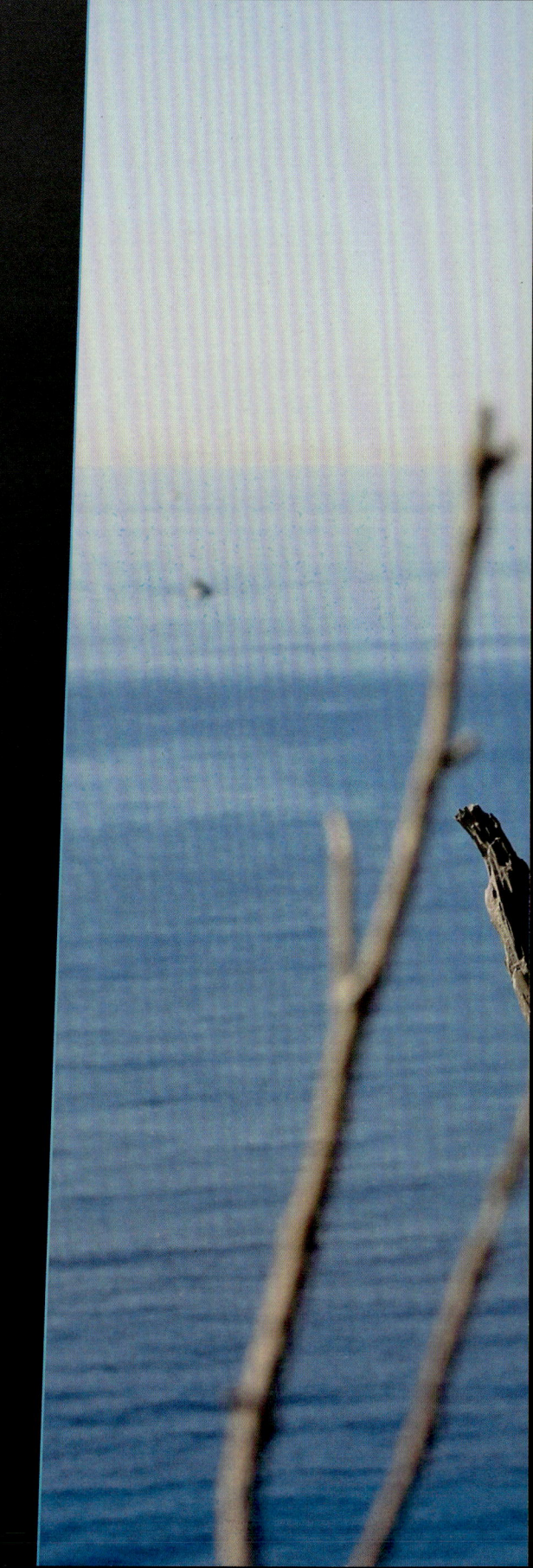

Fish and shellfish
Poissons et fruits de mer

134 Creamed cod
Brandade de morue

134 Creamed cod on toast
Toasts à la brandade de morue

134 Creamed cod pie
Brandade de morue parmentière

134 *Bouchées à la reine* with creamed cod
Bouchées à la reine à la brandade de morue

136 Scallops
Coquilles Saint-Jacques

138 Provençale-style baked sea bream
Dorade provençale au four

140 Oysters
Huîtres

142 Mussels in white wine
Moules marinières

144 Salmon parcels with herb sauce
Saumon en papillote et sauce aux herbes

146 Trout with almonds
Truite aux amandes

Warning !
Some recipes contain alcohol.

Fish and shellfish Poissons et fruits de mer

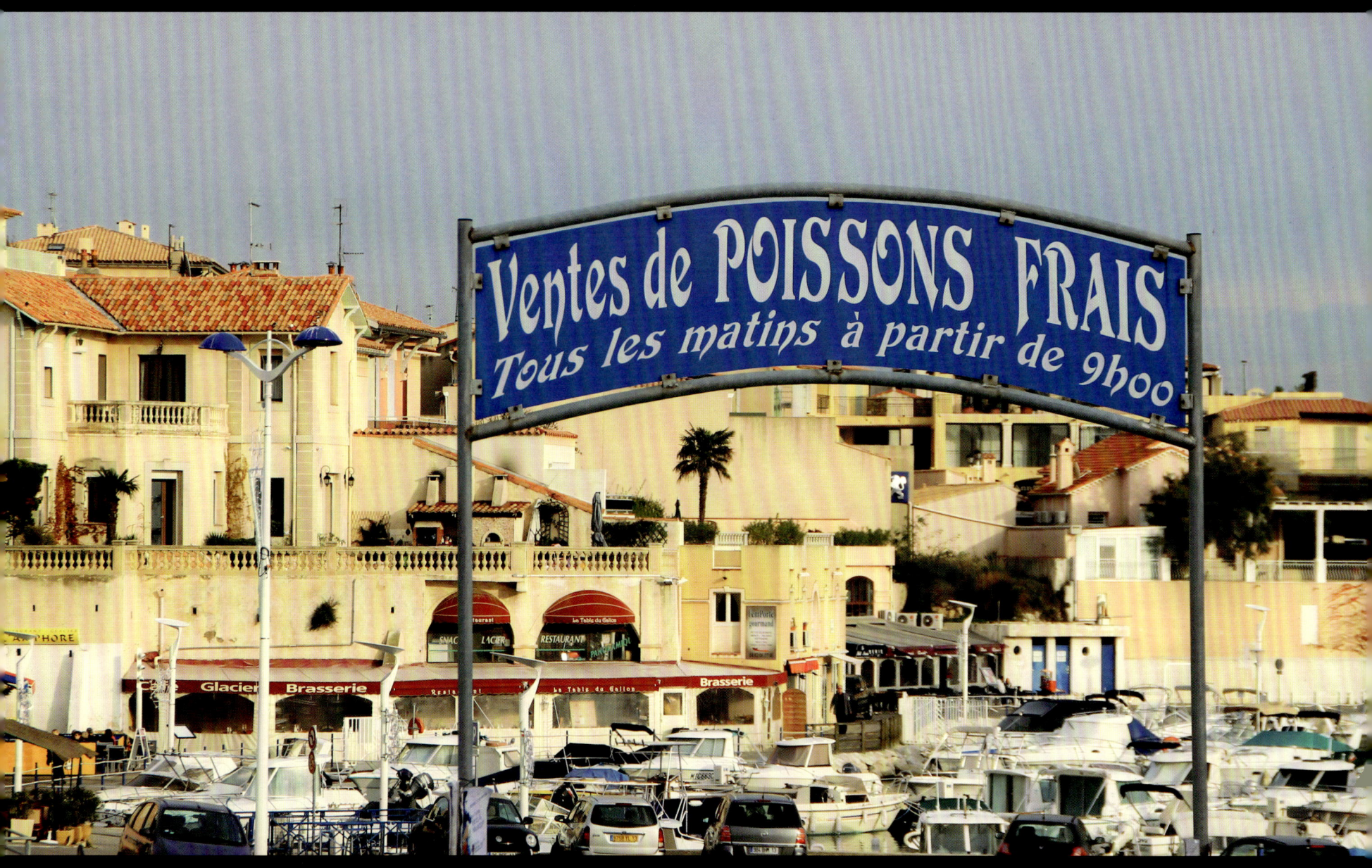

Ventes de POISSONS FRAIS
Tous les matins à partir de 9h00

From the Atlantic to the Mediterranean...

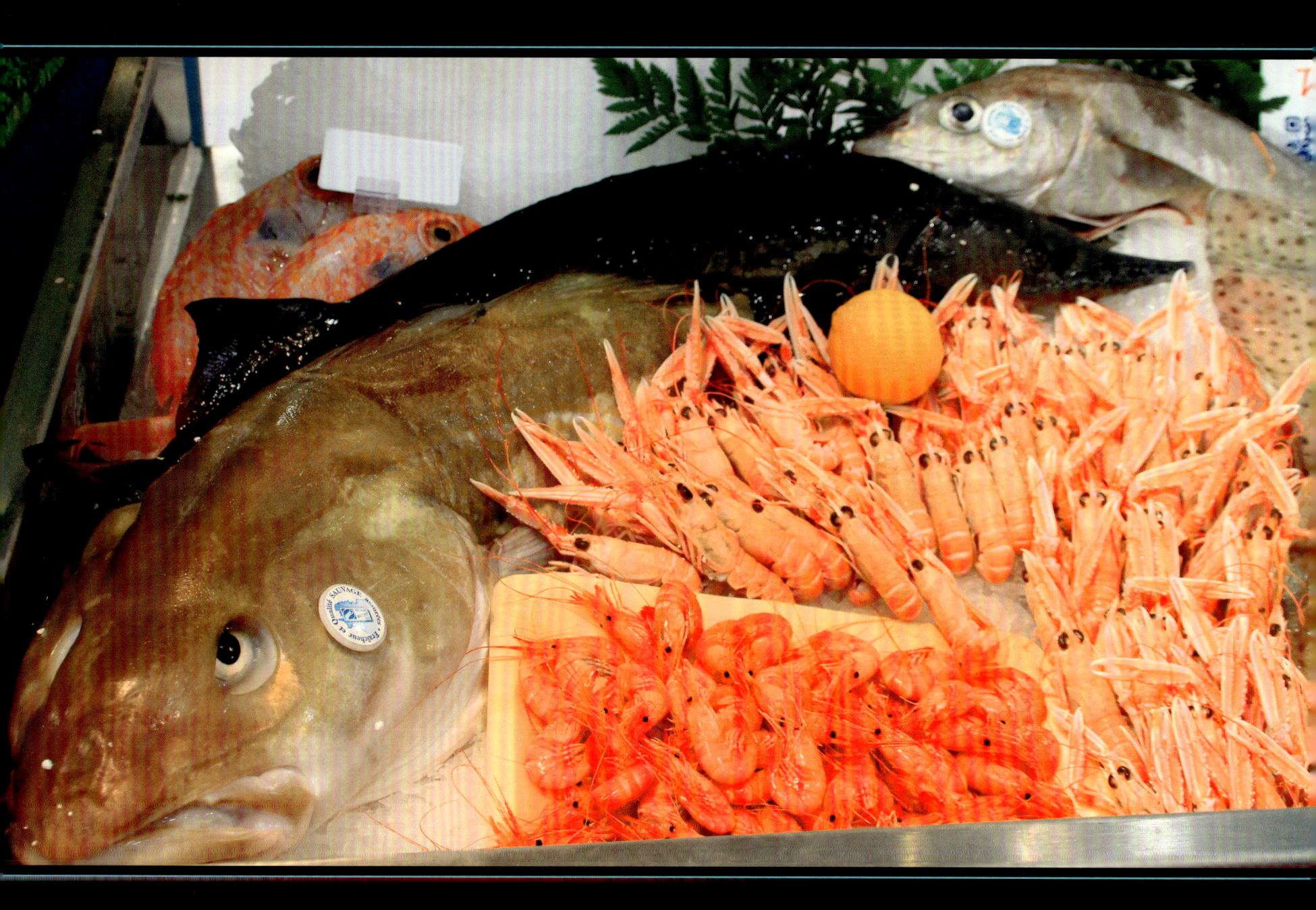

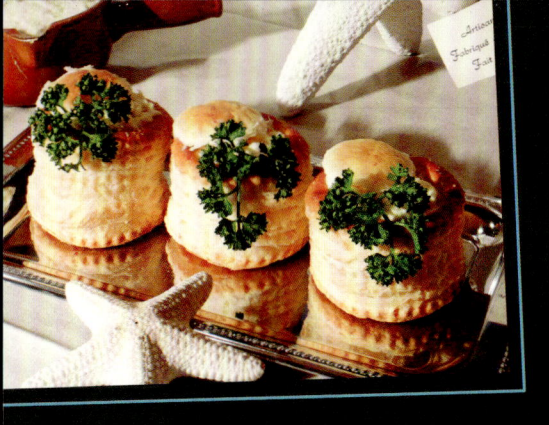

Creamed cod
Brandade de morue

Soak the cod in cold water for about 12 - 24 hours to draw out the salt. The water will need to be changed several times.

Bring a large saucepan of water to the boil. Add the fish and bay leaf. Poach for about 15 minutes. Drain and discard the water and bay leaf.

Put the cooked fish into a liquidiser with the garlic clove. Heat the milk and oil together and pour into the liquidiser. Mix to obtain a smooth paste. Chill before using. (Makes approx. 650 g.)

SERVING SUGGESTIONS:
Creamed cod on toast
Toasts à la brandade de morue

Spread *brandade de morue* on toast and serve cold or spread onto buttered bread, heat in the oven for about 5 – 10 minutes and serve hot.

Creamed cod pie
Brandade de morue parmentière

Mix together the mashed potatoes and parsley with the *brandade de morue* and place in an ovenproof dish. Sprinkle a few breadcrumbs over and dot with the butter.

Cook for about 30 minutes or until golden. Serve hot with *tomates à la provençale.*

Bouchées à la reine with creamed cod
Bouchées à la reine à la brandade de morue

Make the *sauce béchamel* according to the recipe, using 50 g of plain flour instead of 30 g.

Mix the *brandade de morue* with the *sauce béchamel.*

Cook the *bouchées-à-la reine* then fill with the *brandade de morue* mixture. Heat in a hot oven before serving.

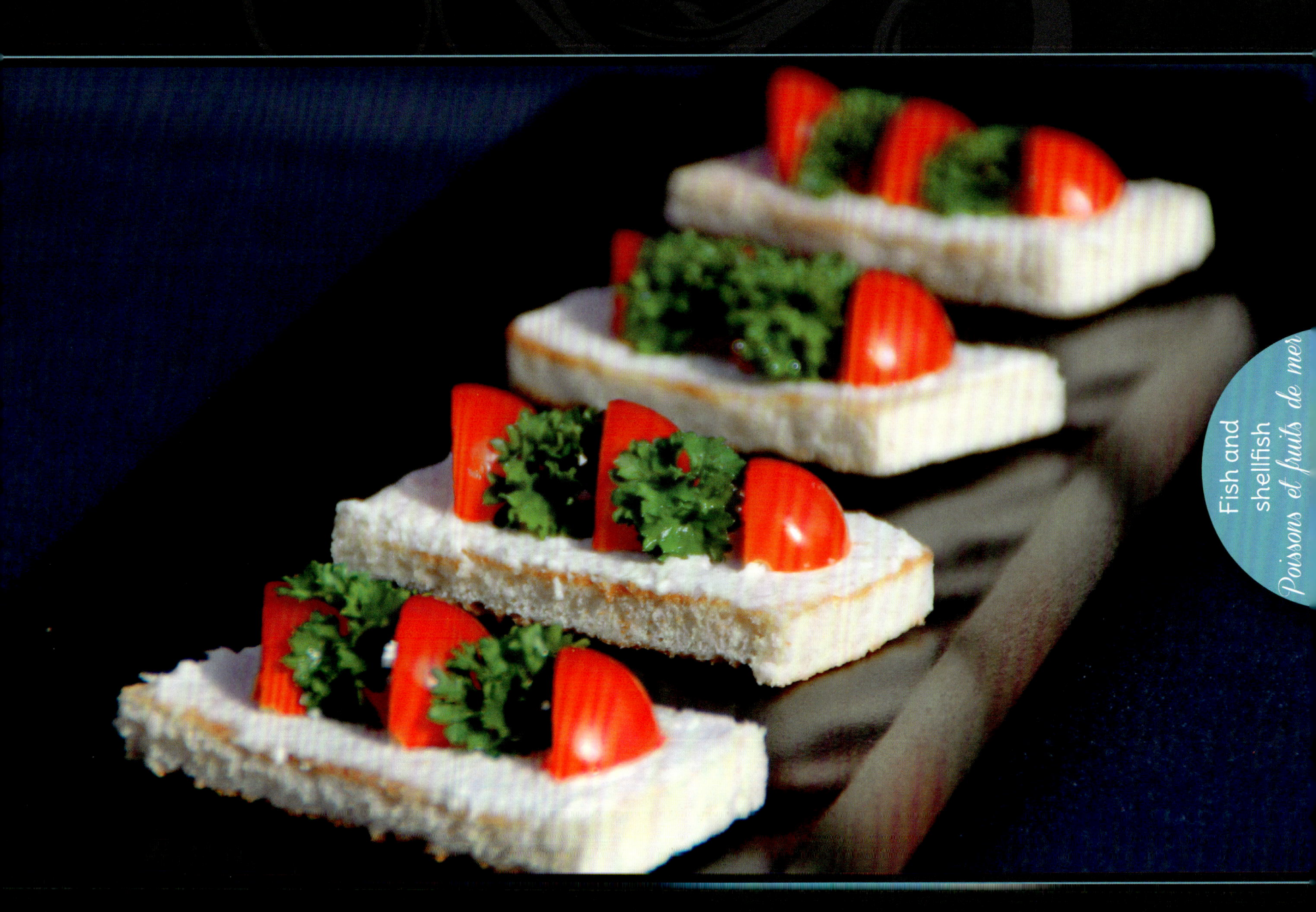

Brandade de morue is a speciality from Nîmes made with salt cod.
There are many versions of this very popular recipe, some of which don't include garlic.

Fish and shellfish
Poissons et fruits de mer

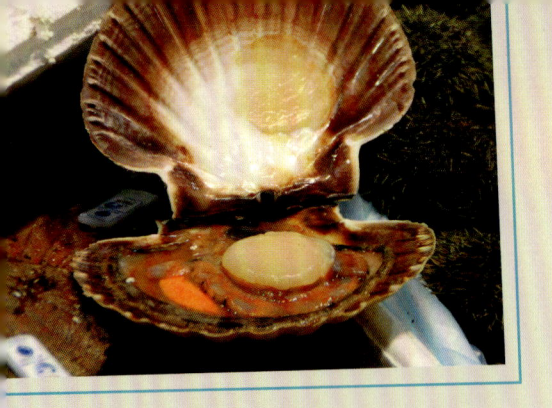

Scallops
Coquilles Saint-Jacques

PREPARE THE STOCK: Pour the wine into a saucepan, with 500 ml water, the onion, carrot, bay leaf and peppercorns. Bring to the boil and allow to simmer for about 20 minutes. Strain and pour into a clean saucepan.

COOK THE SCALLOPS: Reheat the stock and add the scallops. Poach them for about 2 minutes. *Be careful not to overcook them at this stage or they will become tough.* Remove the scallops from the stock, strain them and place in the clean shells. Discard the stock.

MAKE THE SAUCE: Melt the butter in a heavy-based saucepan and add the shallots. Cook for about 3 minutes, stirring from time to time. Add the flour and stir until smooth. Continue cooking for about 2 minutes, stirring all the time.

Take off the heat and add the milk, a little at a time, stirring until it becomes a smooth sauce. Put back on the heat and simmer for 3 minutes, stirring until the sauce thickens. Remove from the heat and stir in the grated cheese. Season with the salt and pepper.

Pour the sauce over the scallops and sprinkle with the breadcrumbs.

Place in the oven and cook until the topping turns golden.

Serve immediately.

The fluted, lower shell serves as an attractive plate for the scallop. Wash and store for use again.

Makes 12 individual shells

Oven: 180°C

- 400 g scallops*
- 12 scallop shells

Stock:
- 250 ml white wine
- 1 onion, chopped
- 1 carrot, chopped
- 1 bay leaf
- 4 peppercorns

Sauce:
- 50 g butter
- 3 shallots, finely chopped
- 25 g plain flour
- 400 ml milk
- 125 g grated cheese
- Salt and pepper
- Breadcrumbs for the topping

If using frozen scallops, defrost them in milk—they will be as good as fresh ones!

Fish and shellfish
Poissons et fruits de mer

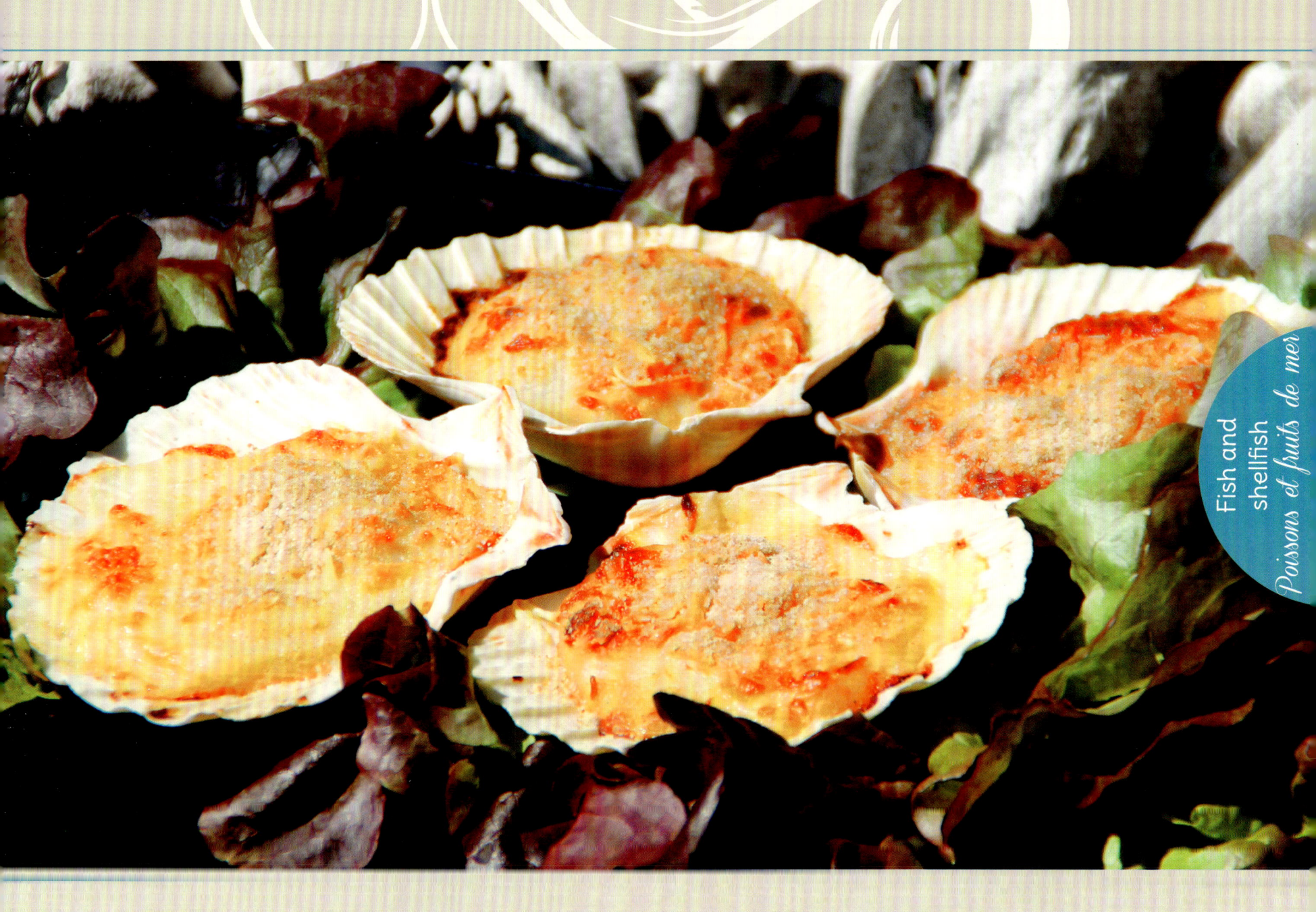

Mediterranean *coquilles Saint-Jacques* are seldom on the market as most French production comes from the Atlantic. They are a good source of proteins, rich in vitamins B12, B2, B6, folic acid, trace elements of sulphur, potassium, sodium, iron, copper, zinc, calcium, phosphorus, magnesium, iodine...

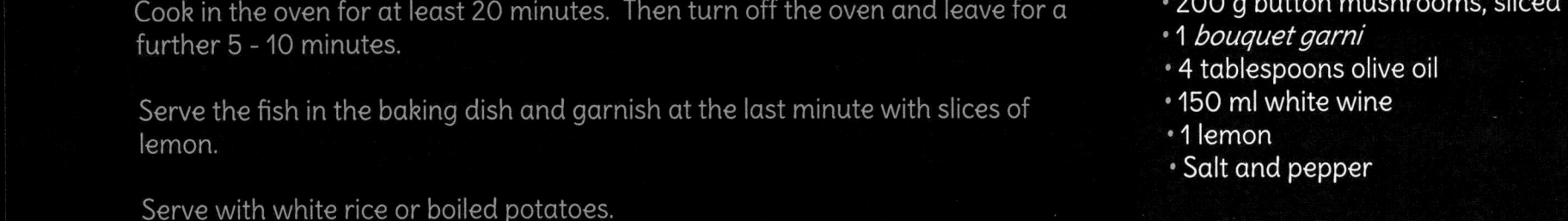

Cook in the oven for at least 20 minutes. Then turn off the oven and leave for a further 5 - 10 minutes.

Serve the fish in the baking dish and garnish at the last minute with slices of lemon.

Serve with white rice or boiled potatoes.

- 200 g button mushrooms, sliced
- 1 *bouquet garni*
- 4 tablespoons olive oil
- 150 ml white wine
- 1 lemon
- Salt and pepper

Fish and shellfish
Poissons et fruits de mer

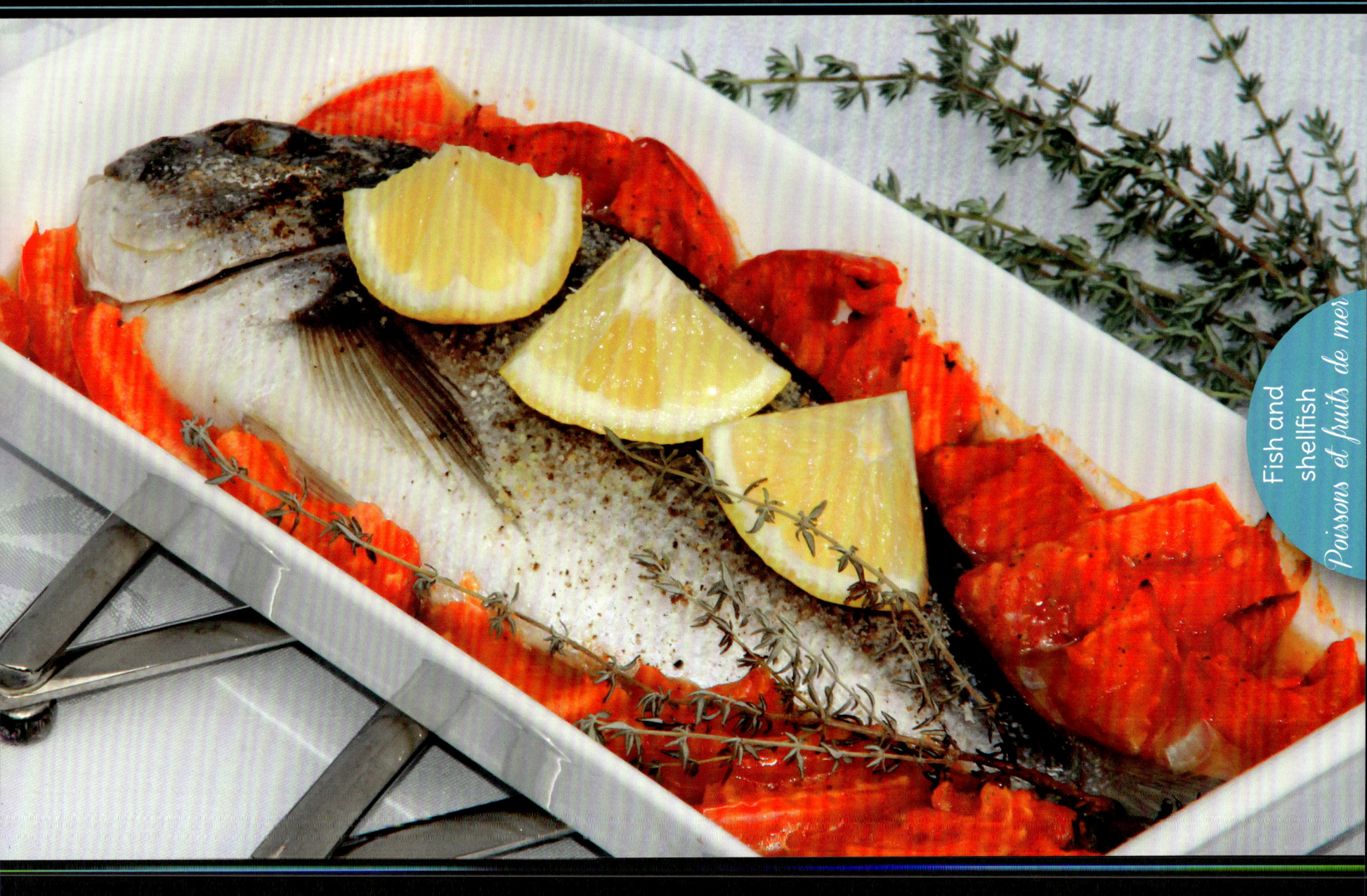

Fish cooked whole are always tastier than fillets, and they are not so dry as they are cooked in their skins and the inside of the fish can be flavoured with herbs

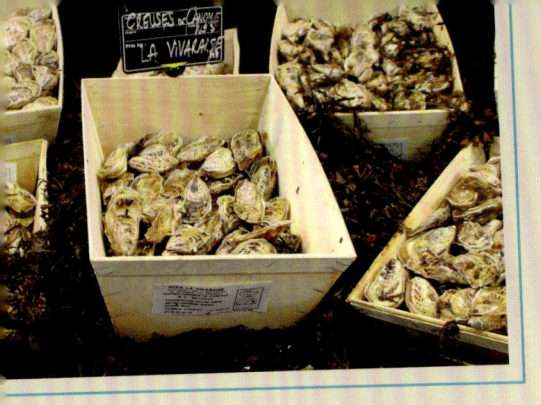

Oysters
Huîtres

PREPARE THE OYSTERS: Ensure that the oysters are properly closed. If there is one slightly ajar, tap the shell and wait until it completely closes. Discard any that fail to close. *A live oyster should feel heavy as it's a sign that it has kept its water.*

Open the oysters by holding one in the left hand with a cloth, rounded side underneath. Slide an oyster knife in next to the hinge and twist to prise the shell open. Then slide the blade horizontally in order to cut the base.

Detach the oyster from the shell by cutting the abductor muscle with the knife and discard the top shell. When opening, always place it rounded side down so that it preserves all of its internal fluids.

SERVE THE OYSTERS: Place the half shells on a plate of coarse salt or seaweed and serve cool (about 8°C).

Mix together the shallot, red wine vinegar and black pepper in a small bowl. Place in the centre of the plate and decorate with the lemon quarters.

Serve with buttered rye bread and *sauce cocktail* (see *recettes de base*). Do not drown the flavour with too much vinegar and lemon—just a hint is enough.

Serves 4 persons

- 24 oysters
- 1 shallot, finely chopped
- 2 tablespoons red wine vinegar
- Pinch black pepper
- 1 lemon, cut in quarters

Storage: Opened oysters should be consumed immediately.

Unopened oysters can be kept in a deep container in the fridge for up to about 1 week, covered with a damp tea towel. Avoid storing them in a plastic bag or container. They should be laid rounded side down.

Fish and shellfish
Poissons et fruits de mer

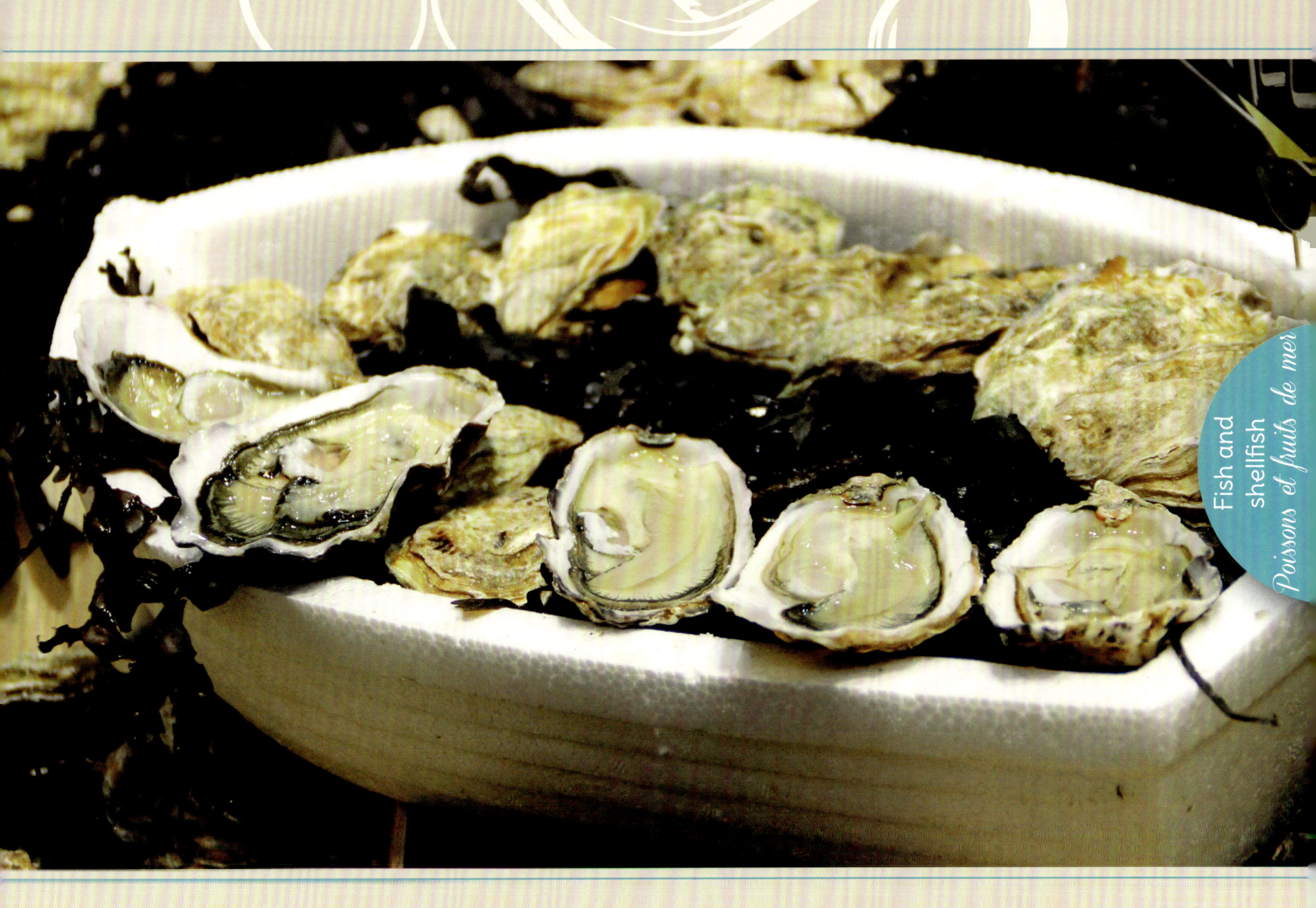

Oysters are full of minerals, vitamins (B12 and D), trace elements of phosphorus, iron, copper, omega 3, selenium, zinc, lipid, etc.
As well as being rich in proteins they are also low in calories.
Generally speaking, the quality of oysters depends more on their habitat than their type, and therefore, eaten raw like this, the differences in flavour become more noticeable.
There are two main types of oysters: the flat oyster or the rounded hollow type.

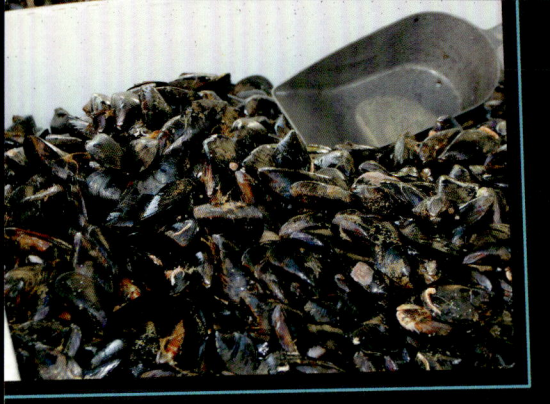

Mussels in white wine
Moules marinières

PREPARE THE MUSSELS: Wash the mussels under a cold tap, scrubbing them well. Do not leave to soak. Scrape off any barnacles with a knife. Press lightly between two fingers any opened mussels. They should slowly close. Discard any that remain open. Pull out and discard the fibrous 'beard' that sprouts between the two halves of the shell.

COOK THE MUSSELS: Heat the olive oil in a saucepan and add the onion and garlic. Sauté gently until cooked.

Add the white wine and parsley and bring to the boil. Add the mussels and leave them to open. Cooking time is very quick—several minutes should be enough—just long enough for them to open. Stir 2 or 3 times during cooking. *Do not add salt; there is enough salt found naturally in the mussels to season the dish.*

MAKE THE SAUCE: Strain the liquid through a sieve into a clean saucepan. Bring to the boil. Mix the cornflour with the water and add to the liquid. Cook for 2 minutes, stirring continuously.

Add the cream and heat (without bringing to the boil).

Place mussels in a serving dish and serve hot with the sauce.

*Do not eat any mussels that have not opened during cooking as they could give food poisoning.
Mussels should be consumed within 48 hours of purchase. They can be stored in the bottom drawer of the fridge in a damp tea towel. Do not store in a plastic bag.*

Serves approx. 4 persons

- 2 kg mussels
- 1 onion, chopped
- 2 garlic cloves, crushed
- 4 tablespoons olive oil
- Bunch of chopped parsley
- 400 ml sweet white wine

Sauce:
- 200 ml double cream
- 30 g cornflour
- 4 level tablespoons water

Fish and shellfish
Poissons et fruits de mer

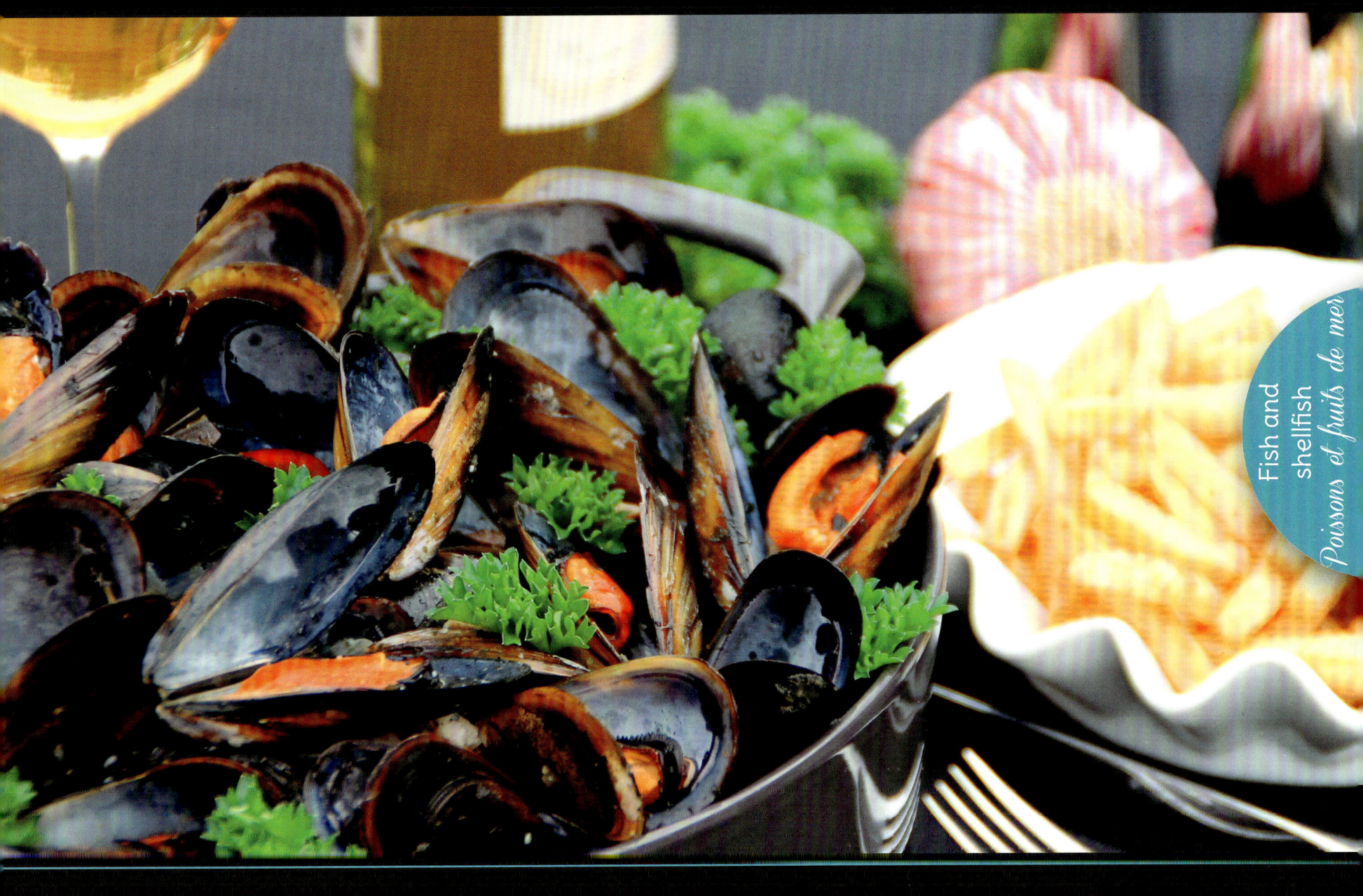

There are mussel farms *les moules de bouchot* all around the French coasts but the best are those cultivated on oak posts planted across large

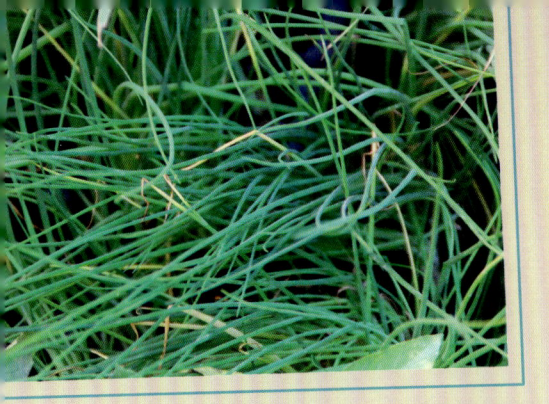

Salmon parcels with herb sauce
Saumon en papillote et sauce aux herbes

PREPARE THE SALMON: Remove any bones from the salmon fillets using a small pair of tweezers.

Cut out 4 large rectangular pieces of greaseproof paper. Fold each rectangle in half, then open again and brush with the melted butter. Place a fillet of salmon on one half of the rectangle, and decorate with 4 half slices of lemon. Sprinkle with salt and pepper and fold the other half of greaseproof paper over the salmon to make a parcel. Seal by carefully folding over the edges.

Place on an oven tray and cook for about 10 - 15 minutes (depending on the size of the fish) or until the salmon is tender but firm to touch.

MAKE THE SAUCE: Heat the olive oil in a saucepan and cook the shallot until soft. Pour in 100 ml of water and the wine. Bring to the boil.

Mix together the cornflour with the remaining 50 ml of water and pour into the saucepan, stirring thoroughly until it boils.

Add the cream and bring back to the boil, stirring continuously.

Add the chopped herbs and salt and pepper to taste.

Serve with the salmon.

As a variation, use a whole salmon fillet instead of individual ones. Place a large piece of greaseproof paper on a baking tray. Continue the recipe then cover with a smaller piece of greaseproof paper. Wrap the bottom layer around the salmon and keep in place with cocktail sticks pierced through the greaseproof paper into the salmon.

Serves 4 persons

Oven: 200°C

- 4 x 200 g salmon fillets
- 10 g butter, melted
- 1 lemon, sliced

Sauce aux herbes :
- 1 - 2 shallots, finely sliced
- 1 tablespoon olive oil
- 150 ml water
- 75 ml white wine
- 1½ tablespoons cornflour
- 110 ml double cream
- 2 tablespoons chopped fresh herbs (parsley, chives, chervil, tarragon or sorrel)

Fish and shellfish
Poissons et fruits de mer

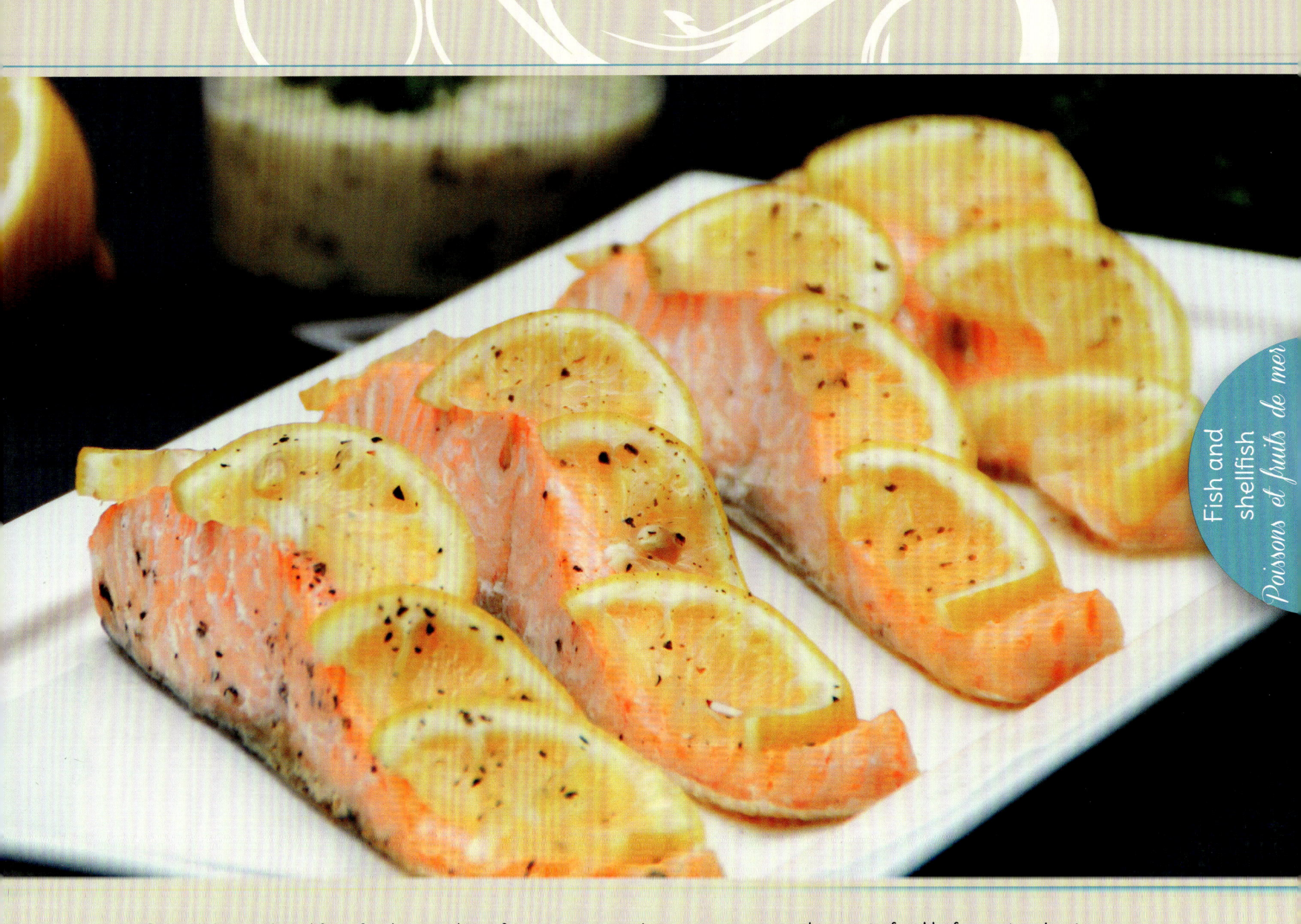

Salmon begin their life in freshwater but after two years migrate upstream to the sea to feed before returning to spawn in the rivers where they were born.
Known as the 'king of the fish', there are many species found throughout the world, but the finest is the Atlantic salmon. Fortunately, they can be farmed successfully, making them more affordable.

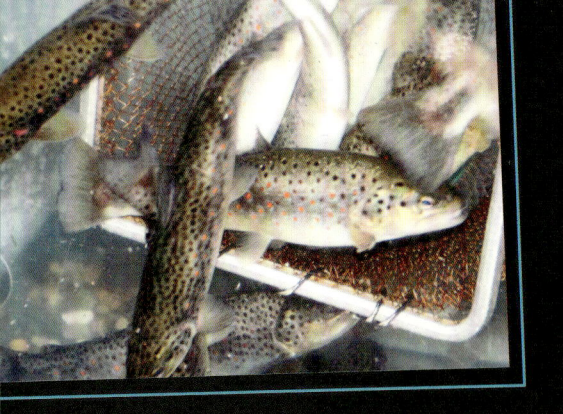

Trout with almonds
Truite aux amandes

PREPARE THE TROUT: Using a tablespoon, make sure the cavity is empty, and remove any blood vessels adjacent to the backbone. Wash the cavity thoroughly, and then pat the fish dry with kitchen paper.

Season the cavity with salt and pepper then soak the fish in the milk, with plenty of salt and pepper. Drain well, then toss them in the flour.

COOK THE TROUT: Heat the oil in a large frying pan. Add 20 g of the butter. Once the butter begins to froth add the trout. Carefully fry the trout on a low to medium heat for about 7 - 8 minutes on each side.

Fry the almonds in a small saucepan in 20 g of butter until they are golden. Sprinkle them over the trout just before serving.

Decorate with half slices of lemon.

Place on a warm serving plate and cover with foil to keep warm.

Fish and shellfish
Poissons et fruits de mer

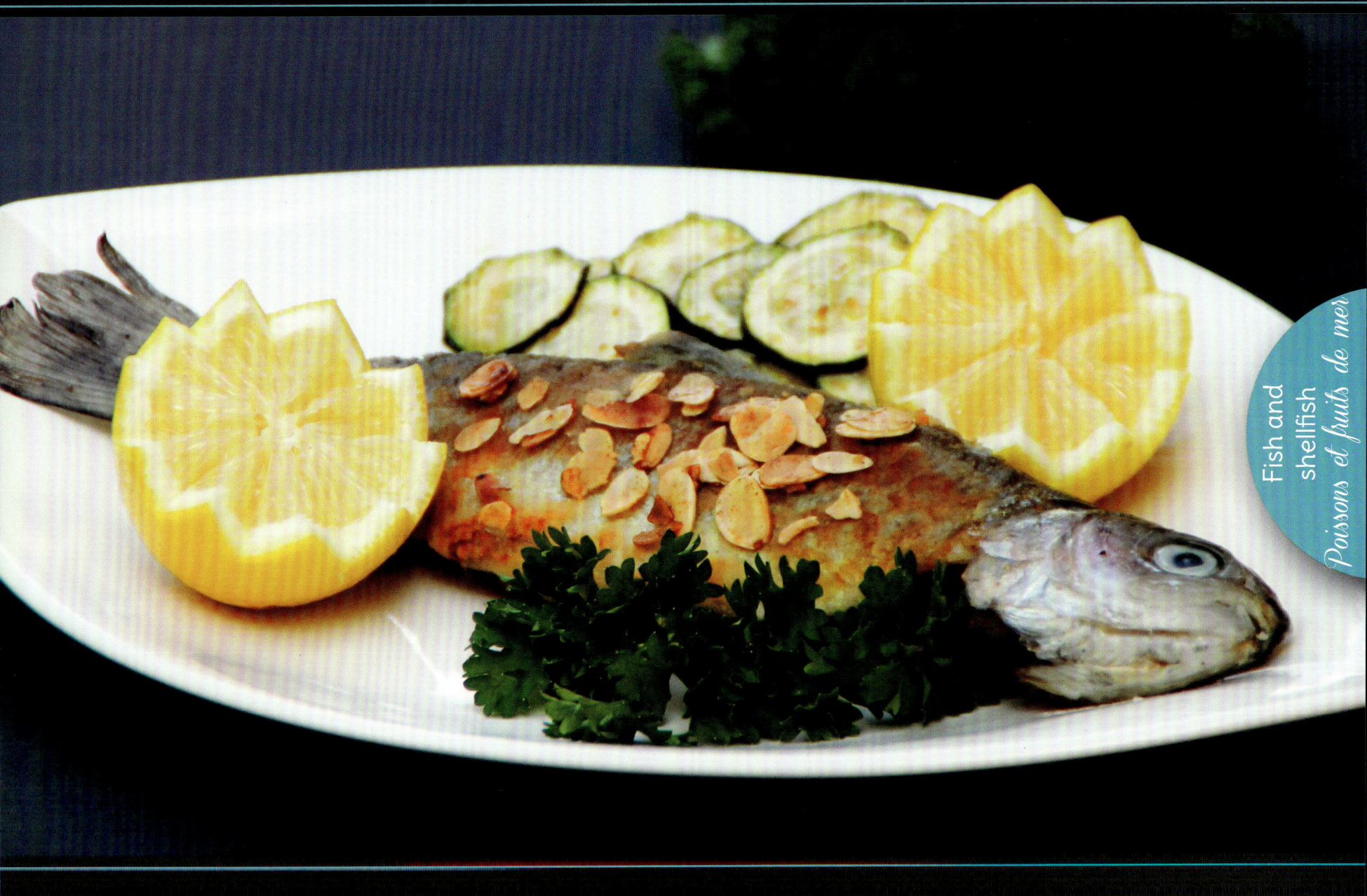

A classic French dish, elegant, yet simple to prepare, perfect for special occasions.
Trout are the best-known of all freshwater fish. The two main species are brown trout and rainbow trout.
Rainbow trout are successfully farmed and are usually available all year round.
In Normandy, they are often baked *en papillotte* with apples, cider and cream.

Meats
Viandes

152 Veal blanquette
Blanquette de veau

154 Beef stew
Boeuf bourguignon

156 Meatballs with cabbage
Caillettes au chou

156 Meatballs with green vegetables
Caillettes aux légumes verts

158 Duck with orange
Canard à l'orange

160 Coq au vin
Coq au vin

162 Beef fondue
Fondue bourguignonne

164 Accompaniments for a beef fondue
Accompagnements pour fondue bourguignonne

166 Rabbit in mustard sauce
Lapin à la moutarde

168 Cooking the duck breast
Cuisson du magret de canard

170 Duck breast with honey and pears
Magret de canard au miel et aux poires

170 Duck breast with cocoa
Magret de canard au cacao

172 Hot pot
Pot au feu

174 Peppered steaks
Steaks au poivre

Warning !
Some recipes contain alcohol.

Meats *Viandes*

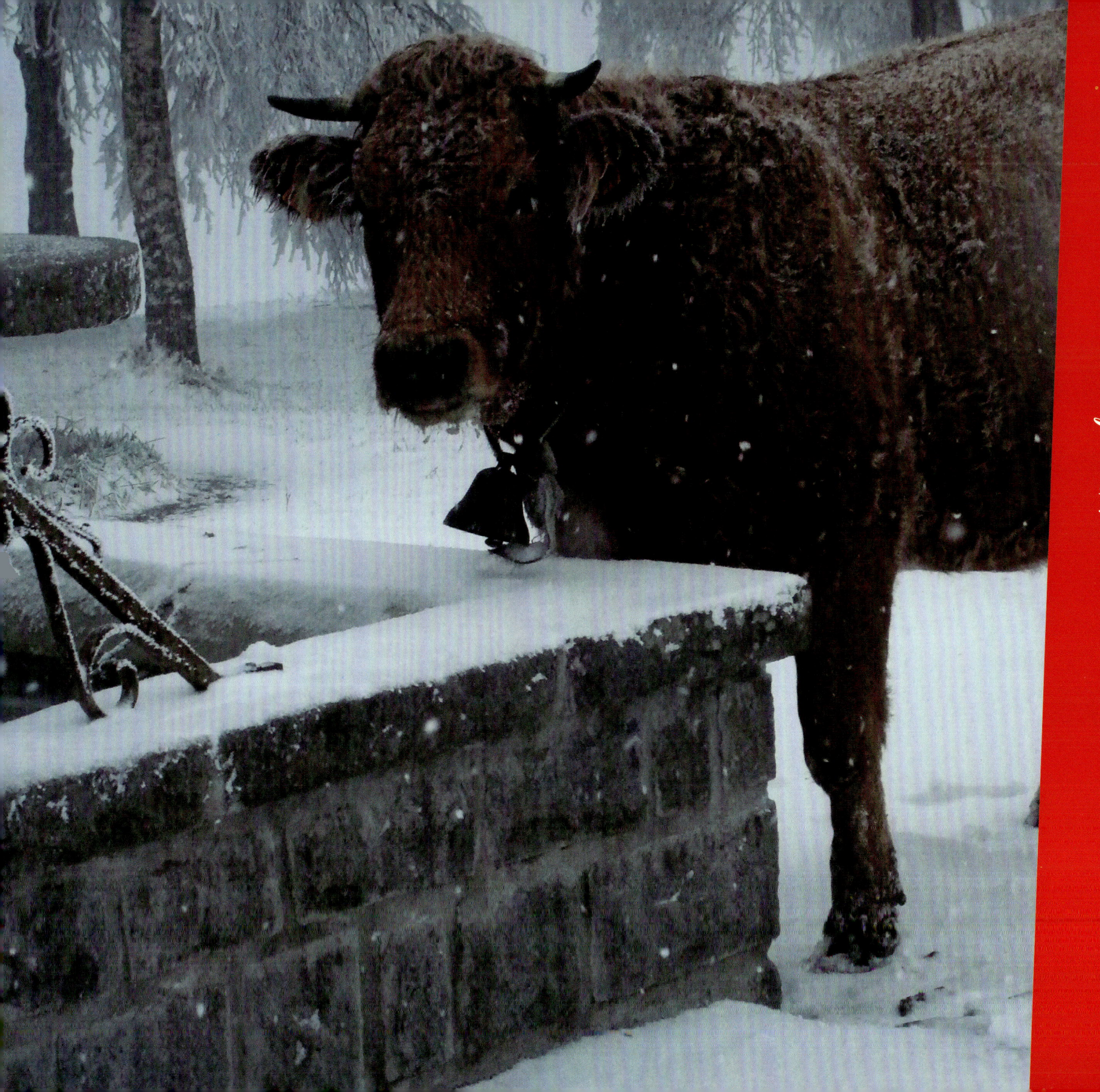

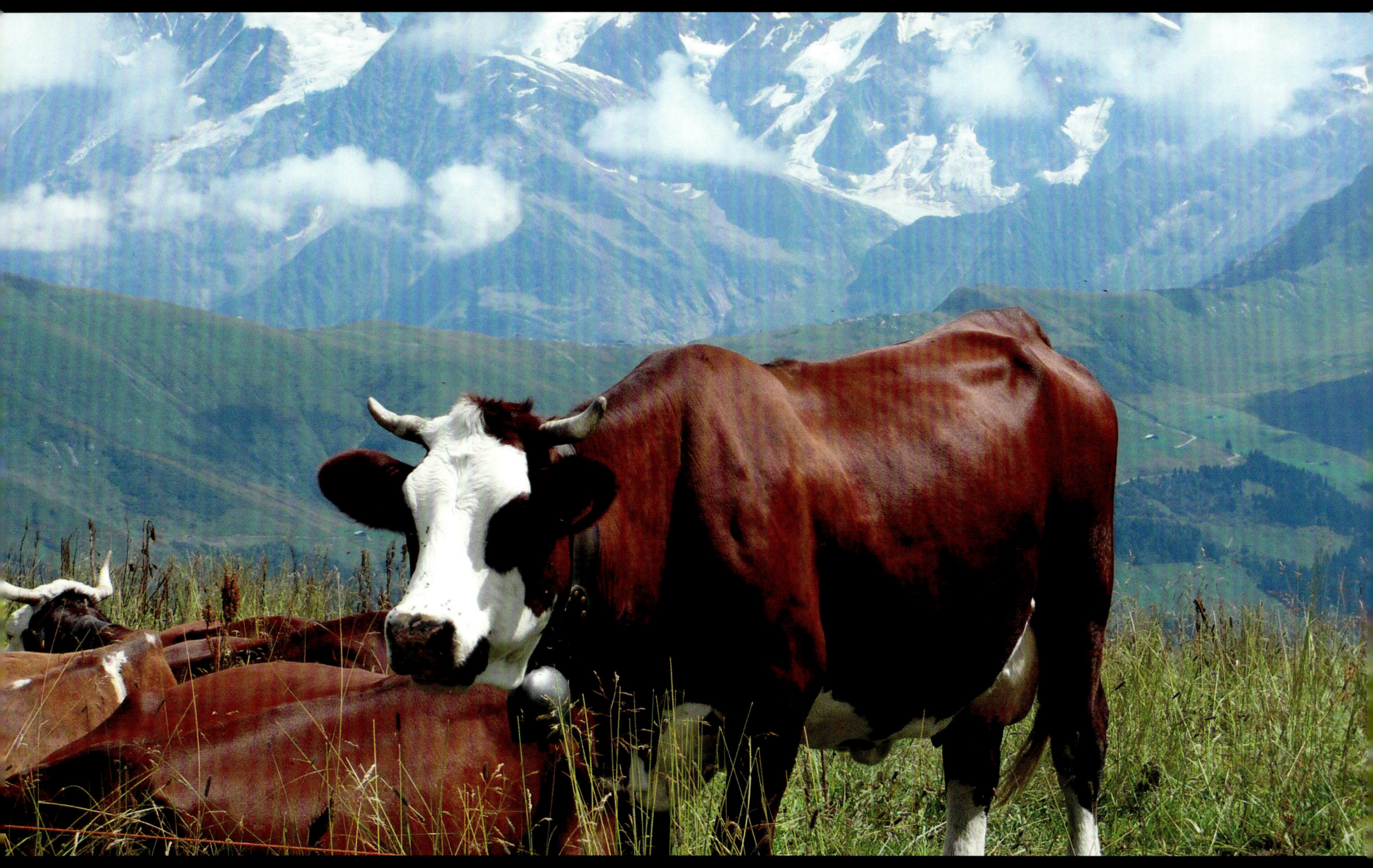

Dining in style...

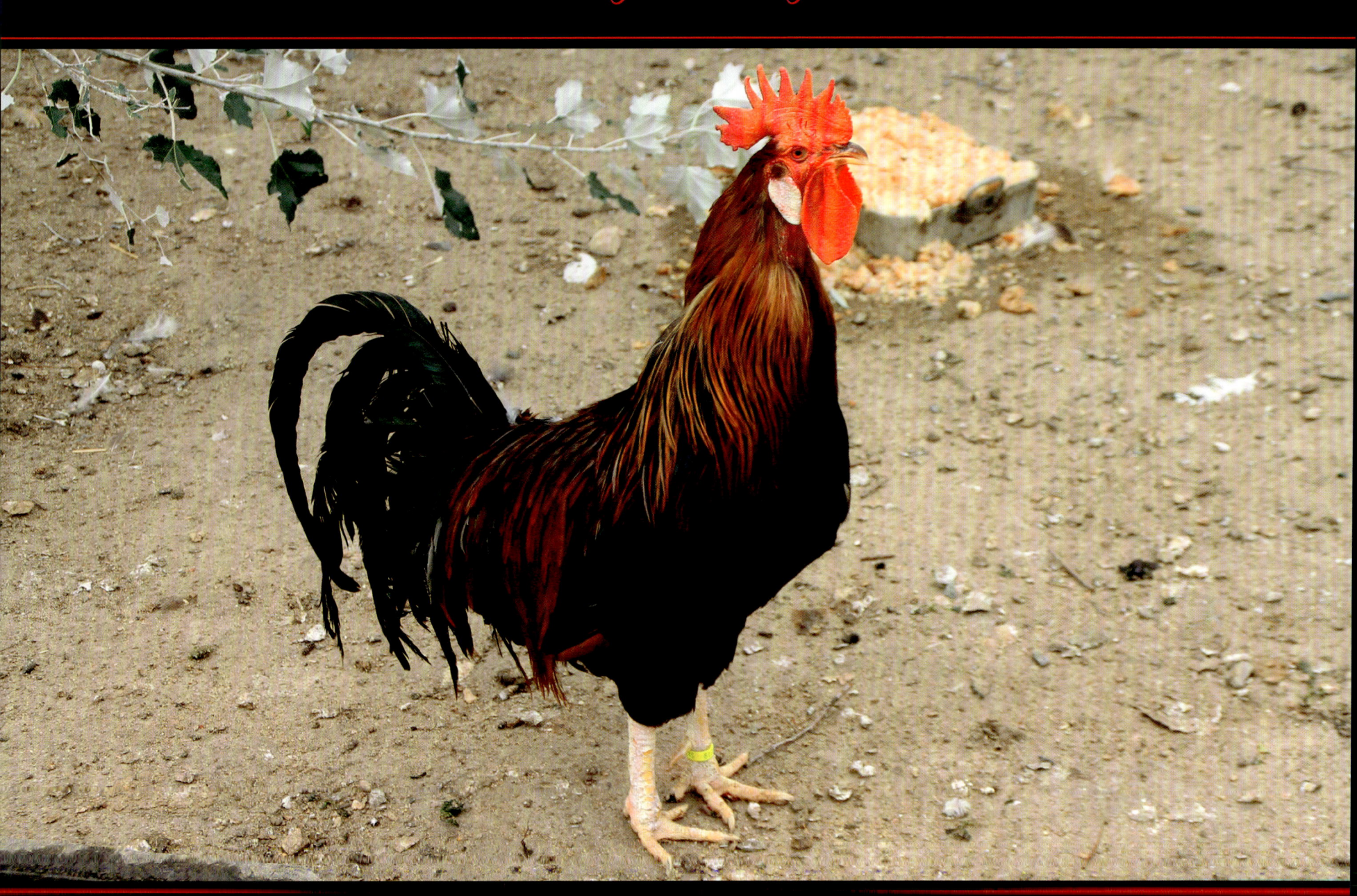

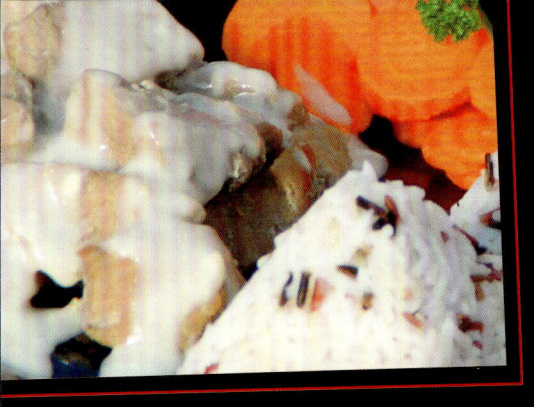

Veal blanquette
Blanquette de veau

Peel and slice the carrots.

Peel the onion and prick the clove into it.

Bring to the boil 2 litres of water in a large saucepan. Plunge the veal pieces into the boiling water and leave for about 1 minute to blanch them. Drain the meat and rinse with cold water. Discard the cooking water and rinse the saucepan.

Place the veal back into the saucepan with the wine and 1 litre of water (or enough to cover the meat). Add the carrots, onion, *bouquet garni*, salt and freshly ground pepper. Bring to the boil, cover and simmer for about 1½ hours.

Remove the pieces of meat and reserve in a shallow dish. Discard the *bouquet garni*. Strain the stock and return to the heat.

Mix together the cream and lemon juice with the flour. *Add a little extra water if the mixture appears too thick.* Add to the stock and cook on a low heat, whisking all the time.

Take off the heat and add the egg yolk. Mix together.

Serves approx. 6 persons

- 1.5 kg stewing veal
- 3 carrots
- 1 large onion
- 1 clove
- 1 *bouquet garni*
- Salt and freshly ground pepper
- 800 ml dry white wine
- 4 tablespoons double cream
- Juice of ½ lemon
- 70 g plain flour*
- 1 egg yolk

Adjust the quantity of flour if a thicker sauce is desired.

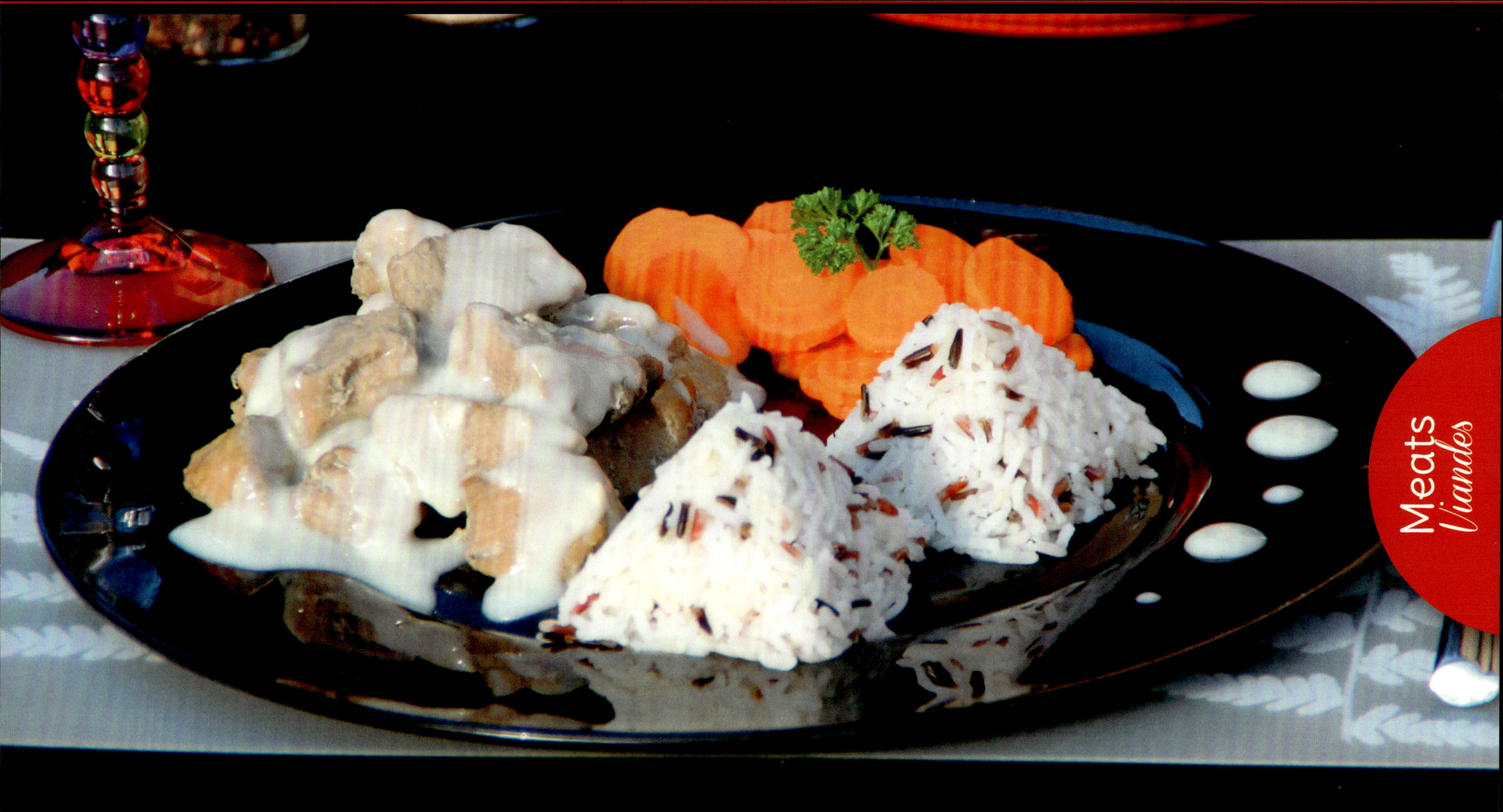

Blanquette de veau was originally a humble dish made from leftovers but was soon transformed into *haute cuisine*.
It appeared on the menus of the very first Parisian restaurants.
This delicious meat that melts in the mouth is served in a thick and creamy sauce and is a very popular dish in the winter.
Classic accompaniments are rice or boiled potatoes.

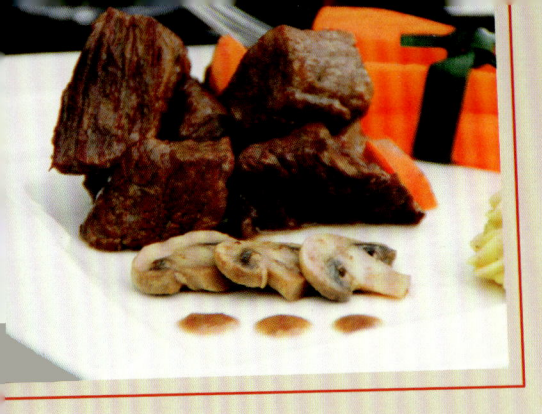

Beef stew
Boeuf bourguignon

Season the pieces of meat with the salt and pepper and roll in the flour. *To make this process easier, place together in a mixing bowl, cover with a plate and shake to allow the flour to evenly coat the meat.*

In a heavy-based saucepan, heat the oil, and lightly fry the meat on all sides. Remove the pieces of meat and reserve in a shallow dish.

In the same saucepan, add a little more olive oil if necessary and fry the onion and carrots until the onion is beginning to soften. Add the meat, covering it with 700 ml of red wine. Add the *bouquet garni* and bring to the boil. Cover and leave to simmer for about 2½ hours, adding more wine during the cooking if it appears to be drying out.

Fry the chopped mushrooms in a frying pan with the bacon.

Discard the *bouquet garni* and sprinkle the mushrooms and bacon over the meat just before serving.

Serves 4 persons

- 1 kg stewing steak
- 2 tablespoons olive oil
- 2 carrots, sliced
- 1 onion, chopped
- 30 g plain flour
- 1 *bouquet garni*
- 700 ml - 1 litre red wine
- 150 g smoked bacon, finely chopped
- 150 g mushrooms
- Salt and freshly ground pepper

For a more economical and lighter version, use half wine, half water.

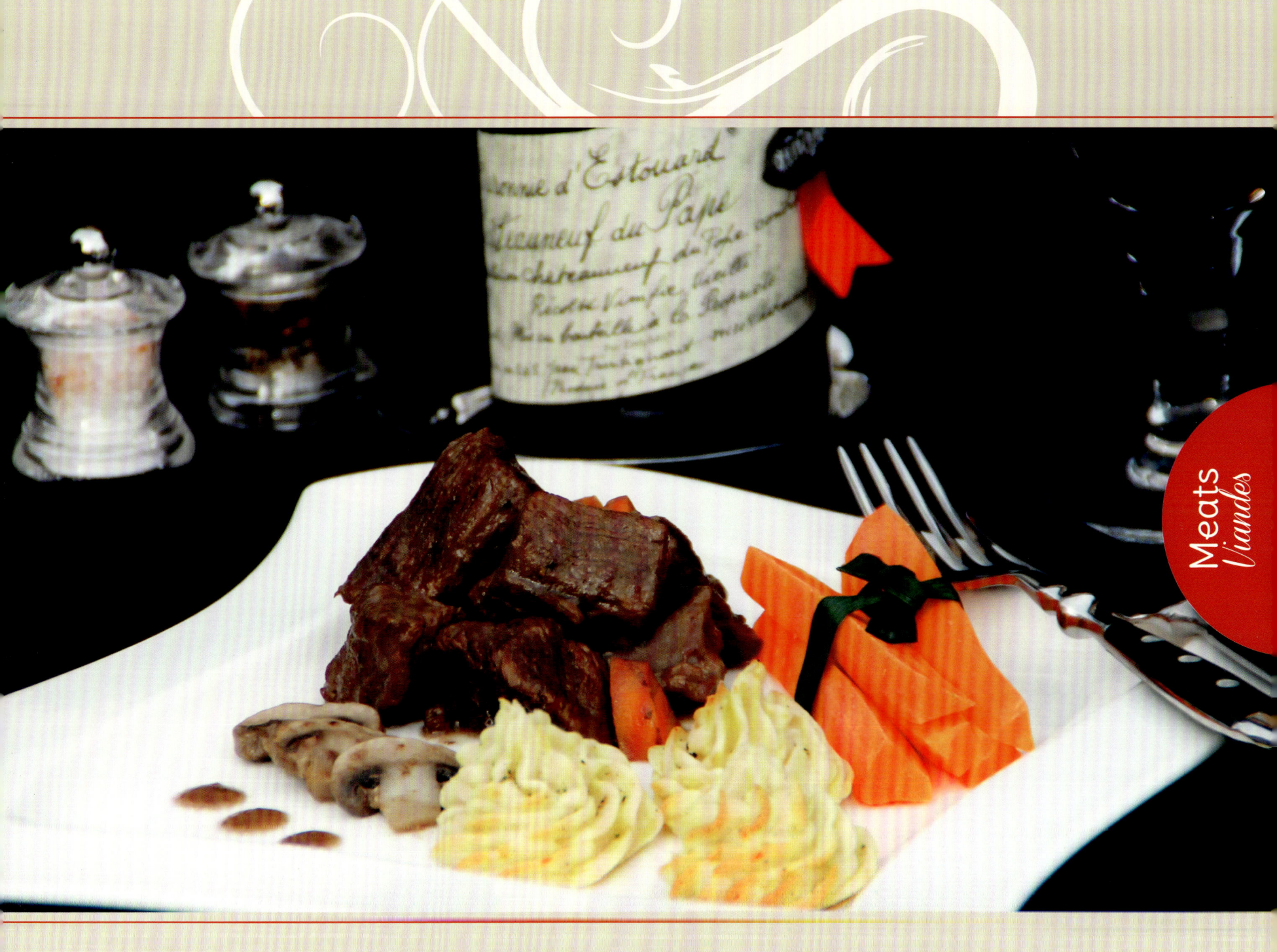

Nearly every region has its own way of cooking beef stewing steak but the *Bourguignon* style is the most famous. Preparing it the day before will help develop the flavours.

Meats
Viandes

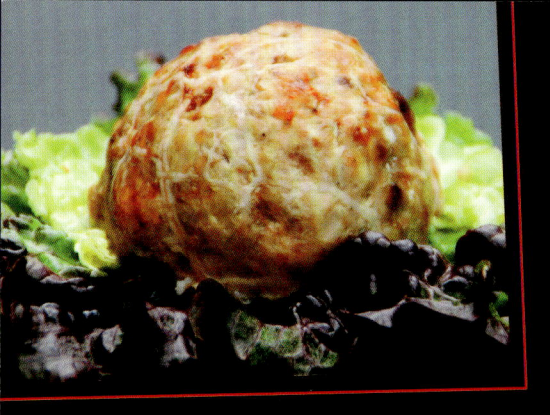

Meatballs
Caillettes

With cabbage
Au chou

Bring a large saucepan of water to the boil. Add a little salt and the shredded cabbage. Once it has returned to the boil, continue cooking for about 5 minute... Drain well, squeezing hard to remove as much of the water as possible. Leave to cool.

Mince together the shredded cabbage with the pork as finely as possible. Ad... the 25 g of salt and crushed garlic cloves. Season with pepper and mix well w... your hands. Make into about 6 individual balls. Wrap with a caul. *Use gloves ... this stage if wished!*

Cook for about 1-1½ hours, or until golden brown.

Serve hot with steamed potatoes.

With green vegetables
Aux légumes verts

Prepare in the same way as for *caillettes au chou* replacing the cabbage wi... green vegetables using the quantity as indicated.

Serve either cold as a starter with gherkins or warm with a green salad, *ravioles*, boiled potatoes or a tomato sauce.

Meats
Viandes

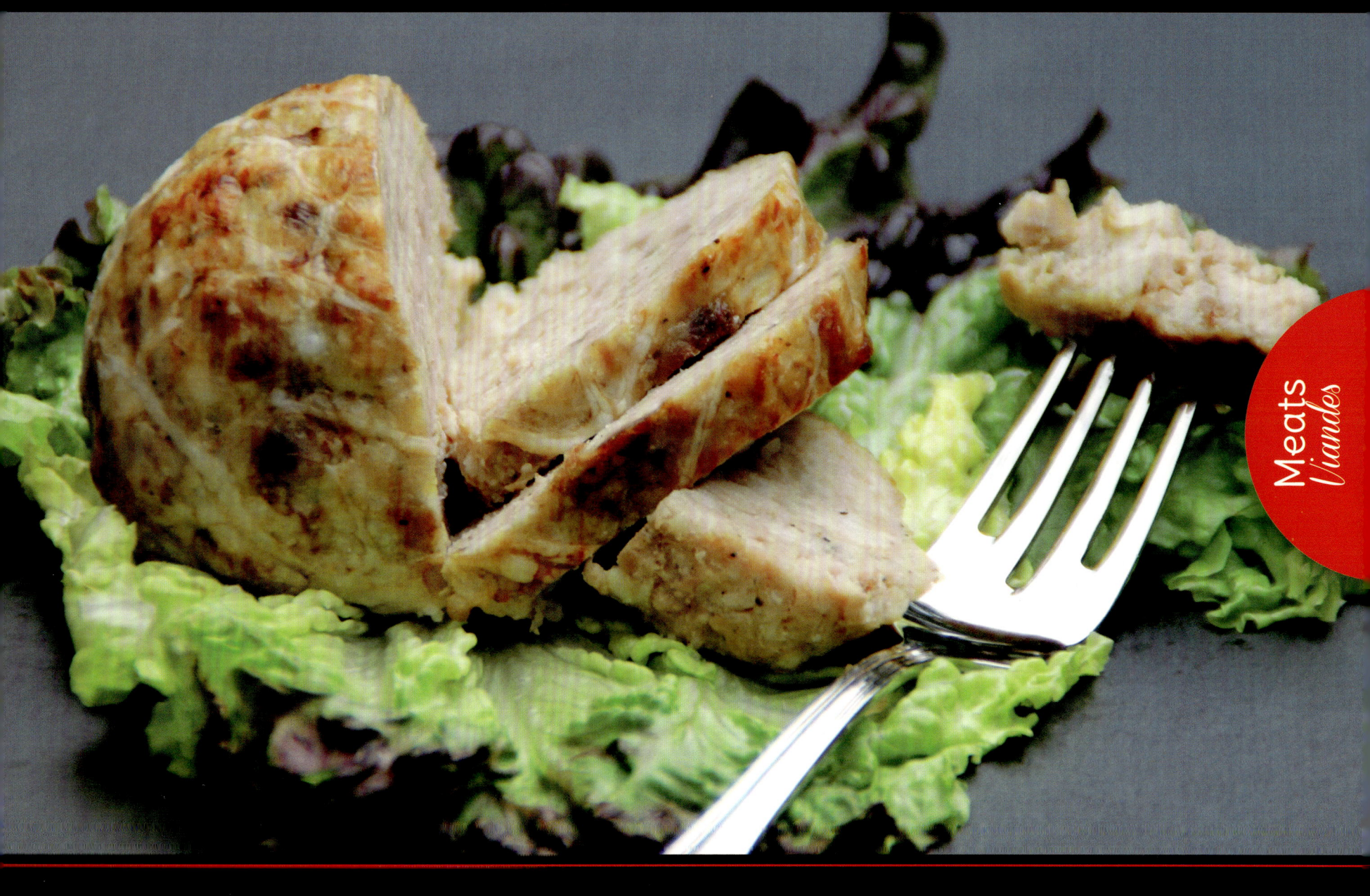

Caillettes were traditionally served at village fêtes after the annual slaughter of the family pig.

In *Ardèche, caillettes* are made with a generous proportion of vegetables and served warm with potatoes and chestnuts. In the *Drôme,* they are often served as a starter with cured meats or even as an *aperitif.*

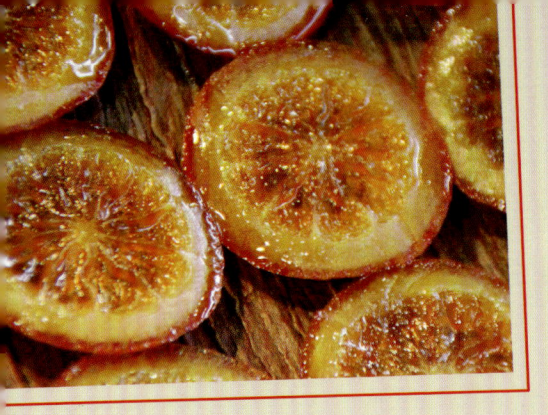

Duck with orange
Canard à l'orange

Heat the oven to 150°C.

Cut two of the oranges in half and rub them over the surface of the duck. Then place them inside the cavity with the cinnamon sticks. Prick the duck all over with a fork. *This helps to release some of the fat.*

Place the duck on a wire rack in the oven with a baking tray underneath. Cook for about 45 minutes, turning halfway through cooking. *Make sure the tray underneath is catching the fat!*

Remove the zest of the other 3 oranges. Reserve. Squeeze out the juice. Heat the sugar in a heavy-based saucepan until it is melted and turns a rich golden brown colour. Stir carefully to ensure that all the sugar is melted evenly. Remove from the heat. Add the vinegar and boil, stirring all the time for about 3 minutes. Add the orange liqueur with the orange juice and leave to simmer for 2 minutes.

Remove the fat from the baking tray. Turn the oven up to 180°C. Place the duck in a roasting tin and baste with some of the orange mixture. Continue cooking for about 45 minutes, basting with the orange mixture every 5 - 10 minutes until it is all used up. *Adjust the cooking time according to the weight of the duck.*

Remove the duck from the oven. Collect all the juice from the bottom of the tin and cool slightly in order to remove the excess fat.

Reheat the juice with the reserved orange zest and the butter. Carefully slice the extra orange (optional) into sections and place on top of the duck. Pour over the hot sauce just before serving.

Serves approx. 6 persons

Oven: 150°C/180°C

- 5 organic or untreated oranges plus 1 extra for decoration (optional)
- 1 duck about 2 kg
- 2 cinnamon sticks
- 95 g brown sugar
- 120 ml cider vinegar
- 80 ml orange liqueur
- 30 g butter

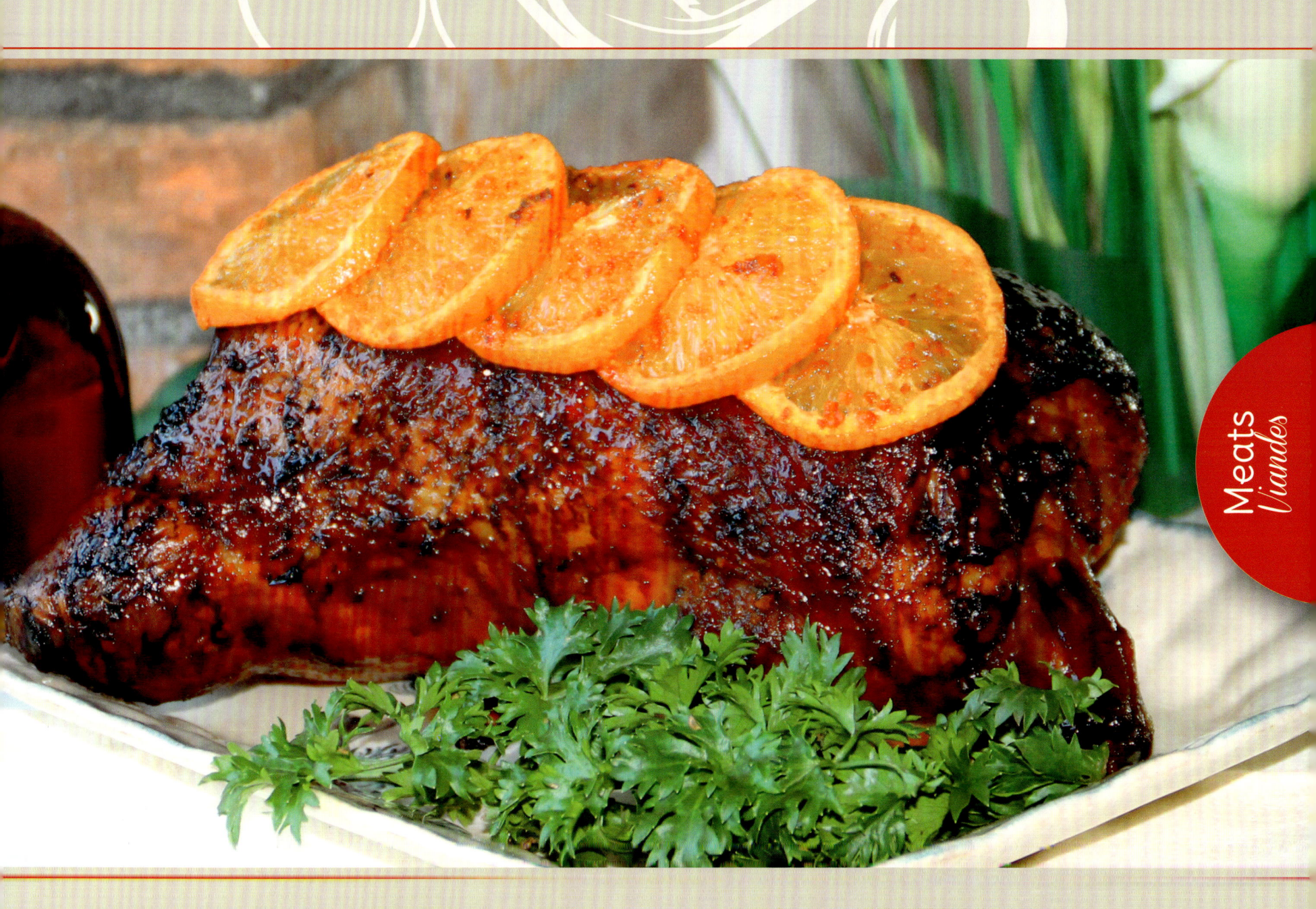

A subtle harmonious combination of sweet and savoury flavours, *Canard à l'orange* displays one of the greatest French gastronomy dishes.

Meats
Viandes

Coq au vin
Coq au vin

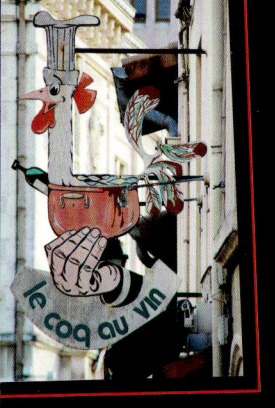

Lightly fry the bacon. Remove from the pan.

Heat the olive oil in a frying pan and add the onions. Sauté until soft. Remove from the pan and leave aside with the bacon.

Chop the chicken into pieces. Fry in the pan with the oil until golden. Remove from the heat. Pour the cognac into a glass and warm slightly. Pour over the chicken pieces. Flame the cognac with a match and leave until the flames have died down. *Be careful! Sometimes the flames can jump up quick—have a saucepan lid ready to put over the flames in case of an emergency!*

Return the onions and bacon to the pan with the chicken. Add the wine, garlic, *bouquet garni*, bay leaf, salt and pepper. Bring to the boil. Cover and leave to simmer for about 1 hour.

Add the mushrooms and cook for another 15 minutes.

Leave to cool. Discard the skin and bones with the *bouquet garni* and bay leaf. Drain the liquid from the pan and leave aside. Keep the meat aside.

Melt the remaining butter in the same pan. Add the flour and stir until smooth. Slowly add the liquid and cook, stirring until smooth and thick. Return the meat to the pan and reheat in the sauce.

Serves approx. 6 persons

- 1 whole chicken approx. 1.75 kg
- 125 g bacon
- 2 tablespoons olive oil
- 2 tablespoons oil
- 3 onions, finely chopped
- 6 - 8 tablespoons cognac
- 1 bottle red wine (700 ml)
- 3 garlic cloves, crushed
- 1 *bouquet garni*
- 1 bay leaf
- Salt and pepper
- 125 g button mushrooms
- 2 tablespoons plain flour

The longer you cook the coq au vin the tastier it will be, and if cooked a day in advance, it is even better!

Meats
Viandes

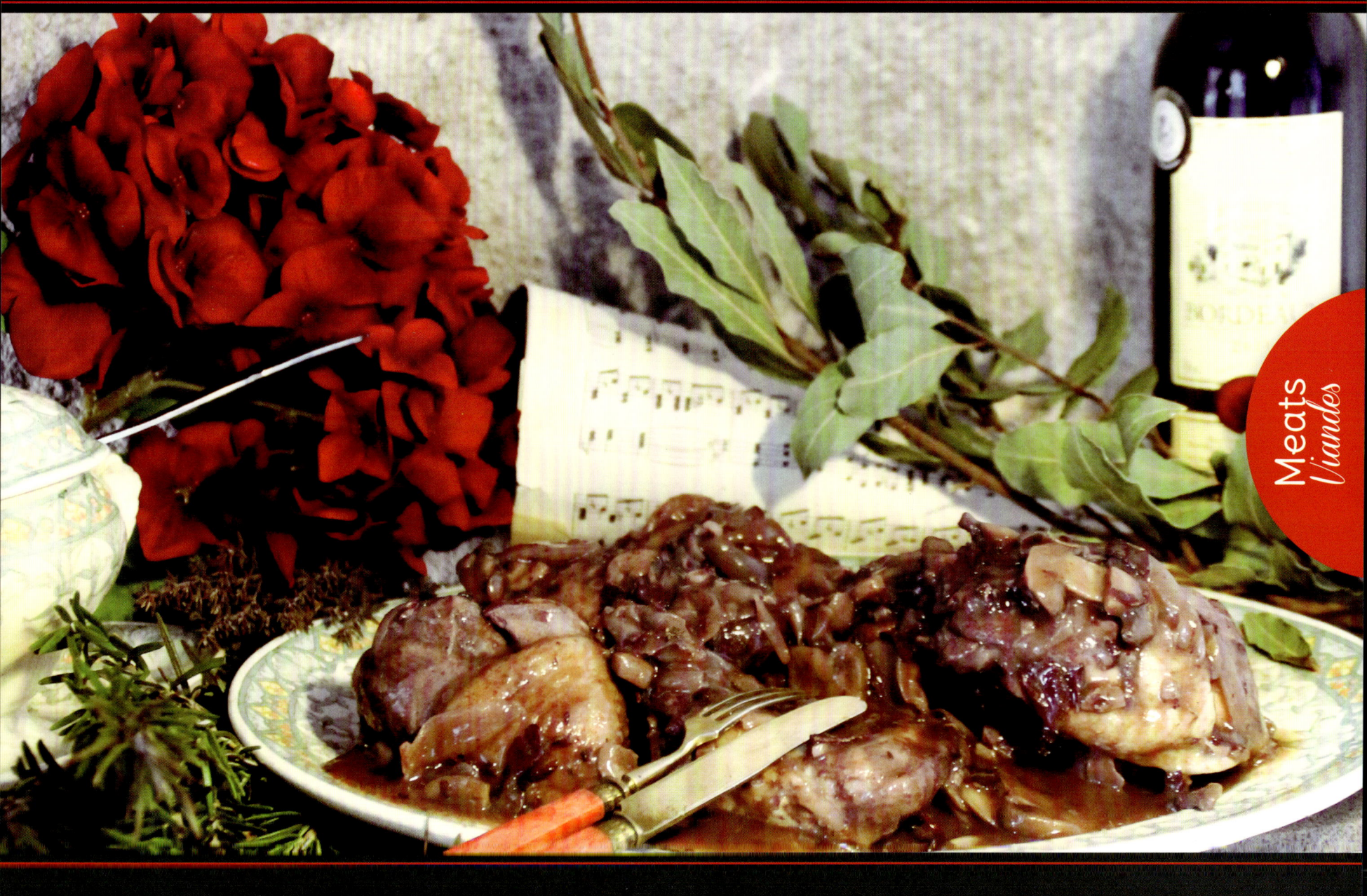

Coq au vin is essentially chicken braised in wine with bacon, mushrooms and garlic.
Many regions claim the originality of this classic French dish: *Bourgogne, Alsace, Champagne* and *Auvergne*.
There are several varieties such as *coq au vin jaune* (chicken braised in white wine from Jura), *coq au riesling* (chicken braised in white wine from Alsace), *coq au pourpre* (chicken braised in new *Beaujolais* wine), *coq au champagne* (chicken braised in champagne), etc.

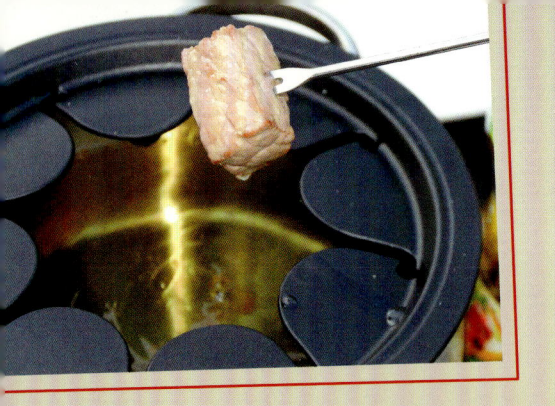

Beef fondue
Fondue bourguignonne

Half fill the earthenware fondue bowl with the oil. Place in the centre of the table in reach of all the guests and heat with the alcohol burner until simmering.

With the special long-handled forks, each guest takes a piece of meat and dips it in the hot oil. When the meat is cooked according to each one's taste (rare, medium or well-done), it is served with the accompanying sauces and crudities, and the fork replaced in the oil with another piece of meat.

- Meat, cut into small cubes
- Oil

IDEAS FOR FLAVOURING THE OIL:
- A garlic clove, cut in half
- 2 shallots
- A sprig of basil or thyme
- A few bay leaves

Simply add a choice of flavourings to the oil in the fondue bowl before heating. Or, for a more pronounced flavour, heat the oil and the flavourings in a saucepan before pouring it into the fondue bowl.

TYPES OF MEAT THAT CAN BE USED:
Tradition always leans towards beef (especially *charolaise* due to its quality, taste and low fat), and its choice pieces such as topside, shoulder, top rump, rump steak, aitch-bone cut, etc.
Veal, turkey or chicken pieces are also delicious.

QUANTITY OF MEAT PER PERSON:
Allow 150 g – 250 g per person (depending on the company).

TYPES OF OIL TO USE:
Be careful as this is the crucial part of the fondue. Some oils are not suitable for a high temperature. The best types are peanut oil or grape seed oil.

See ideas for sauces and accompaniments on the following page.

Meats
Viandes

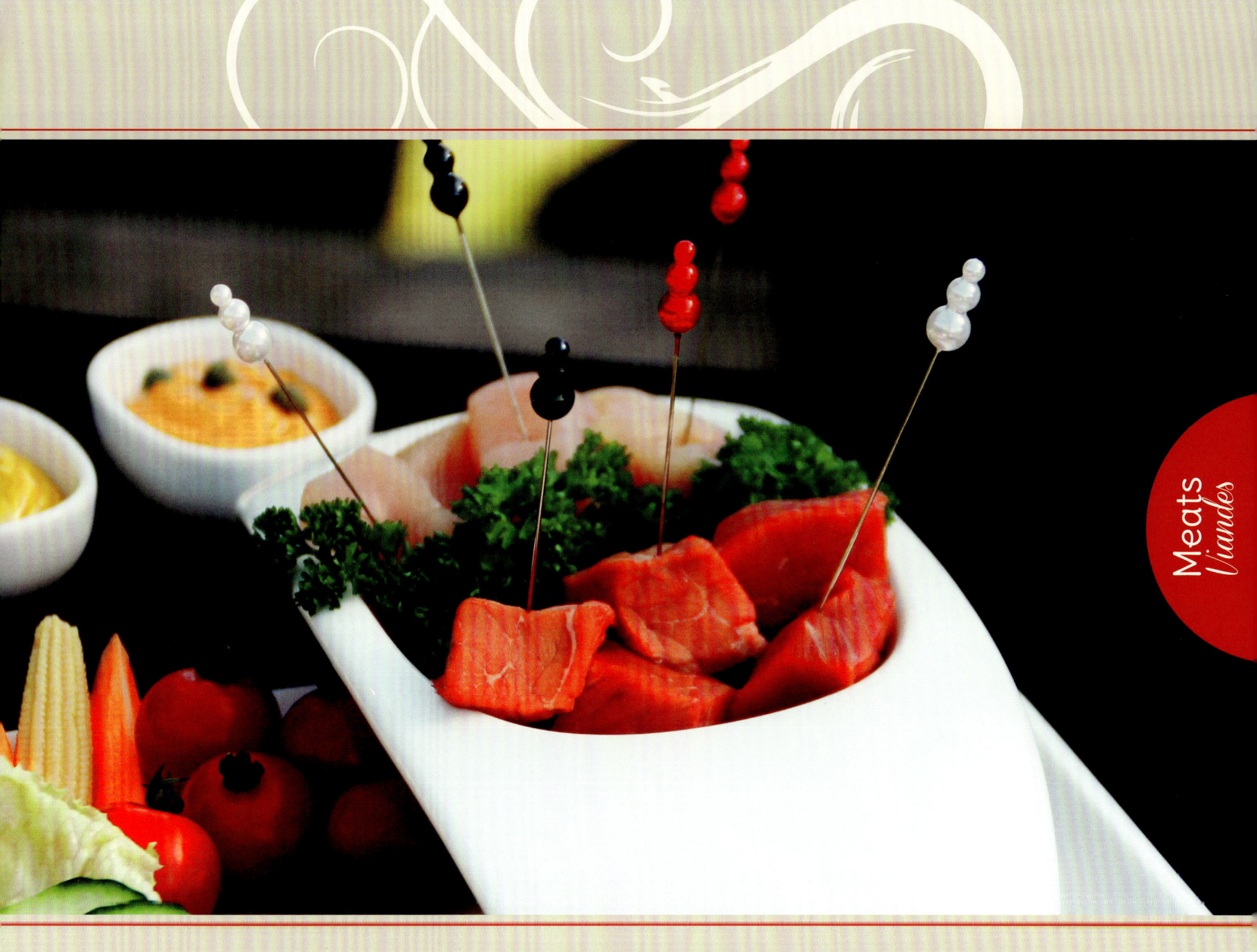

According to legend, *fondue Bourguignonne* is named after the duke of *Bourgogne* who cooked a piece of meat in the boiling oil that was reserved for the enemy during the siege of Dijon in 1652, and shared it with his cavaliers. In 1953, a special skillet was invented which was designed to cook pieces of meat more safely in boiling oil and since then connoisseurs prefer to only cook with quality meat such as *charolais* beef which comes from one of the best races of French cattle. *Charolais* is an area found in the *Bourgogne* region.

163

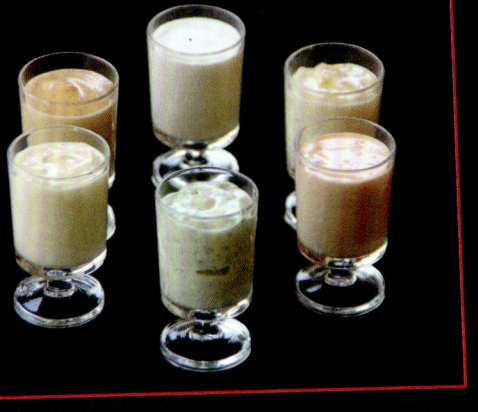

Accompaniments for a beef fondue
Accompagnements pour fondue bourguignonne

Garlic sauce / Sauce à l'ail
Add half a garlic clove, crushed, into a ½ quantity of mayonnaise (see *recettes de base*).

Shallot sauce / Sauce à l'échalote
Cook 2 finely chopped shallots in 100 ml white wine. Once the wine has evaporated and the shallots are soft, stir into a ½ quantity of mayonnaise (see *recettes de base*).

Andalusian sauce / Sauce Andalouse
Chop 1 red and 1 green pepper into tiny cubes. Add to a ½ quantity of mayonnaise (see *recettes de base*). Add a pinch of cayenne pepper and 1 teaspoon of concentrated tomato purée.

Paprika sauce / Sauce au paprika
Mix together 1 teaspoon of paprika, ½ teaspoon of curry powder, 1 tablespoon of tomato ketchup, 1 teaspoon of Cognac and a few drops of tabasco® into a ½ quantity of mayonnaise (see *recettes de base*).

Moussed sauce / Sauce mousseuse
Carefully mix 6 tablespoons of mayonnaise with 2 tablespoons of whipped cream. Add a few drops of lemon juice.

Tartare sauce / Sauce tartare
Finely chop a bunch of mixed, fresh herbs: eg. parsley, chervil, tarragon and chives. Mix into a ½ quantity of mayonnaise (see *recettes de base*). Add a quarter of a finely chopped garlic, a few capers and some chopped gherkins with 1 teaspoon Dijon mustard.

IDEAS TO ACCOMPANY A *FONDUE BOURGUIGNONNE*

- A selection of mustards
- Small serving bowls of gherkins and pickled onions; baby pickled corn on the cobs
- A selection of chutneys
- An assortment of olives
- Radishes, cauliflower florets and celery sticks
- Asparagus with *vinaigrette* (see recipe *asperges à la vinaigrette*)
- Sweet corn seasoned with *vinaigrette* and mixed with finely sliced grilled (and skinned) red pepper
- Cubes of raw vegetables (button mushrooms, courgettes or aubergines) to cook in the oil
- A green salad with a *vinaigrette* is always appreciated

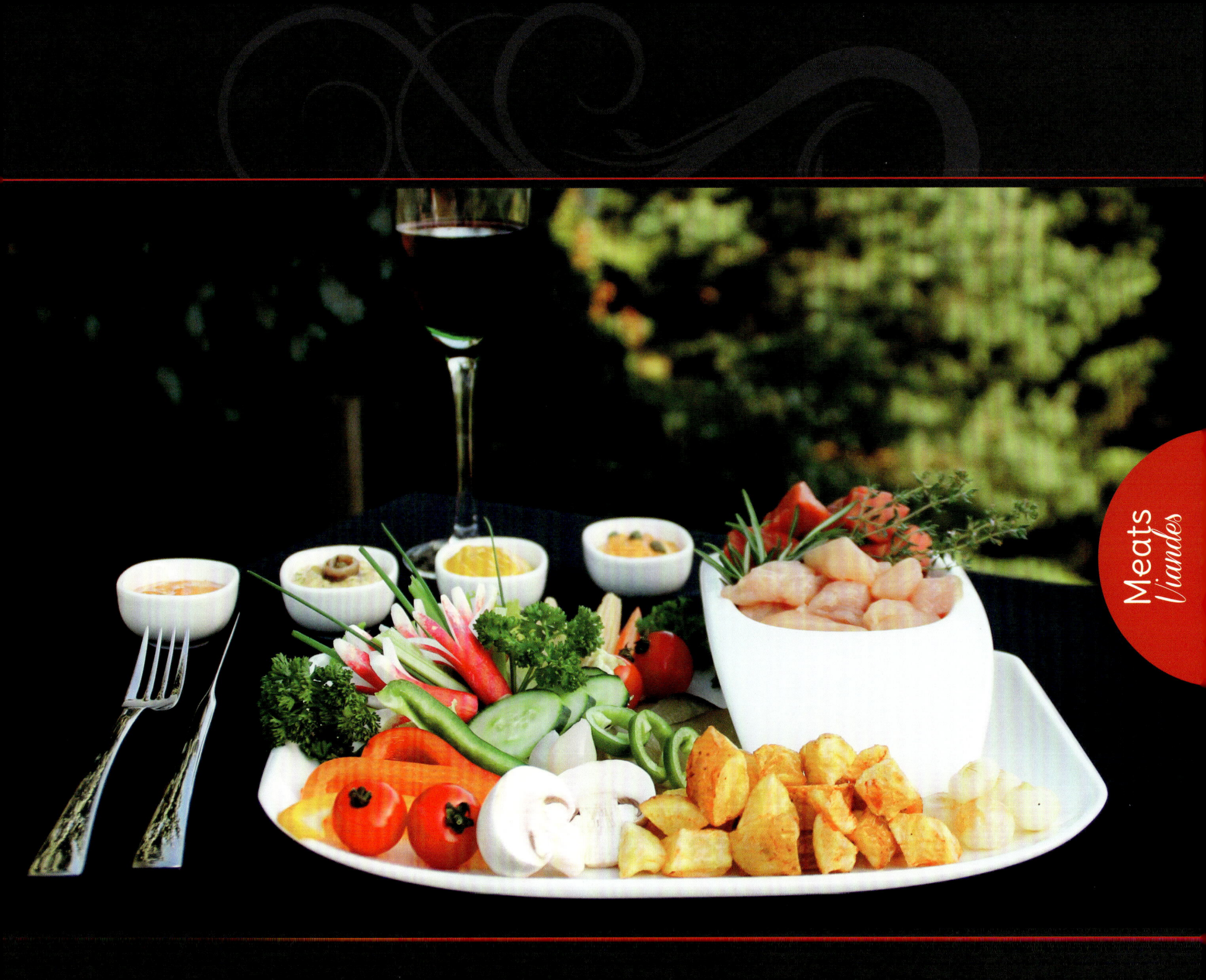

Sometimes it's all the little extras that make a meal so special.

Meats
Viandes

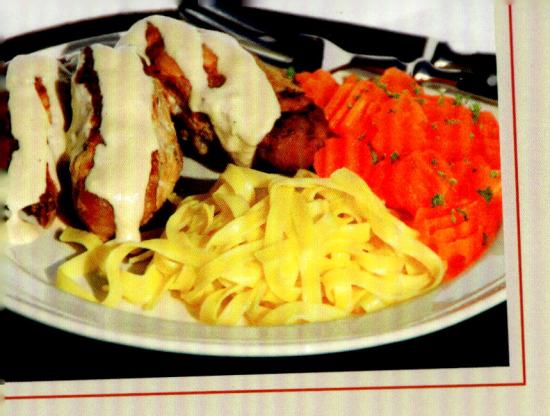

Rabbit in mustard sauce
Lapin à la moutarde

Baste each piece of rabbit with the mustard.

Heat the oil in an ovenproof pan and fry the onion until golden.

Add the rabbit pieces with the salt and pepper and wine. Cover the pan and cook in the oven for at least 45 minutes or until the meat is tender, adding more wine or water during cooking to prevent the rabbit from drying out.

When cooked, remove from the oven and put the rabbit pieces onto a serving dish.

Add the mushrooms and cream to the juice left in the bottom of the pan and cook until soft. Pour over the rabbit pieces and serve.

Serves approx. 6 persons

Oven: 180°C

- 1 whole rabbit, chopped into sections
- 150 g Dijon mustard
- 2 tablespoons olive oil
- 150 ml double cream
- Salt and pepper
- 175 ml white wine plus more if necessary
- 1 onion, chopped
- 150 g button mushrooms.

Tastier if cooked a day in advance!

Meats
Viandes

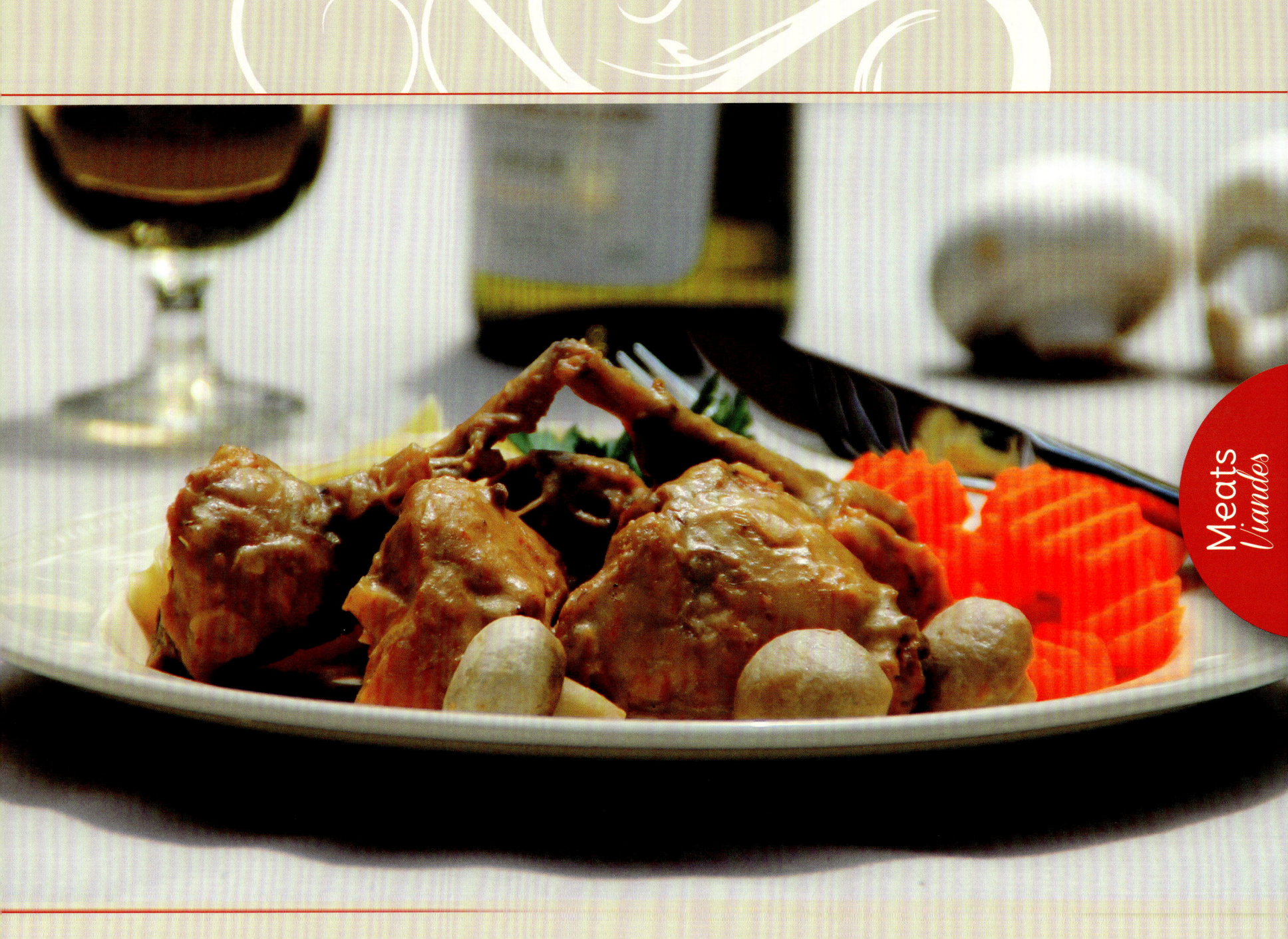

Lapin à la moutarde is a great classic and nobody can deny that the delicate and tender flesh of a rabbit makes a refined dish, appreciated by the finest gourmet.
This dish can be prepared a day in advance, and is even tastier when reheated the next day.

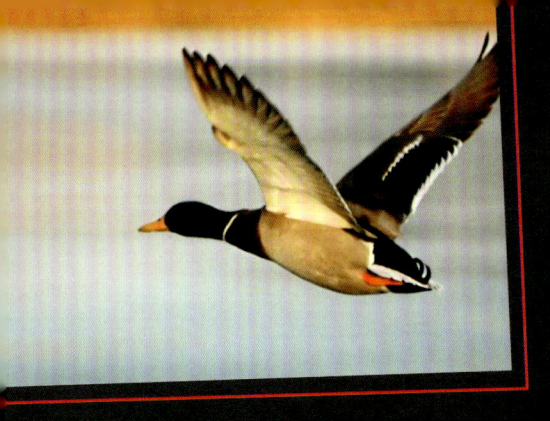

Duck breast
Magret de canard

COOKING THE DUCK BREAST:
Trim off the fat on each side of the breast then score a diamond pattern on the skin with the point of a knife, taking care not to pierce the meat.

Heat a non-stick frying pan and fry the breast skin-side down, for about 15 minutes or until the fat is rendered.

Remove from the pan and discard all but a trace of the fat.

Generously season both sides of the breast with salt and freshly ground pepper and return to the hot frying pan. Cook for another 10 minutes, skin-side up. *The cooking time will depend on whether the meat is preferred rare or well-done.*

Remove from the frying pan, wrap in foil and keep warm.

Duck breast with honey and pears..........................P. 170
Magret de canard au miel et aux poires

Duck breast with cocoa..P. 170
Magret de canard au cacao

Duck breast with cocoa/*Magret de canard au cacao*

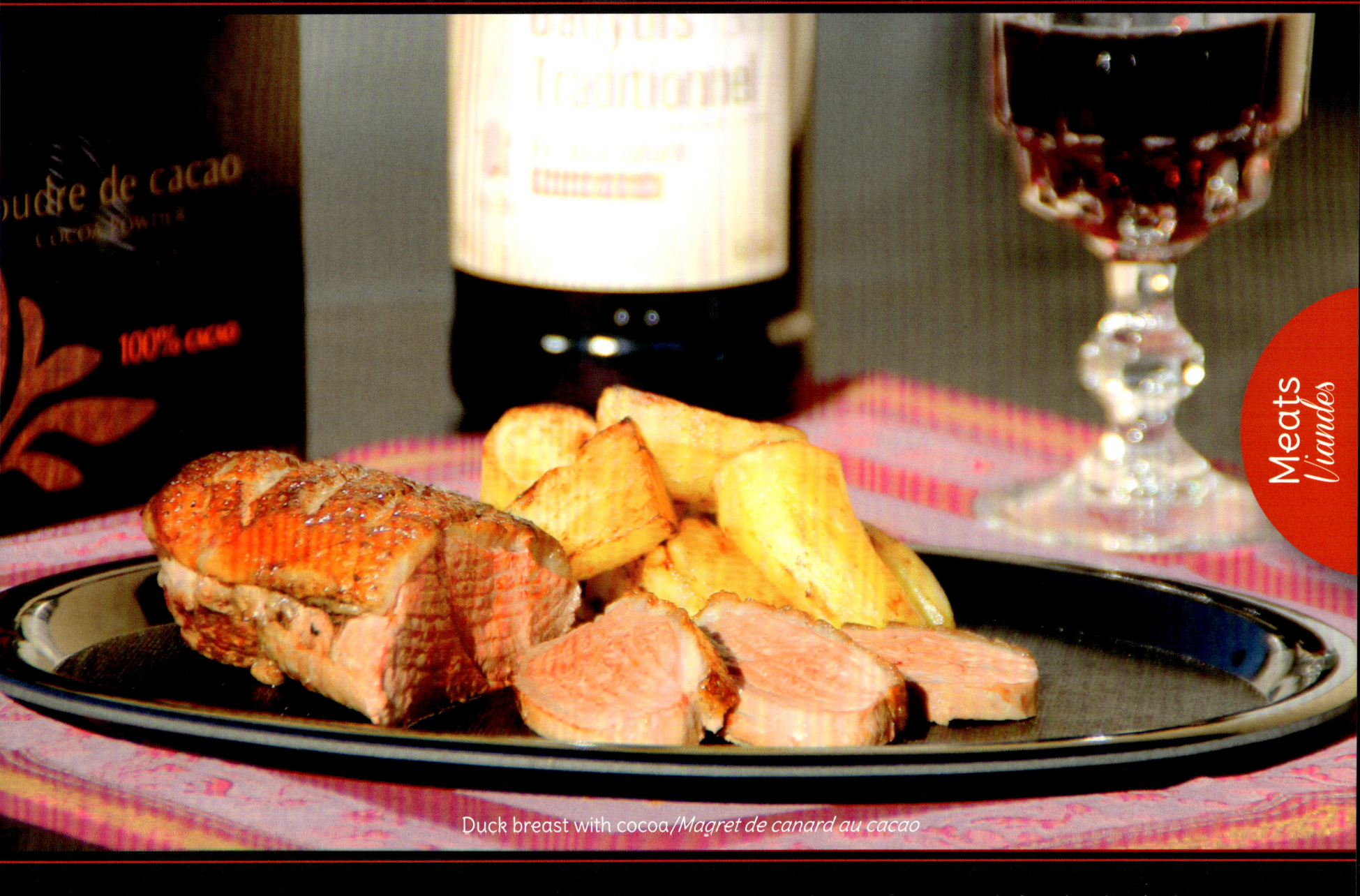

Meats
Viandes

Up until about 1960, duck was always cooked whole or preserved in fat. Apparently, it was a chef in a hotel in *Auch*, *Gers* department, who originally removed the breast of a force-fed duck and cooked it separately. Today, a fried or grilled duck breast, which looks more like red meat than poultry, has become one of the great French classics.

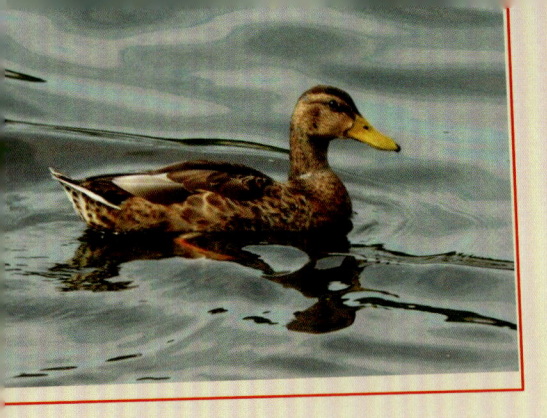

Duck breast
Magret de canard

With honey and pears
Au miel et aux poires

Cook the duck breasts as shown on the previous page.

Drain the fat from the frying pan and add the honey. Cook on a high heat, then deglaze with the wine. Add the sliced pears, salt and pepper and bring to the boil. Simmer until the sauce begins to reduce, basting the pears often.

Slice the meat and place on a warm plate. Add the pear slices. Pour over the sauce and sprinkle with the parsley just before serving.

🍴 Serves approx. 8 – 10 persons

- 3 duck breasts
- 6 pears, peeled, cored and sliced
- 2 tablespoons honey
- 200 ml sweet white wine (eg. *Muscat*)
- 3 sprigs flat-leaved parsley
- Salt and freshly ground pepper

With cocoa
Au cacao

Cook the duck breasts as shown on the previous page.

Drain the excess fat from the frying pan. Mix together the orange juice, zest, honey, cocoa powder and Banyuls and use to deglaze the pan. Do not allow the mixture to boil. Season with salt and pepper.

Slice the meat and serve with the hot chocolate sauce.

Banyuls is a sweet wine produced in Languedoc – Roussillon region, in the South of France. It can be served as an apéritif, or with a fruit or chocolate dessert, and goes particularly well with the pronounced flavour of duck. (Some consider it to be the best and only accompaniment to chocolate!)

🍴 Serves approx. 4 – 6 persons

- 2 duck breasts
- Juice of 1 orange
- Zest of ½ orange, organic or untreated
- 2 tablespoons honey
- 1 level tablespoon cocoa powder
- 100 ml Banyuls
- Salt and pepper

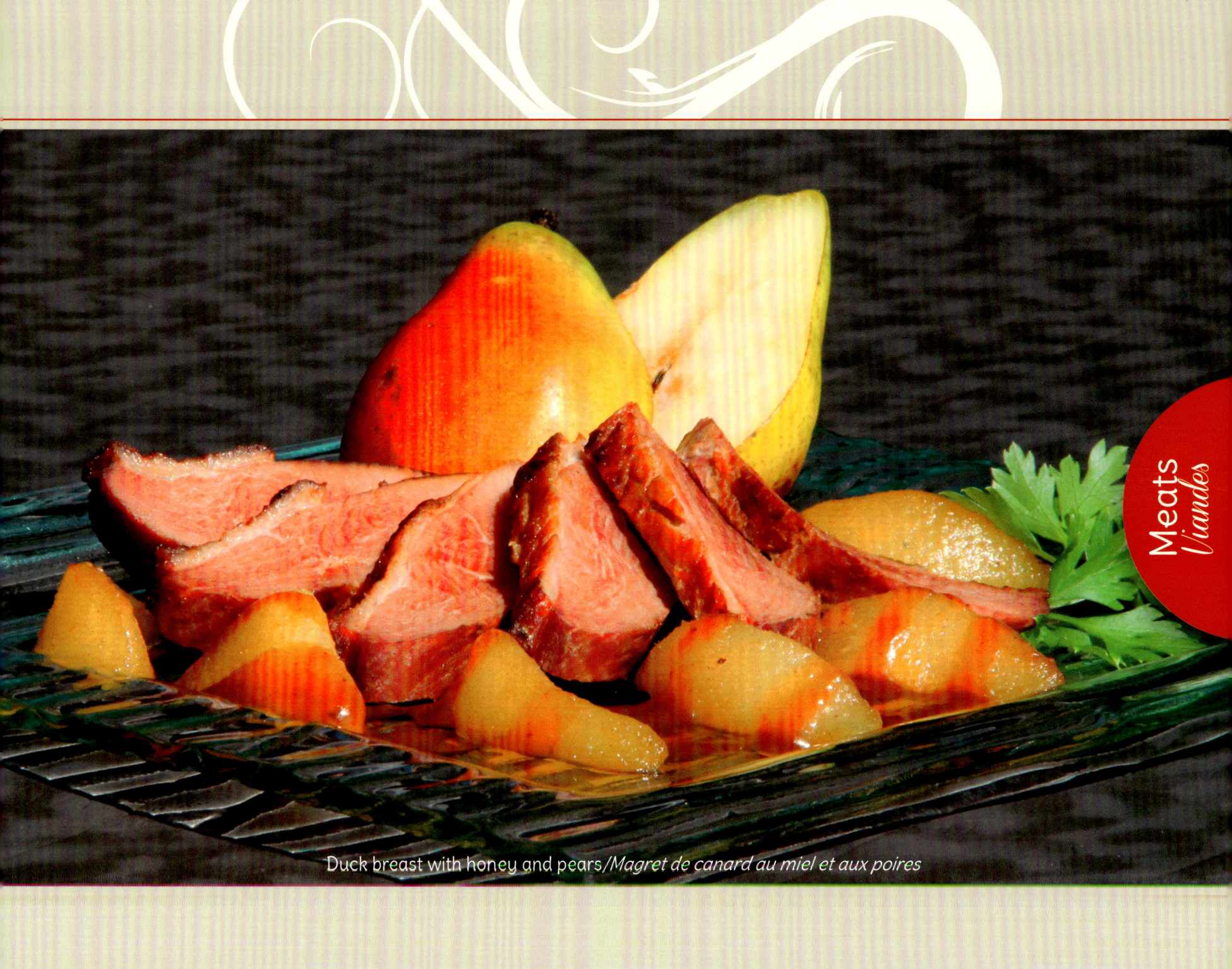

Duck breast with honey and pears/*Magret de canard au miel et aux poires*

Meats
Viandes

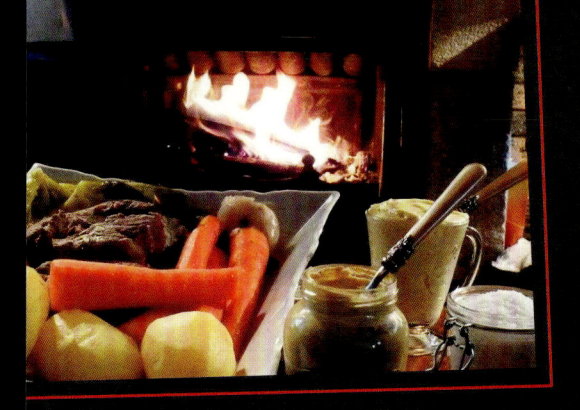

Hot pot
Pot au feu

Place the meat in a large saucepan with 5 litres of cold water and the salt. Add the *bouquet garni* with the celery (including the green leaves), garlic and onions pricked with the cloves. Bring rapidly to the boil. After 5 minutes, reduce the heat and leave to simmer for at least 1 - 1½ hours.

Add the peeled whole carrots and cook for another 30 minutes.

Add the sliced leeks and continue cooking for another hour.

Place the meat and the vegetables into a warmed serving dish.

Strain the stock and pour some over the meat to prevent it drying out.

Serve with boiled potatoes, salt and pepper, gherkins, mustard and mayonnaise (see *recettes de base*).

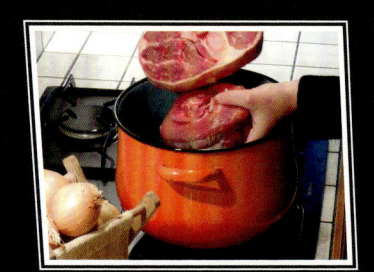

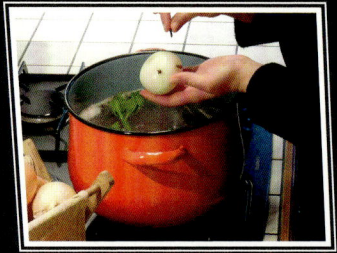

Serves approx. 6 persons

- 1.5 kg shoulder of beef (chuck, middle rib, shin or knuckle with bone) Add a bone if there is none with the meat
- 2 rounded teaspoons coarse salt
- 1 *bouquet garni*
- ½ head celery
- 2 garlic cloves
- 2 onions
- 4 cloves
- 6 carrots
- 4 - 6 leeks (just the white part)

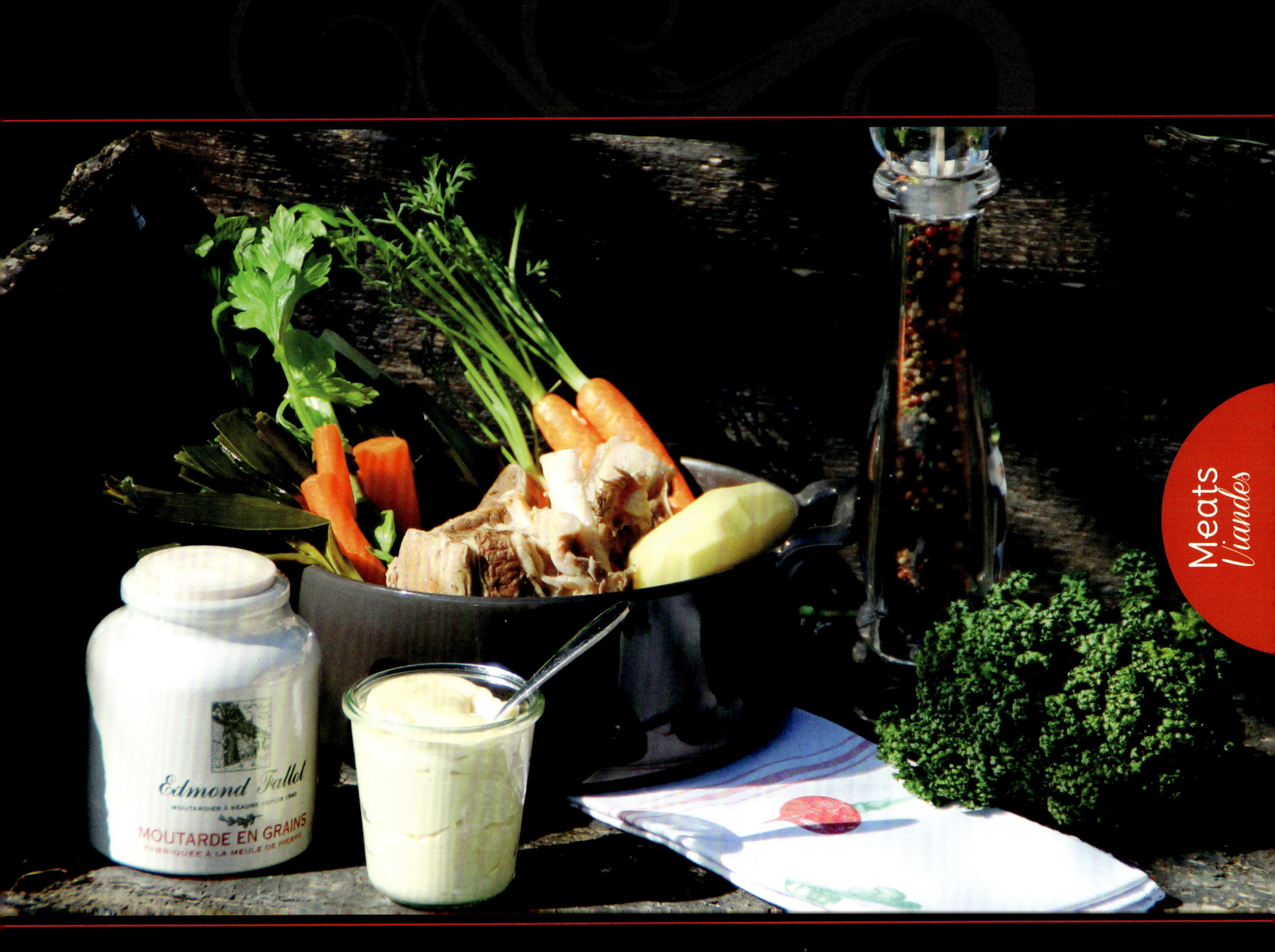

Pot-au-feu is a culinary emblem of France, distinguishing it from other countries as the meat is boiled in water with the vegetables. It is a substantial, homely, country-style meal which requires plenty of cooking time, and is unbeatable on a cold winter's day. Produces a particularly flavoursome stock, ideal for making *soupe à l'oignon* or simply for cooking pasta.

Meats / *Viandes*

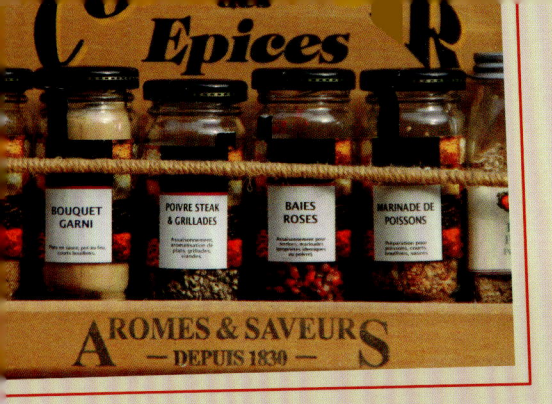

Peppered steaks
Steaks au poivre

Brush the steaks with the olive oil. Place the peppercorns in a shallow bowl and press the steaks firmly onto them, to allow the pepper to penetrate.

Melt the butter in a large frying pan and fry the steaks for about 2 - 4 minutes on each side depending on whether rare or well-done steak is preferred.

Heat the Cognac slightly, pour into the frying pan over the steaks and ignite with a match or a gas lighter. *This should be done with outstretched arms and a frying pan lid to hand in case of an emergency.*

Place the steaks onto a warm plate. Pour the wine into the frying pan and simmer for 1 minute, stirring well to deglaze the pan. Add the cream and heat gently, stirring for 1 - 2 minutes.

Season the sauce and pour over the steaks before serving.

Serves 4 persons

- 4 x 200 g tender fillet steaks
- 2 tablespoons olive oil
- 4 tablespoons crushed peppercorns
- 30 g butter
- 3 tablespoons Cognac, slightly warmed
- 60 ml white wine
- 125 ml double cream

This recipe uses a lot of peppercorns and therefore has a very strong flavour. Use green peppercorns for a light, fresh vegetable flavour. Vary quantities according to taste.

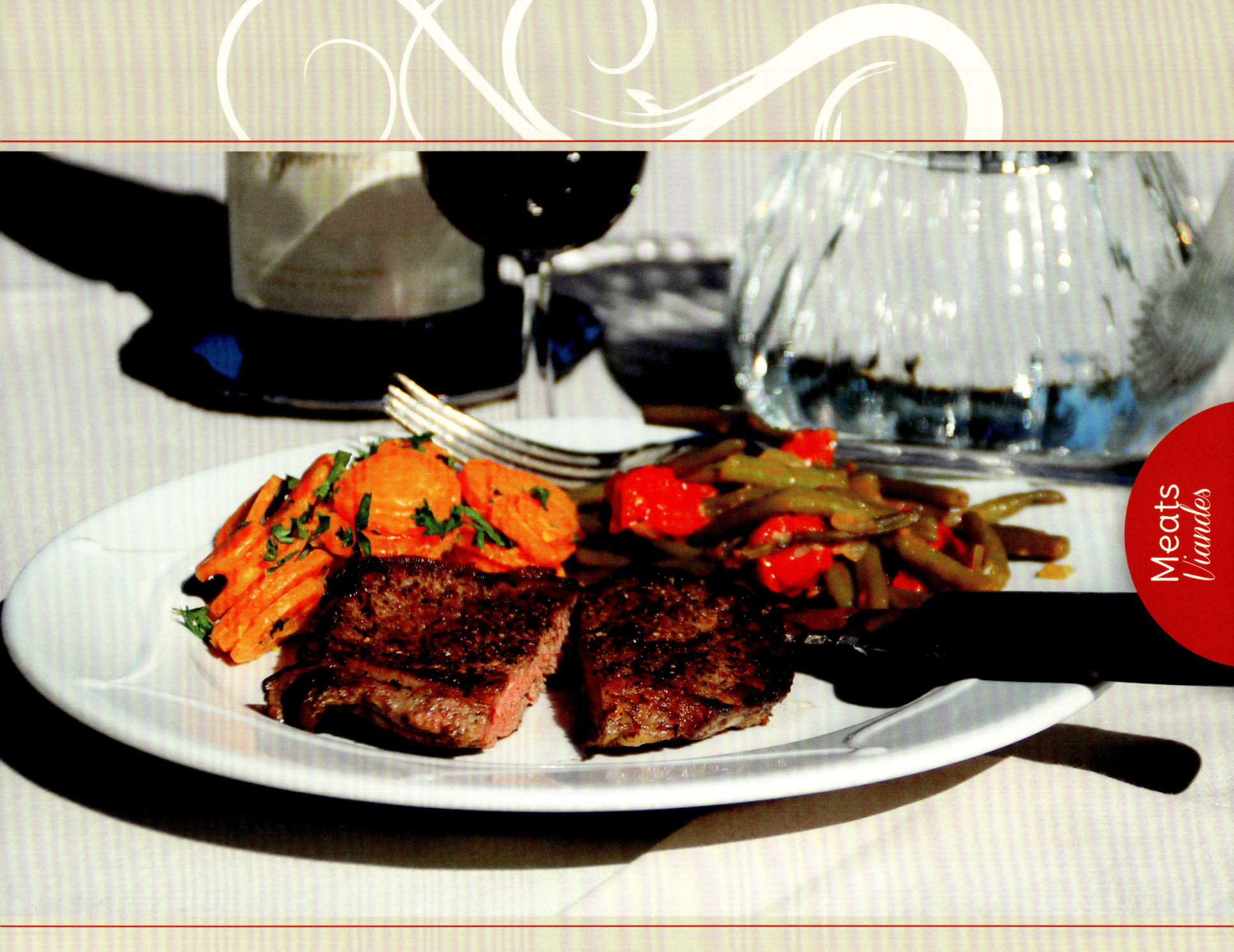

Originating from *Ile de France* where it is served with chips, *steak au poivre* is a refined meal which requires quality ingredients but is very simple to prepare.

Meats
Viandes

Vegetables and starches
Légumes et féculents

180 Vichy carrots
Carottes Vichy

182 Raw sauerkraut
Choucroute crue

184 Sauerkraut from Alsace
Choucroute d'Alsace

186 Carrot bake
Fondant aux carottes

188 Provençale-style bake
Gratin à la provençale

190 Chicory bake with ham
Gratin d'endives au jambon

192 *Gratin Dauphinois*
Gratin Dauphinois

194 Swiss chard bake
Gratin de blettes

194 Swiss chard in tomato sauce
Blettes en sauce tomate

196 Cardoon bake
Gratin de cardons

198 Pumpkin bake
Gratin de potiron

200 Potato and leek bake
Gratin de pommes de terre aux poireaux

202 Potato and tomato bake
Gratin de pommes de terre aux tomates

204 French beans with cherry tomatoes
Haricots verts aux tomates cerises

204 French beans with tomatoes
Haricots verts aux tomates

206 Lentils with sausages
Lentilles aux saucisses

208 Sautéed potatoes
Pommes de terre sautées

208 Duchess potatoes
Pommes duchesses

Warning!
Some recipes contain alcohol.

210 Semolina *quenelles*
Quenelles à la semoule

212 Flour *quenelles*
Quenelles à la farine

214 Grated potato cakes
Rapée de pommes de terre

216 Ratatouille
Ratatouille

218 Courgette soufflé
Soufflé à la courgette

218 Broccoli soufflé
Soufflé au brocoli

220 Semolina soufflé
Soufflé de semoule

222 Provençale-style tomatoes
Tomates à la provençale

224 Stuffed tomatoes
Tomates farcies

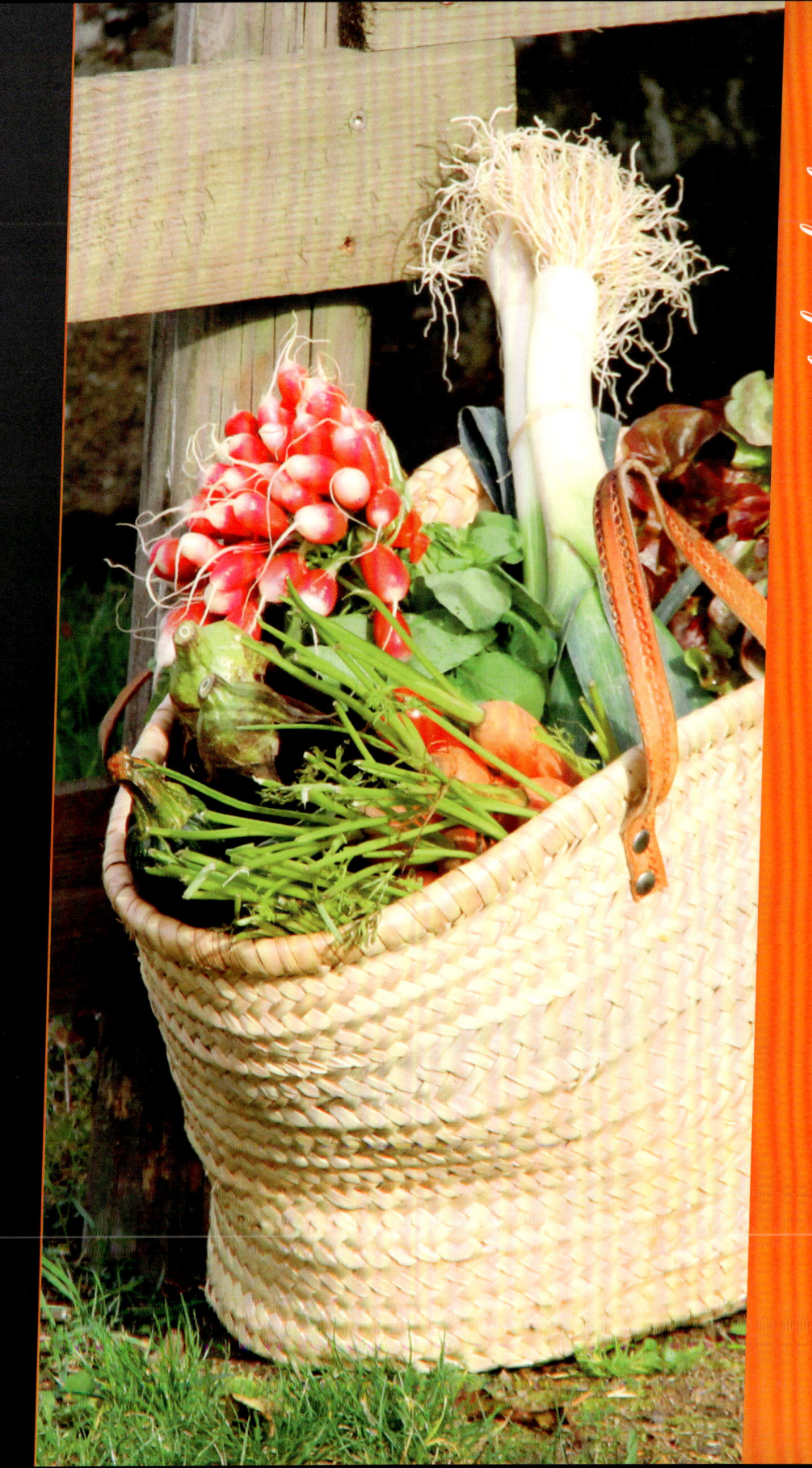

Vegetables and starches *Légumes et féculents*

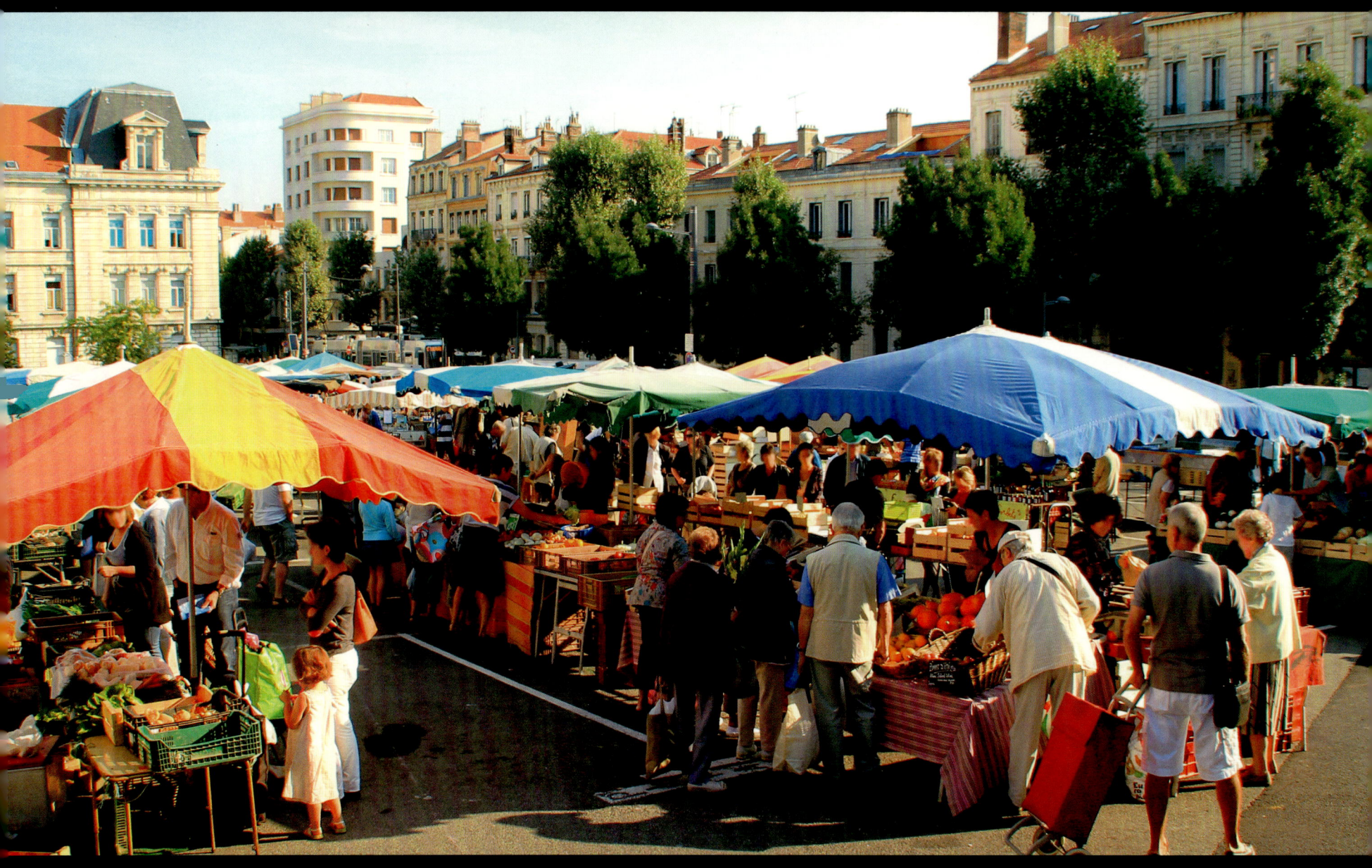

Fresh and nutritious...

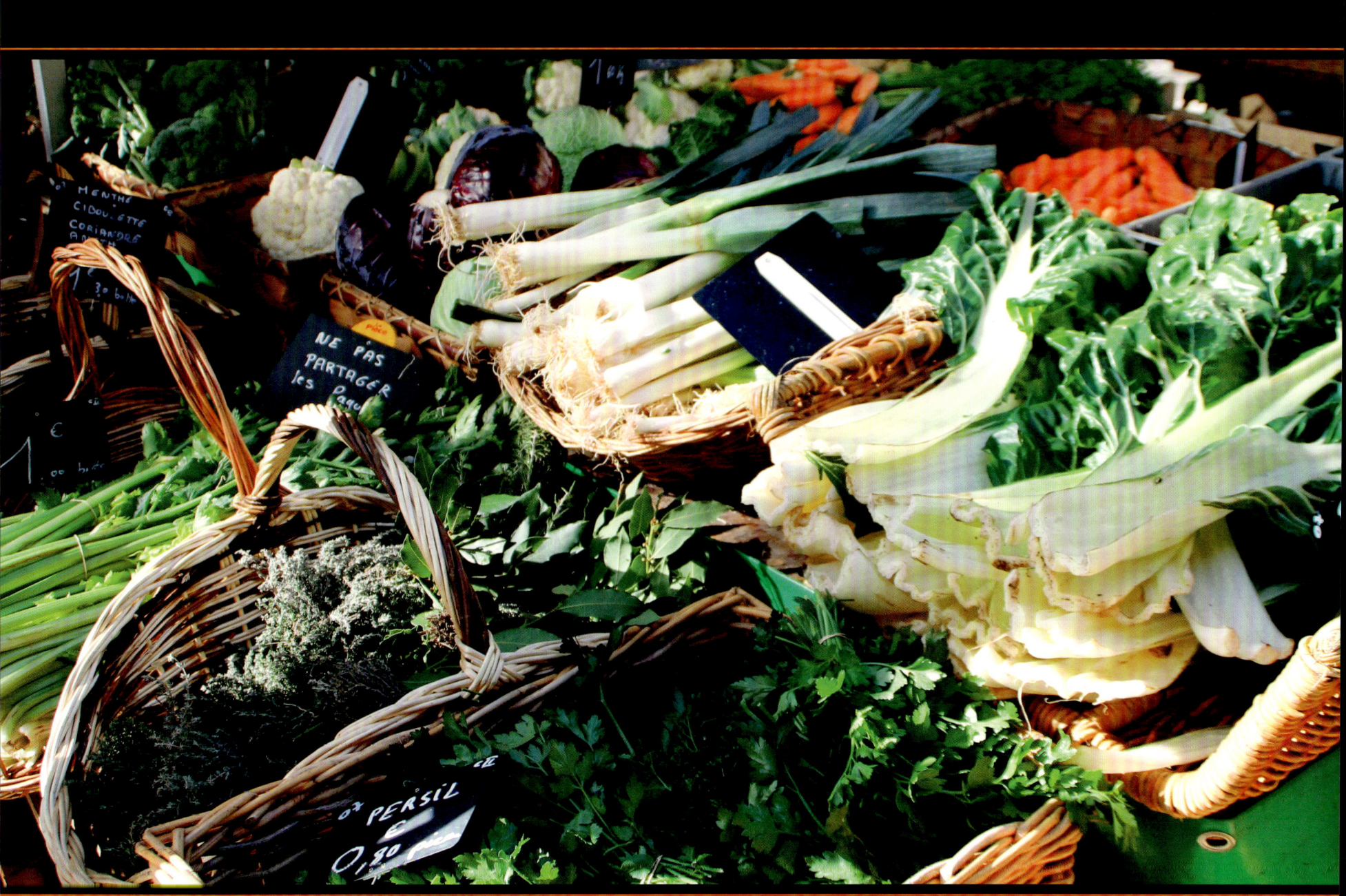

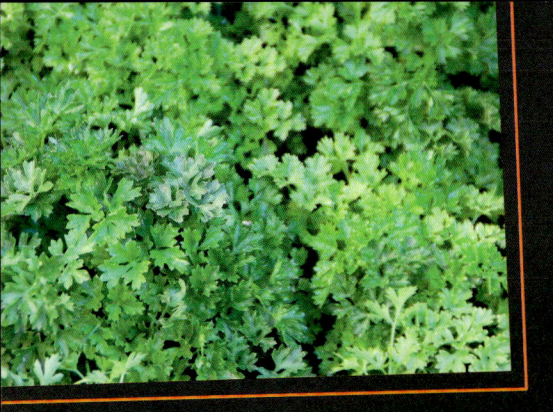

Vichy carrots
Carottes Vichy

Peel and cut the carrots into rings. Heat the butter and sugar in a deep frying pan or a large saucepan.

Once the mixture is hot, add the carrots and stir well to glaze them with the butter. Add the salt.

Cover the carrots with 100 ml of the stock. Cook uncovered on a medium heat, stirring from time to time, until the carrots are cooked and the water evaporated. If the stock has evaporated and the carrots are not yet cooked, either cover the saucepan and continue cooking or add the rest of the stock and continue cooking. At the end of cooking, the carrots should have absorbed the liquid.

If using new carrots, they will cook quicker and need less liquid to cook in. If any stock is left after the carrots are cooked, drain well.

Shake the saucepan to glaze all the carrots, add the chopped parsley and pepper.

Toss and serve hot.

For a healthy alternative, replace the butter with 30 ml olive oil and lightly fry a

Vegetables and starches
Légumes et féculents

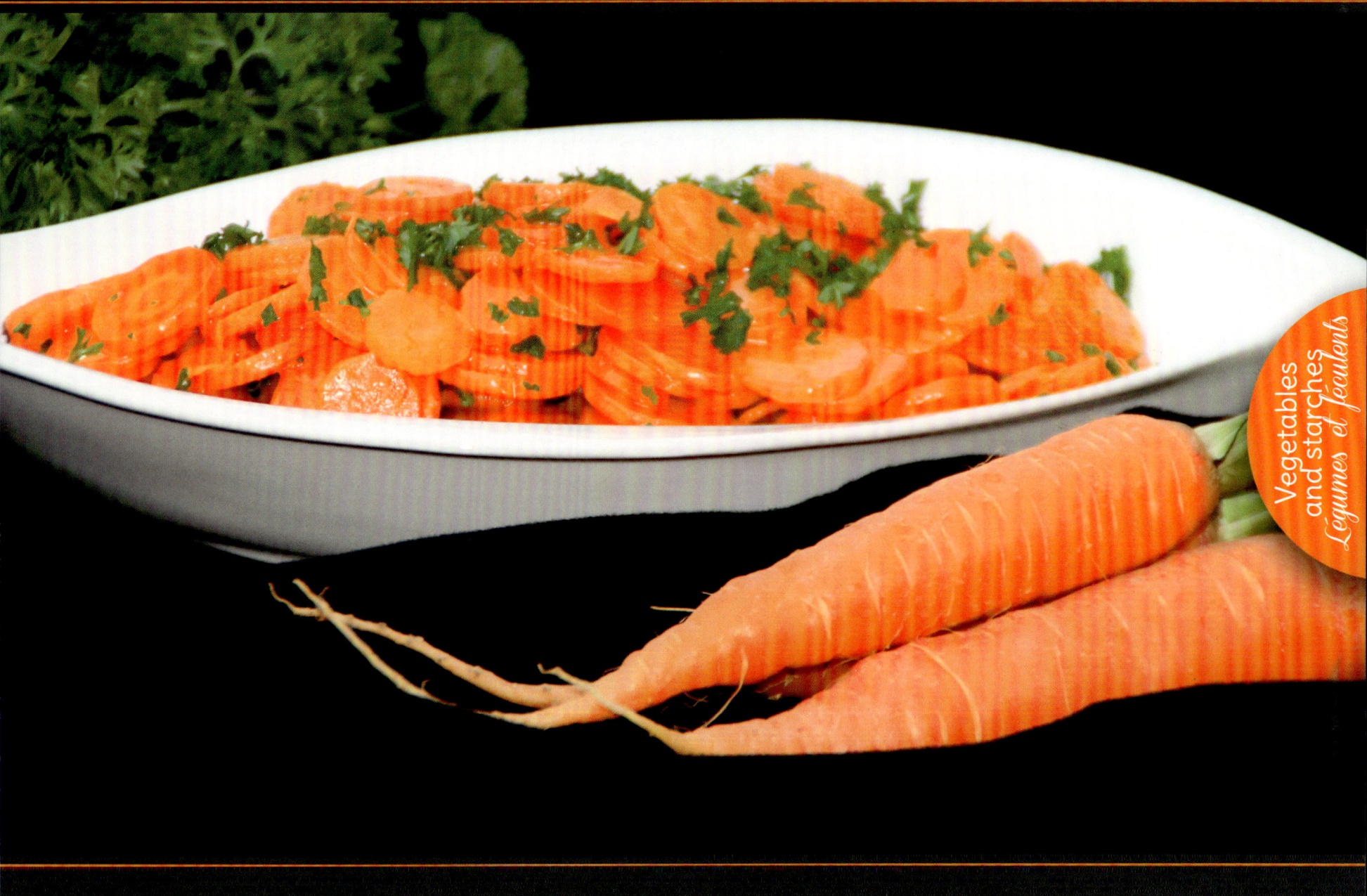

This simple, economic yet delicious recipe is supposed to date back to the 16th or 17th century. During this epoch spas in *Vichy* were very much the fashion, where they were treating rheumatism and digestive disorders. The restaurant chef in a spa created this recipe using the famous natural spring water from *Vichy* to cook the carrots in, as a light accompaniment to grilled or roasted meats.

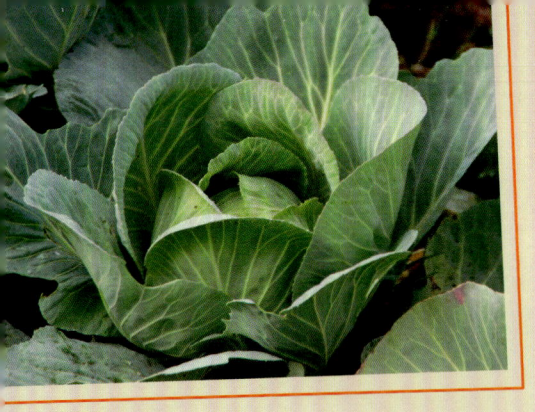

Raw sauekraut
Choucroute crue

Wash the cabbage and peel off the outer leaf. Reserve. Shred the rest of the cabbage finely with a very sharp knife or with a food processor.

Place layers of finely chopped cabbage with salt and juniper berries into an airtight jar, pressing down very firmly between each layer. Ensure that the jar is completely full. Cover with some of the reserverd outer leaf, pressing down firmly. Close the lid. *It is very important that there is no air space as this will prevent fermentation.*

Leave to ferment at room temperature for 1 - 2 days.

Presently the cabbage will be soaking in its own juices. Some bubbles will appear round the lid. This is normal—just leave the jar on a tray.

Place in a cooler temperature (12°C - 15°C) and leave to ferment for a minimum of 3 weeks. *The reaction between the salt and the sugars found in the cabbage produces enough lactic acid to preserve the cabbage throughout the whole winter.*

Drain the *choucroute* and rinse under clean running water before using for the following recipe *choucroute d'Alsace*.

- 5 kg white cabbage
- 25 g coarse salt
- 10 g juniper berries

Vegetables and starches
Légumes et féculents

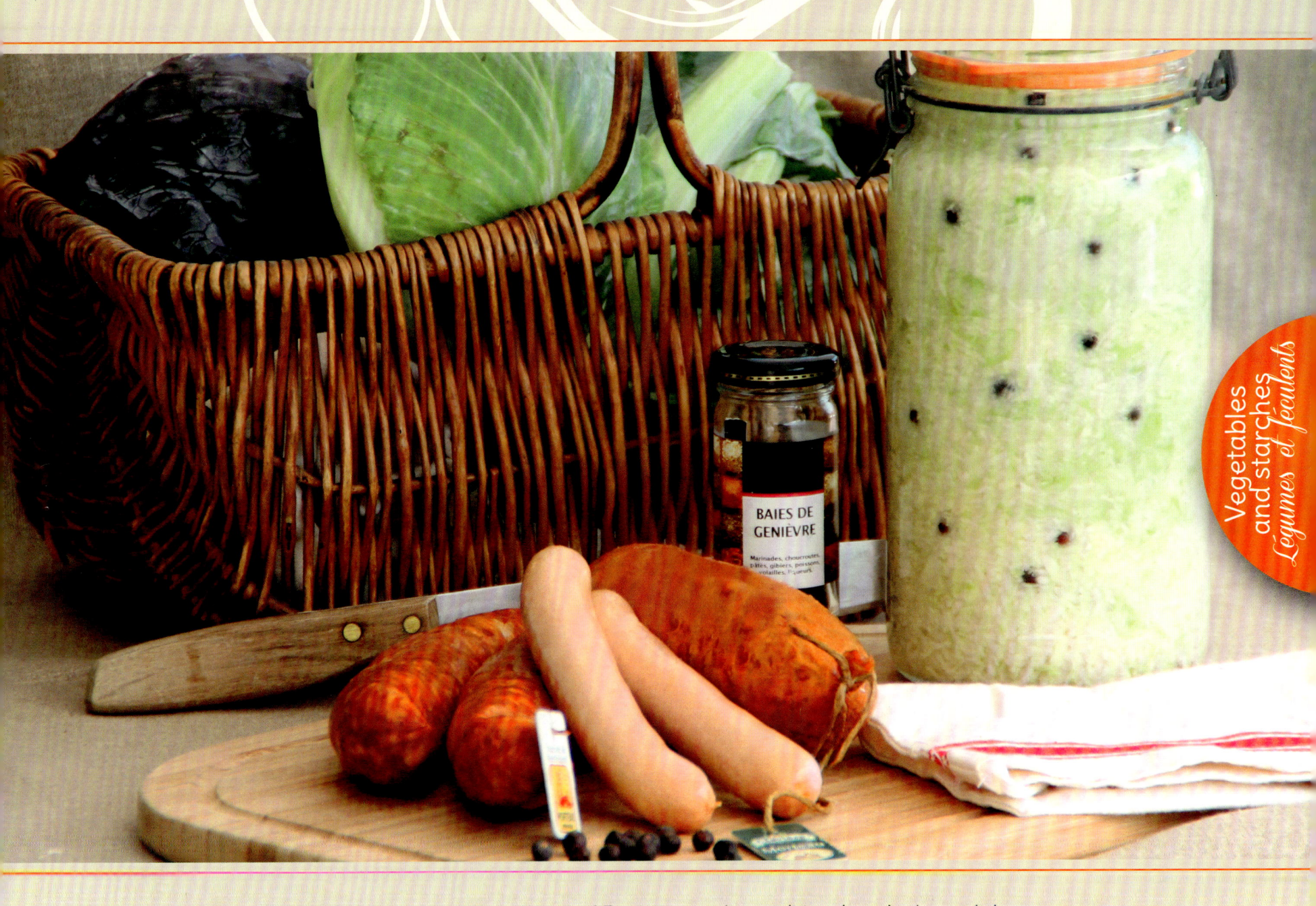

Fermentation is at the base of some of France's proud specialities—bread, wine and cheese.
Over the last 100 years, most traditionally fermented foods have been eliminated from our diet, but recent research has proved that these foods provide good bacteria which are very beneficial for the health.
Although fermentation is done commercially, mostly food is pasteurised destroying beneficial bacteria therefore homemade fermented food is far healthier—*choucroute* is one way of enjoying real fermented food.

183

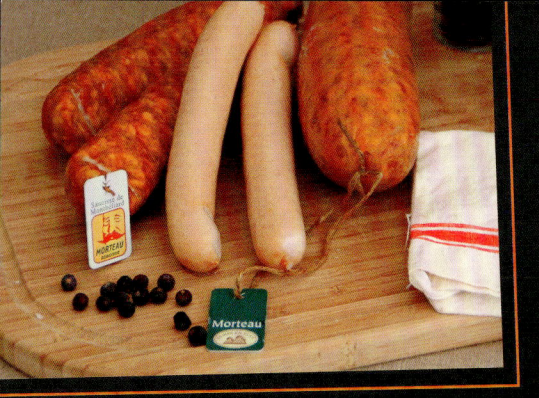

Sauerkraut from Alsace
Choucroute d'Alsace

Place the uncooked sauerkraut in a colander and rinse with fresh cold water, until the water runs clear.

Pour half the wine into a pressure cooker along with half the cloves and juniper berries. Place half the sauerkraut on top. Lightly season with salt and 1 tablespoon of stock. *Do not add too much salt if adding bacon later.*

Cut the Montbéliard sausages into quarters, and slice the Morteau sausage. Place them on top of the sauerkraut.

Place the rest of the sauerkraut on top of the sausages. Lightly season with salt and add the remaining stock, cloves, juniper berries, wine and the water.

Close the lid and bring up to pressure. Cook on a medium - low heat for about 45 minutes.

Add the rashers of bacon and the loin chops. Bring up to pressure again and cook for another 10 minutes.

Cook the Alsace sausages with the Saveloys in a saucepan of simmering water for about 5 minutes.

Strain the sauerkraut before serving and serve with the sausages.

Choucroute d'Alsace is served with boiled potatoes and a white wine from *Alsace* (such as *Riesling*) or beer.

Serves approx. 8 persons

- 1.5 kg uncooked sauerkraut
- 20 cloves
- 20 juniper berries
- Salt
- 2 tablespoons concentrated vegetable stock
- 700 ml white wine (preferably Riesling)
- 600 ml water
- 2 - 3 Montbéliard sausages
- 1 Morteau sausage
- 6 - 8 Alsace sausages, halved
- 6 - 8 thick rashers of bacon
- 3 - 4 loin chops, halved
- 2 Saveloy, quartered

This recipe can be adapted by adding more sauerkraut or more meat depending on the company. This recipe is just a guide.

Vegetables and starches
Légumes et féculents

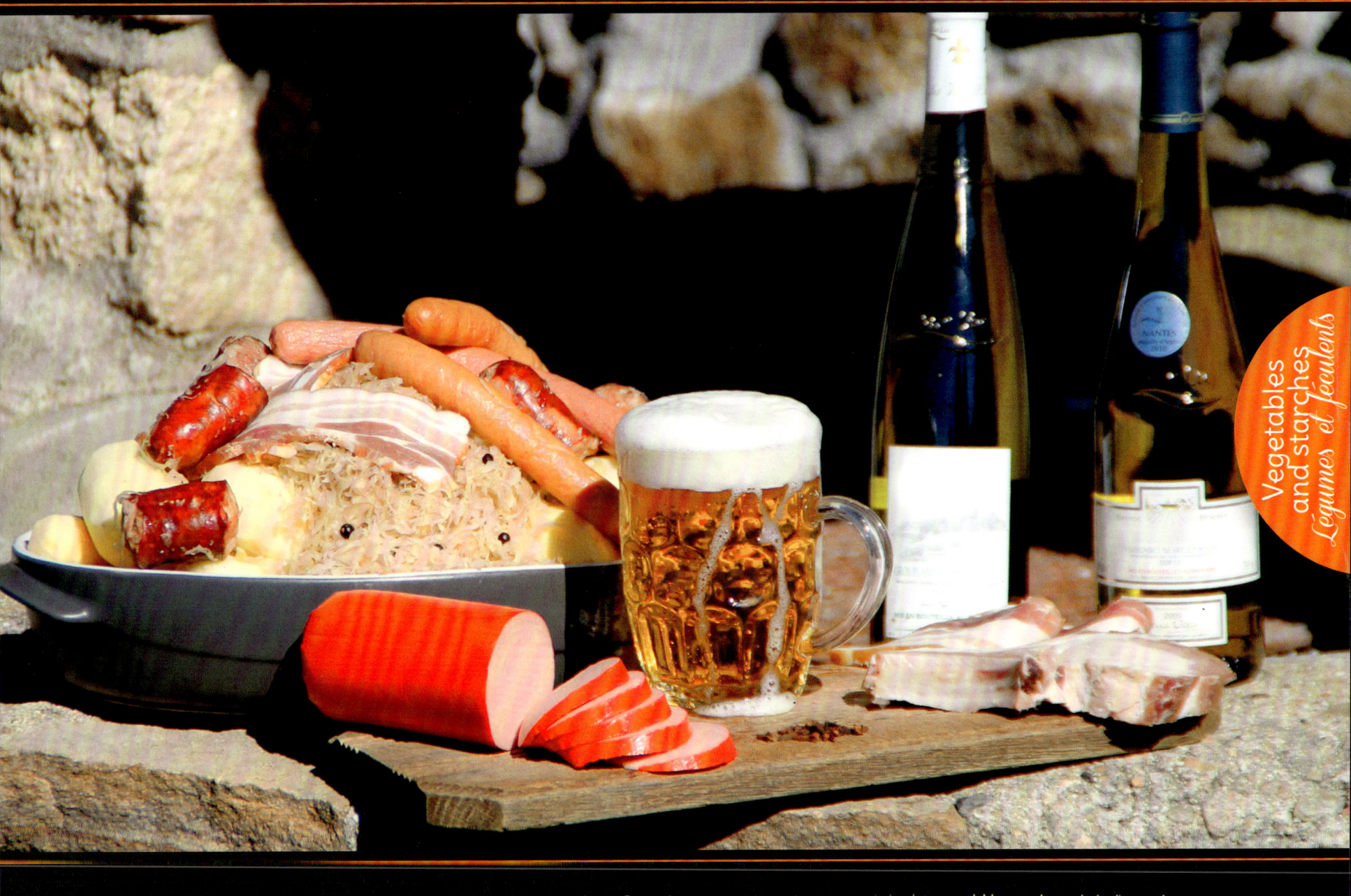

It is said in *Alsace* that there are as many recipes for *choucroute* as there are inhabitants! Nowadays it is found in every region of France and not only in *Alsace*. This recipe is one example showing the types of meat and sausages used. If preferred, choose a selection of these meats.

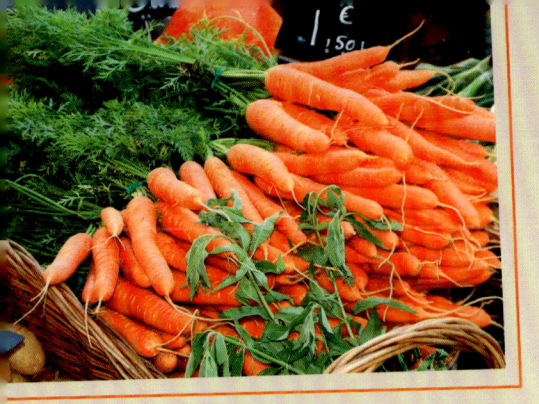

Carrot bake
Fondant aux carottes

Cut the carrots into slices.

Heat the olive oil in a frying pan and add the carrots. Cook on a medium heat for about 5 minutes, stirring from time to time.

Add the vegetable stock and cook uncovered on a medium heat for about 20 minutes or until the carrots are soft and the liquid has almost evaporated. *Stir from time to time especially at the end of cooking, so that the carrots don't burn dry.*

Drain off any excess liquid and leave to cool slightly then liquidise with the eggs, grated cheese, cream and herbs until smooth. Season with salt and pepper according to taste.

Pour into a well-greased baking dish (29 x 20 cm). Place the dish into a roasting tin and half fill with hot water.

Cook for about 35 minutes or until a knife inserted in the centre comes out clean. Leave to cool.

Cut into squares and serve hot.

Makes 24 squares (5 x 5 cm)

Oven: 170°C

- 1 kg carrots, peeled
- 50 ml olive oil
- 600 ml vegetable stock
- 6 eggs
- 150 - 200 g grated cheese
- 2 tablespoons double cream
- 1 teaspoon *herbes de Provence*
- Salt and pepper

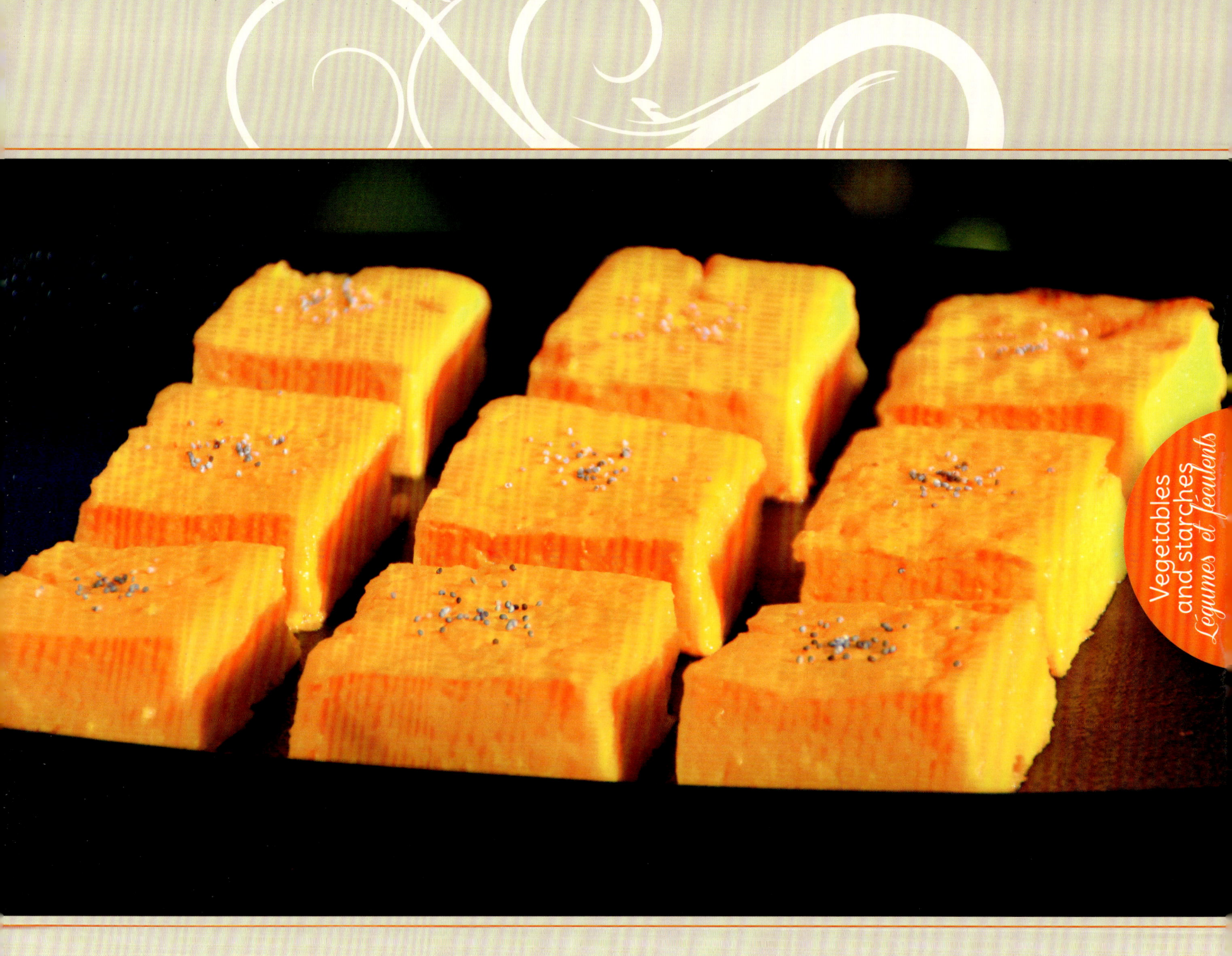

This original savoury delicacy attracts everyone by its striking orange colour and by its special melt-in-the-mouth texture.

Vegetables and starches / Légumes et féculents

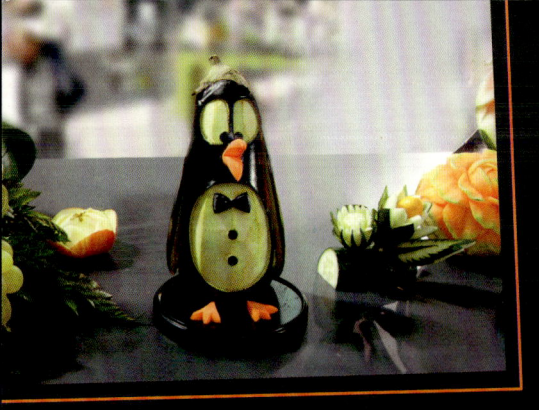

Provençale-style bake
Gratin à la provençale

Wash and dry all the vegetables. Peel the aubergines. Peel alternate lines on the courgette, leaving a stripy effect.

Slice the courgettes and tomatoes into thin rounds.

Cut the aubergines into 1 cm cubes.

Pour 2 tablespoons of olive oil into an ovenproof gratin dish (dimension 20 x 25 cm).

Layer the aubergines over the base of the dish. Pour over 4 tablespoons of olive oil. Sprinkle generously with salt.

Peel and slice the onion finely and place over the aubergines with 1 tablespoon of olive oil.

Layer the courgettes over the onion slices then pour over 3 tablespoons olive oil.

Salt generously again. Sprinkle over the crushed garlic clove.

Finish with a layer of tomatoes and 2 tablespoons of olive oil. Sprinkle with salt, pepper and *herbes de Provence*.

Cook uncovered for approximately 1 hour 15 minutes.

Sprinkle with the cheese and cook until golden.

Serves approx. 8 - 10 persons

Oven: 180°C

- 500 g tomatoes
- 500 g courgettes *(zucchini)*
- 400 g aubergines (eggplant)
- 1 medium sweet onion
- 1 garlic clove, crushed
- 1 teaspoon *herbes de Provence*
- 80 g grated cheese
- Olive oil
- Salt and pepper

Vegetables and starches
Légumes et féculents

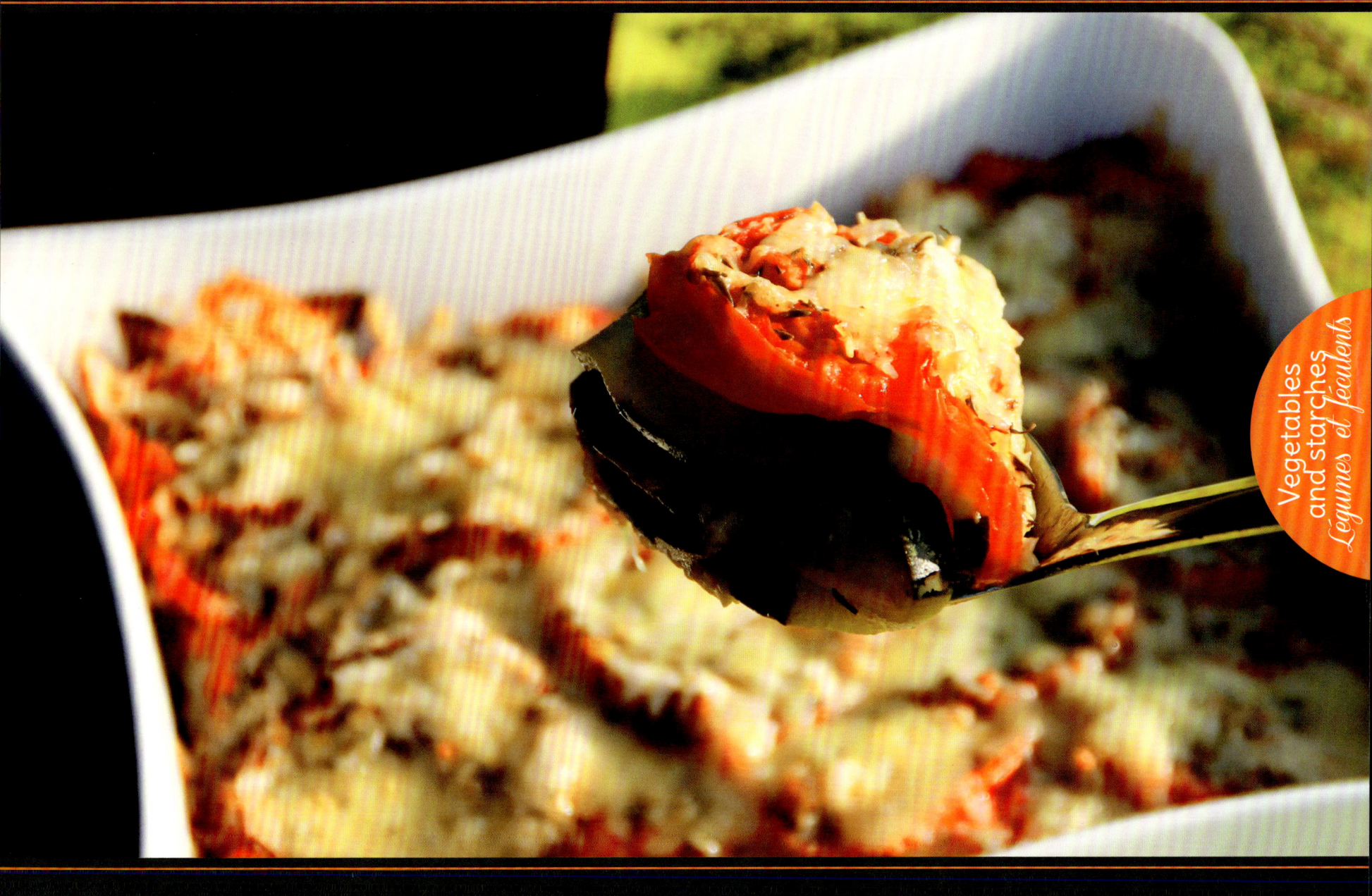

This delicious dish, laden with flavours from *Provence*, is best made during the summer months when vegetables are wonderfully sun-kissed. There is hardly anything simpler and more flavoursome for accompanying grilled or barbecued meat.

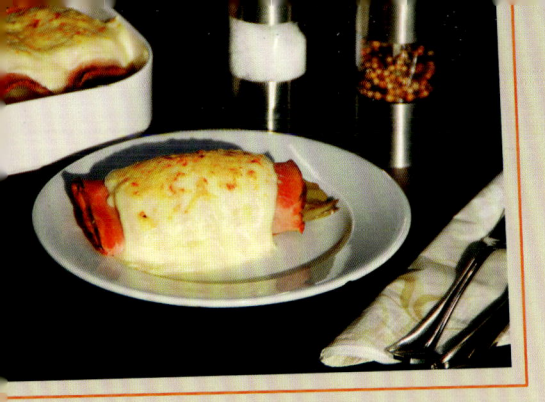

Chicory bake with ham
Gratin d'endives au jambon

Remove the outer layer of leaves from the chicory and trim the stalk. *To reduce the bitterness of chicory, remove the hard, central core.*

Cook in boiling, salted water for about 30 minutes or until soft. *To preserve the whiteness of chicory, sprinkle with lemon juice before cooking.*

Drain well through a colander and if necessary on a clean tea towel. *It is important to drain chicory well or the sauce will curdle.*

MAKE THE *SAUCE BÉCHAMEL* according to the recipe.

Roll a slice of ham around each cooked chicory and place in an ovenproof dish. Pour the sauce over and sprinkle with the grated cheese.

Cook for about 30 minutes or until the top is golden and crispy.

Serves 4 - 6 persons

Oven: 190°C

- 6 chicory heads
- 6 slices of ham
- 120 g grated cheese

- 1 quantity *sauce béchamel* (see *recettes de base*)

Vegetables and starches
Légumes et féculents

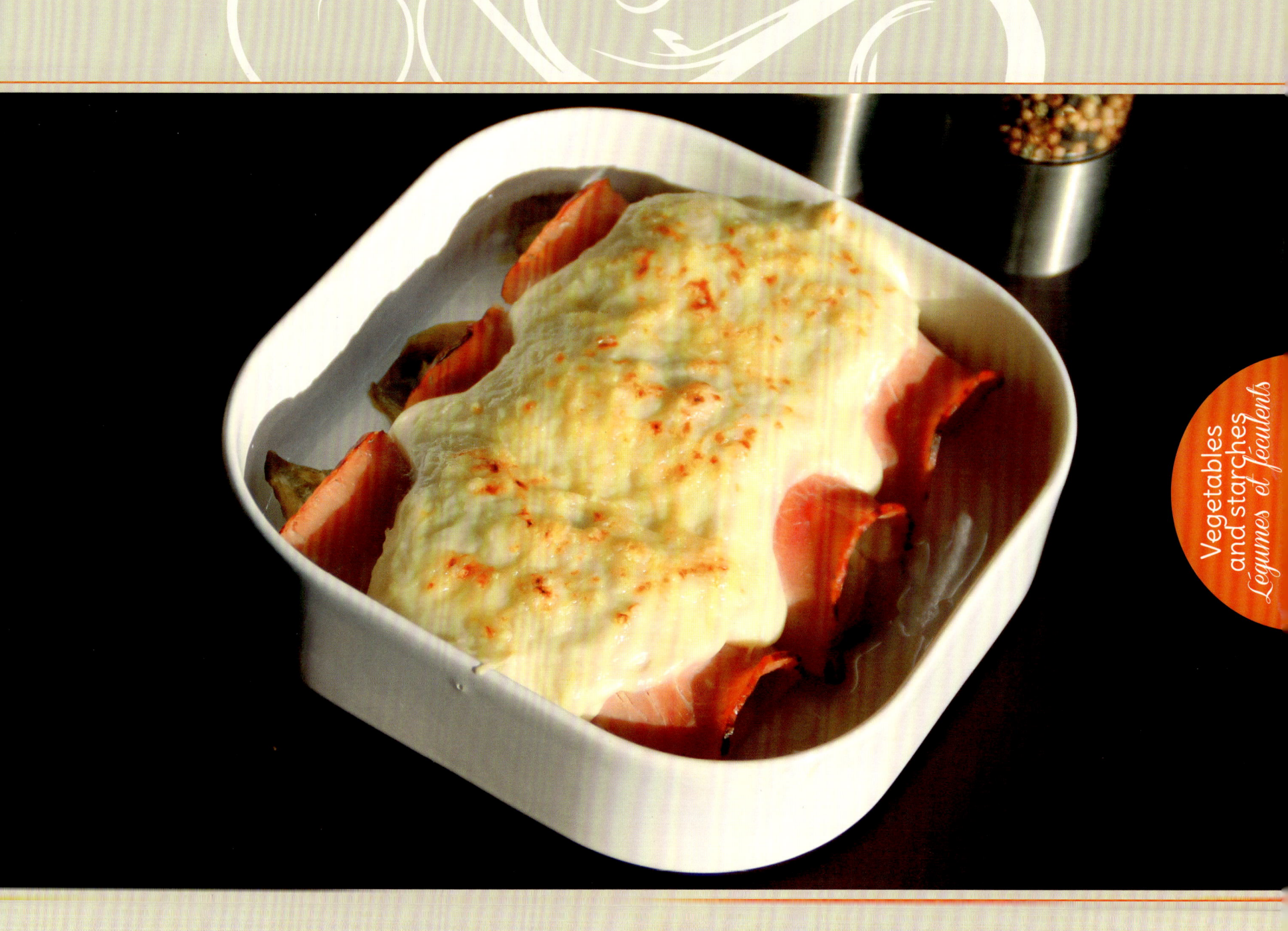

Apparently, chicory was discovered in the middle of the 19th century by a botanical gardener in Brussels. To avoid paying extra taxes on his crops, he hid his wild chicory heads under a little earth in his cellar. Several weeks later a white cone shaped vegetable had appeared: the chicory!

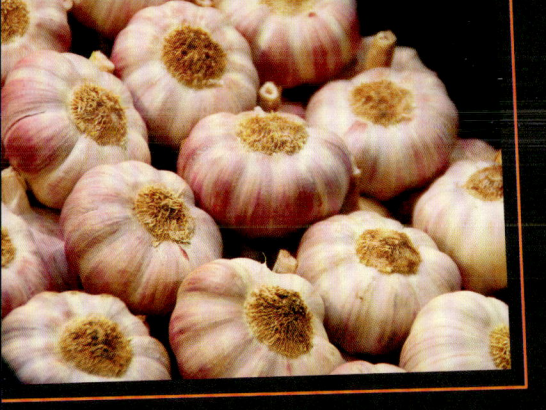

Gratin Dauphinois
Gratin Dauphinois

Peel and rinse the potatoes. Slice them very finely, using a food processor or mandolin if available. *Do not rinse them after they have been sliced as the starch found in the potatoes helps to thicken the gratin.*

Place the cream, nutmeg, salt and pepper in a large frying pan. Add the potatoes. Bring to the boil and cook on a low heat for about 20 minutes, stirring from time to time to prevent the cream and the potatoes from sticking to the bottom of the pan.

Rub the garlic over the base of a greased ovenproof dish and pour in the warm, creamy potatoes.

Dot with some butter.

Cook for at least 1- 1½ hours or until the potatoes are soft and the topping golden brown. The cooking time will vary according to the thickness of the potatoes and the size of the dish! *The slower and longer the cooking, the tenderer and tastier the gratin will be.*

Gratin Dauphinois doesn't have a cheese topping, however for the *Savoyard* version, sprinkle with grated *emmental* or *beaufort* cheese towards the end of cooking.
For a *Lyonnais gratin Dauphinois*, add sliced onions to the potatoes.
To make a lighter *Lyonnais* or *Savoyard gratin Dauphinois*, replace part or all of the cream with chicken or vegetable stock.

Vegetables and starches
Légumes et féculents

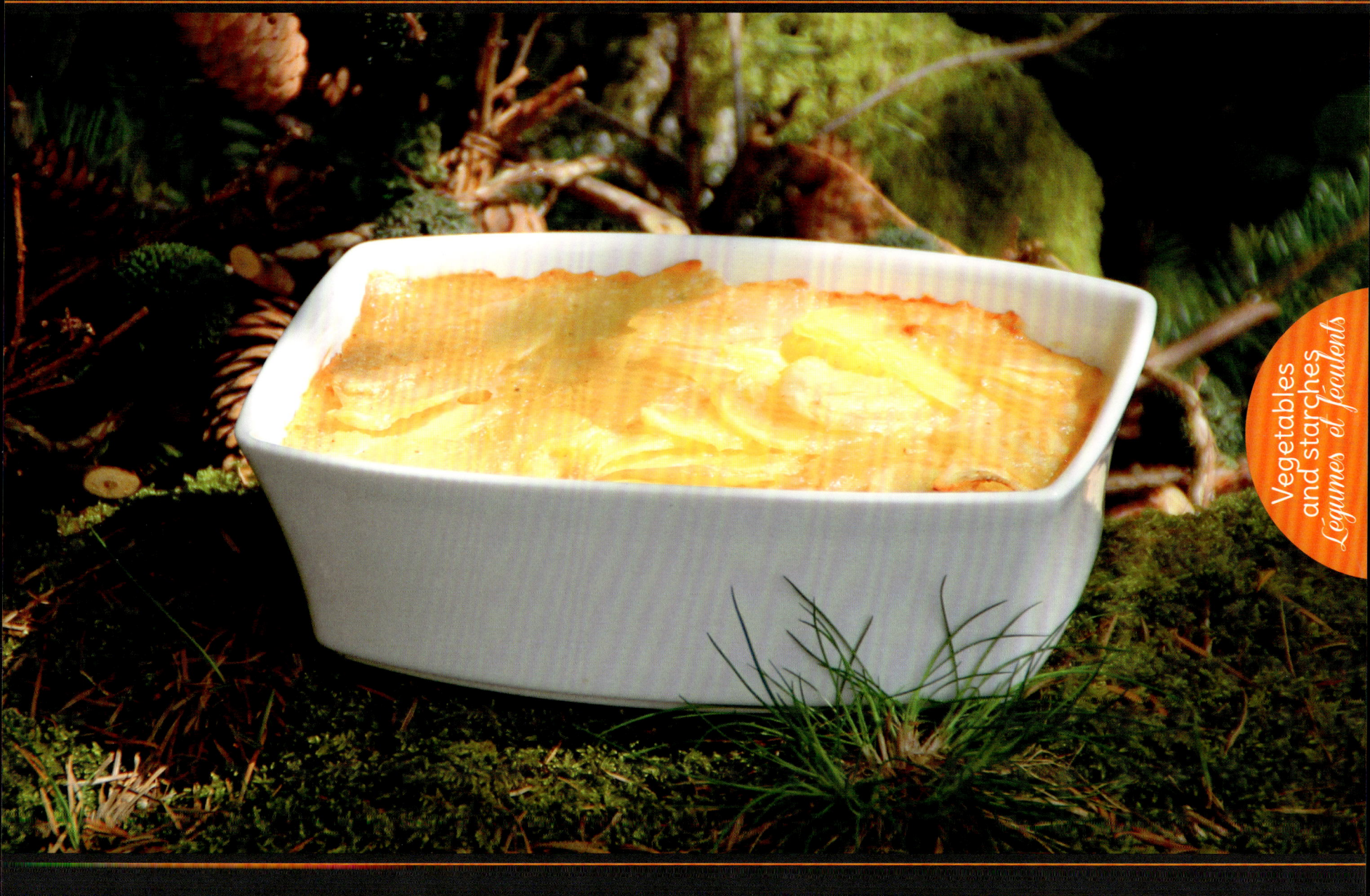

Gratin Dauphinois dates back to the 18th century in the region known as *le Dauphiné*, (which is now the *Isère*, *Drôme* and *Hautes-Alpes* departments). It was very popular with the country people as it was so tasty and filling, and yet so cheap to make.

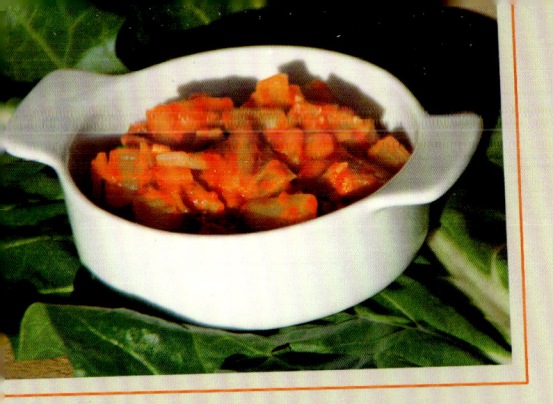

Swiss chard bake
Gratin de blettes

Heat a large saucepan of water. Add salt. Separate the leaves from the stalks of the Swiss chard. Clean the stalks under running water and cut them into chunks of about 2 - 3 cms. Cook them in boiling water for about 15 - 20 minutes. *The cooking time will vary according to the age and thickness of the Swiss chard*. Wash the leaves and cook them in a separate saucepan of boiling, salted water for 5 minutes.

Grease the insides of an ovenproof dish with butter. Once the stalks and greens are cooked, leave to drain in a colander, pressing down well with your hands to extract as much liquid as possible.

MAKE THE *SAUCE BÉCHAMEL* according to the recipe.

Roughly chop the greens and mix together with the stalks and the sauce and pour into the prepared dish. Sprinkle with grated cheese. Cook in the oven until the cheese is melted and golden.

Serves 6 persons

Oven: 200°C

- 400 g white Swiss chard stalks
- 150 g Swiss chard leaves
- Cheese, grated

- 1 quantity *sauce béchamel* (see *recettes de base*)

Swiss chard in tomato sauce
Blettes en sauce tomate

Cook the white Swiss chard stalks as above. Drain and leave aside.

Fry the onion lightly in the olive oil. Add the cooked Swiss chard and continue cooking to allow some of the juice to evaporate. Add the crushed garlic clove and the *coulis de tomates*. Continue to cook until the sauce has thickened.

Serves 6 persons

- 800 g white Swiss chard stalks
- 300 g *coulis de tomates* (see *recettes de base*)
- 4 tablespoons olive oil
- 1 large onion, finely chopped
- 2 garlic cloves, crushed

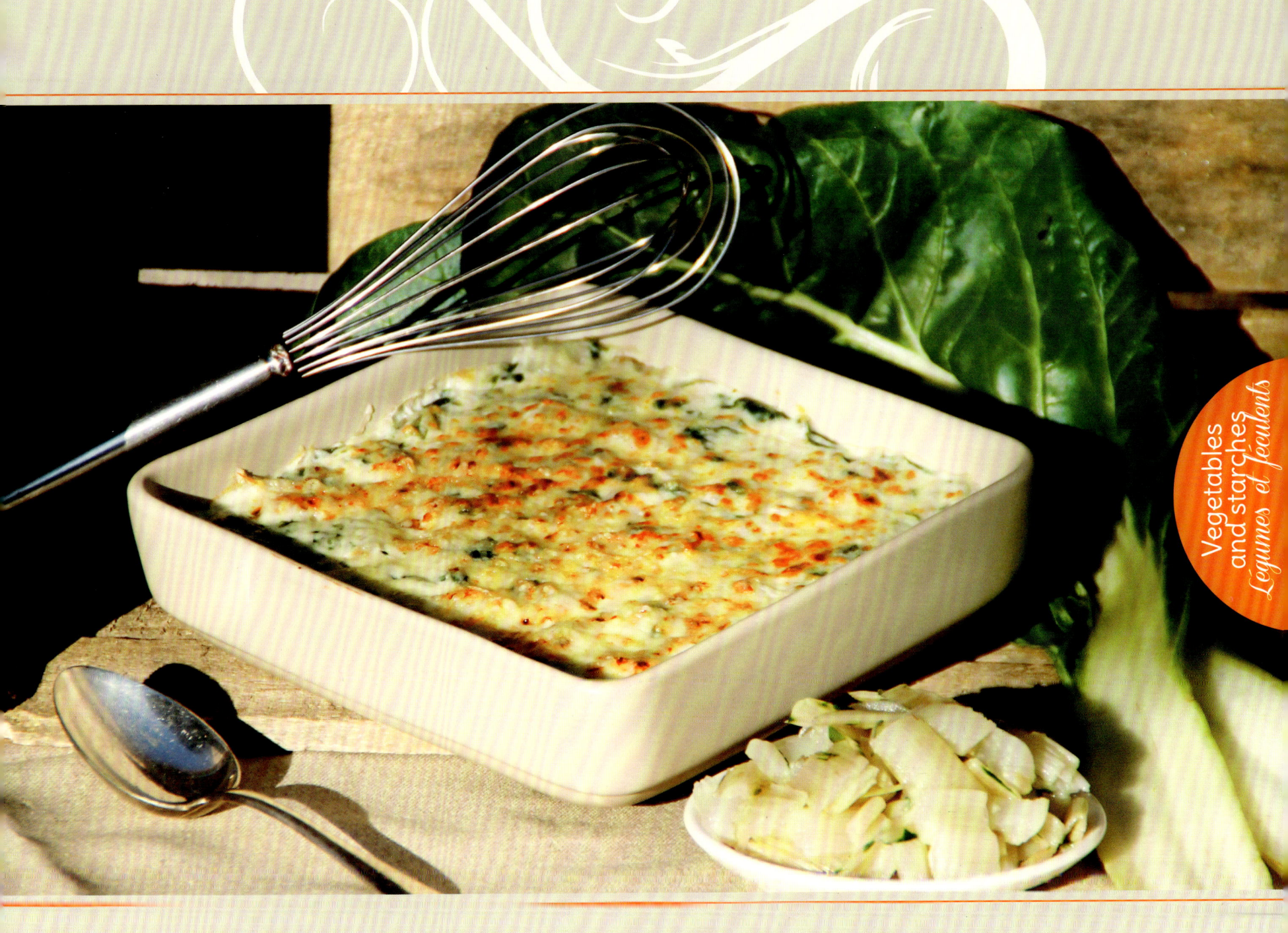

Swiss chard (silver beet) is rich in calcium and fibres and also an excellent source of vitamin A. When buying, look for bright, almost shiny leaves and white, crisp stalks.

Vegetables and starches
Légumes et féculents

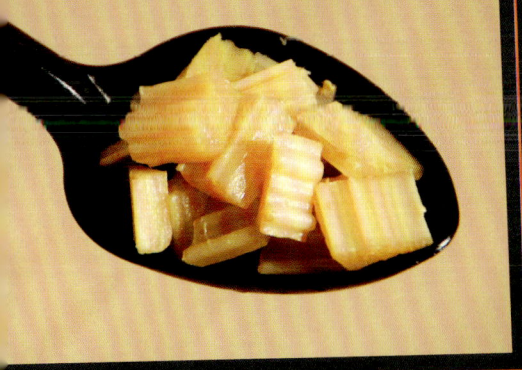

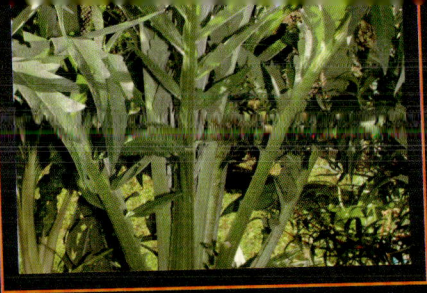

Cardoon bake
Gratin de cardons

Fry the bacon until it is lightly cooked.

Heat the oil in a saucepan. Add the onion and cook until soft and beginning to turn golden.

Add the flour and stir well with a wooden spoon. Cook for about 1 minute. Slowly add the beef stock, a little at a time. Cook on a medium heat, stirring continuously until it thickens slightly and boils. *This makes a fairly thin sauce.*

Drain the cardoons and rinse with water.

Stir the cooked bacon and the cardoons into the sauce.

Pour into a greased ovenproof dish.

Sprinkle with the grated cheese and cook in the oven for about 1½ hours. *The longer the baking time, the better the flavour and texture will be.*

Serve hot.

Serves approx. 6 persons

Oven: 180°C

- 40 ml olive oil
- 1 large onion, chopped
- 30 g plain flour
- 1 beef stock cube, diluted in 600 ml water or 600 ml beef stock
- 100 g bacon, diced
- Jar of bottled cardoons (approx. 700 ml)
- Cheese, grated

Vegetables and starches
Légumes et féculents

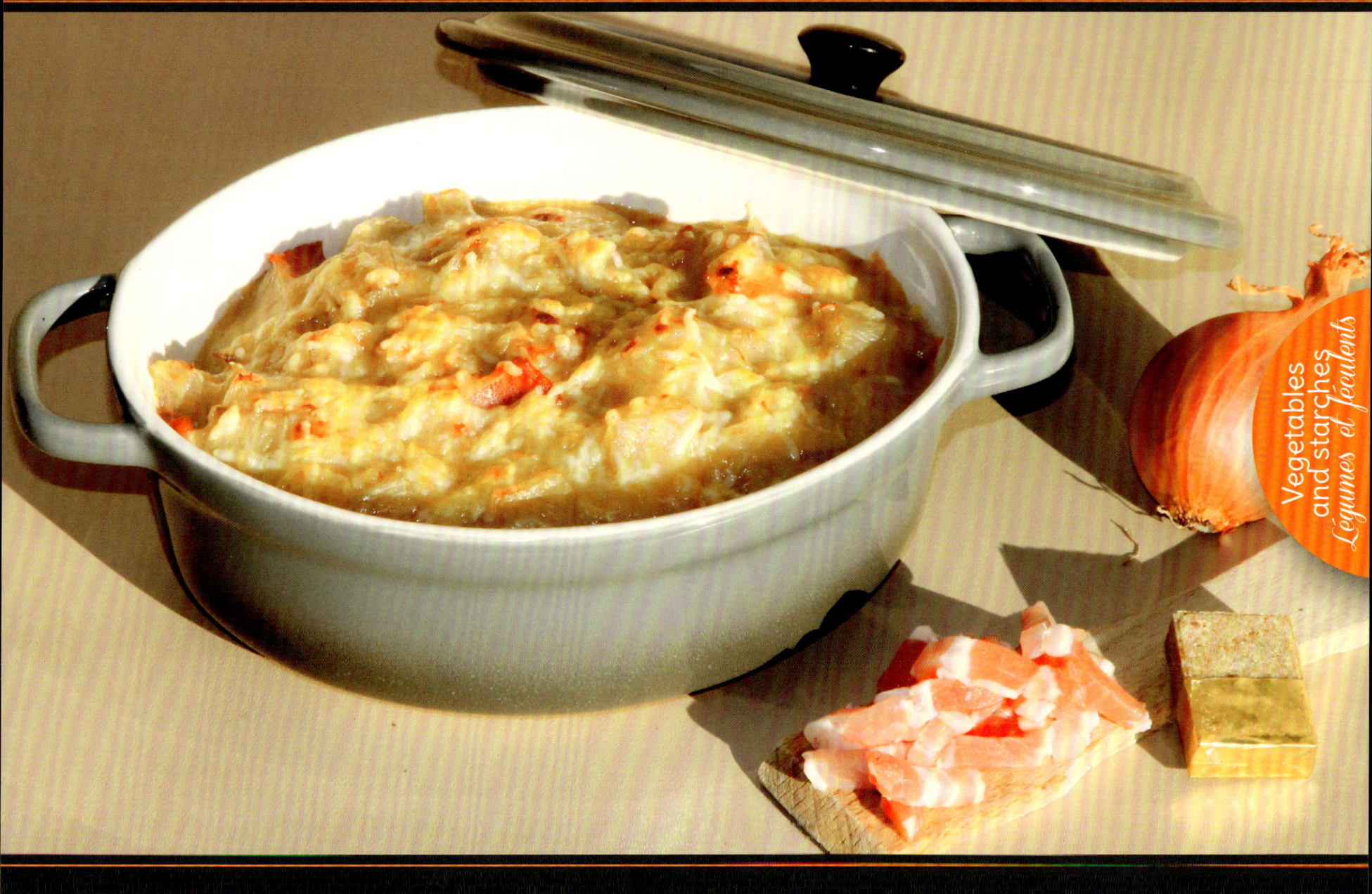

Cardoon is actually an edible thistle and closely related to the artichoke family. It has prickly outer leaves and silvery stalks, which are whitened before harvesting by covering the plants with an opaque cover.
The whiter they are, the better! They are particularly popular in the *Lyon* and *Savoie* region.

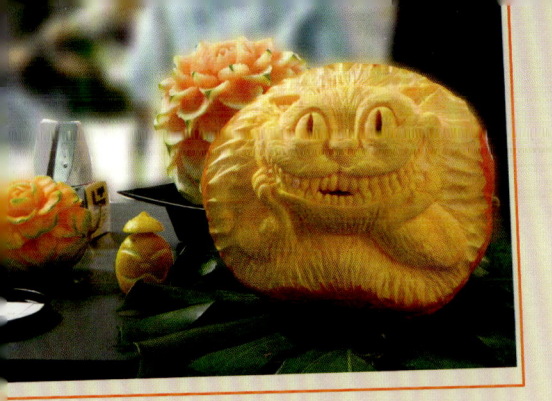

Pumpkin bake
Gratin de potiron

Heat the olive oil in a large saucepan and fry the onion until transparent.

Cut the pumpkin into 3 - 4 cm cubes and place in the saucepan with the onions. *Do not be tempted to add any water.* Cover with the lid and cook gently until the pumpkin is soft. Drain well. *When cooked, pumpkin produces water. It is better to leave it to drain for several hours in a colander for the gratin to have the right consistency.*

MAKE THE *SAUCE BÉCHAMEL*: Melt the butter or heat the oil. Add the flour and stir until smooth. Cook for 2 to 3 minutes, still stirring. Remove from the heat and add the milk a little at a time, whisking until smooth. Place back on a moderate heat and cook until the sauce is thick, stirring continuously. Allow to boil for 1 - 2 minutes, still stirring. Remove from the heat, add the cream, salt, pepper and grated nutmeg. Leave the sauce to cool a little then add the eggs.

Mash the pumpkin with a fork and add to the sauce. Pour into a well-greased ovenproof dish.

Sprinkle with grated cheese.

Place in an unheated oven, then turn the heat on 170°C. Cook for about 40-50 minutes once the oven has reached temperature.

Serves approx. 8 - 10 persons

Oven: 170°C

- 1 large onion, finely chopped
- 3 tablespoons olive oil
- 1 kg pumpkin, peeled

Sauce béchamel:
- 40 g butter or oil
- 50 g plain flour
- 500 ml milk
- 100 ml double cream
- 2 eggs, lightly beaten
- Salt and pepper
- ½ teaspoon grated nutmeg

- Grated cheese for the topping

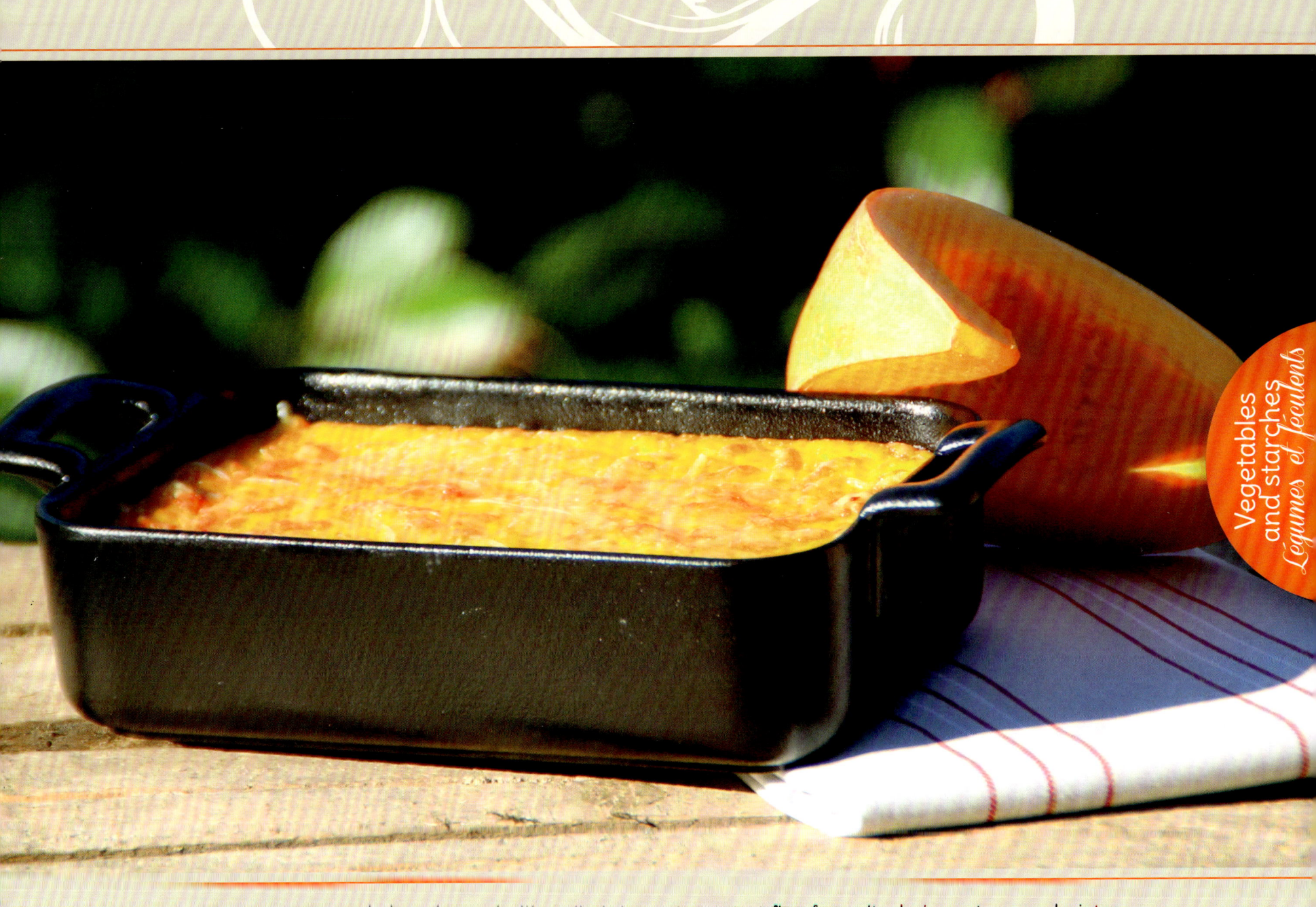

A delicious creamy bake enhanced with melted cheese topping—a firm favourite during autumn and winter.

Certain types of pumpkins are harvested in August, but mostly they are harvested in September and October. If the stalks are left attached and they are kept in a cool, dry place, they can be stored until the end of December. Once cut, remove the seeds and fibres and store in the fridge. Avoid wrapping it in plastic.

Vegetables and starches
Légumes et féculents

199

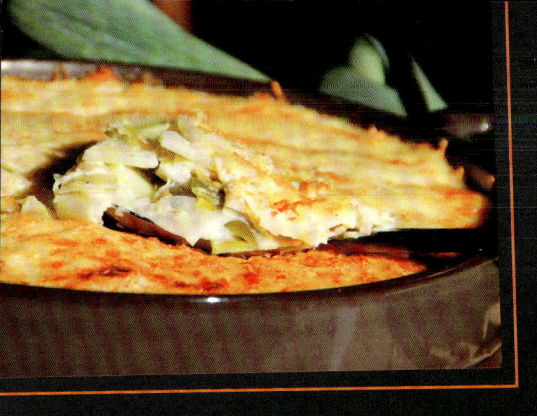

Potato and leek bake

Gratin de pommes de terre aux poireaux

Slice the leeks in half lengthways. *This helps to remove the dirt trapped inside.* Rinse thoroughly and slice.

Heat the oil in a frying pan and gently fry the onion and leeks until soft. Add the garlic and season with salt and pepper.

Finely slice the potatoes. *Do not rinse them after they have been sliced as the starch found in the potatoes helps to thicken the gratin.*

Dissolve the stock cube in the boiling water and stir in the cream.

Layer half the potatoes in a well-greased ovenproof dish (21 x 27 x 5 cm or 27 cm diameter). Pour over some cream mixture. Season with salt and pepper. Cover with the leeks and pour over some more of the cream mixture. Season with salt and pepper. Layer over the rest of the potatoes, pour over the rest of the cream mixture and season with salt, pepper and nutmeg.

Cover with aluminium foil and cook for about 1 hour. Remove the foil and press down the potatoes with a skimming spoon to allow the juices to cover the potatoes. Continue cooking uncovered for at least 30 minutes or until the liquid thickens. *The cooking time will vary according to the thickness of the potatoes.* Sprinkle with cheese and continue cooking until golden.

As a variation, top with raclette *or* reblochon *cheese.*

This bake can be made one or two days in advance omitting the final stage of adding the cheese. Allow to cool and place in the fridge.
For serving, place the cheese on top and cook until the potatoes are warmed through and the cheese melted and golden.

Serves approx. 10 - 12 persons

Oven: 180°C

- 1.2 kg potatoes, peeled*
- 800 g leeks (white part only)
- 4 tablespoons olive oil
- 1 onion, finely chopped
- 2 garlic cloves, crushed
- Salt and pepper
- 380 ml water, boiling
- 1 vegetable stock cube
- 380 ml double cream
- 200 g cheese, grated
- Grated nutmeg

*Choose potatoes that are suitable for baking (such as Agatha in France).

Vegetables and starches
Légumes et féculents

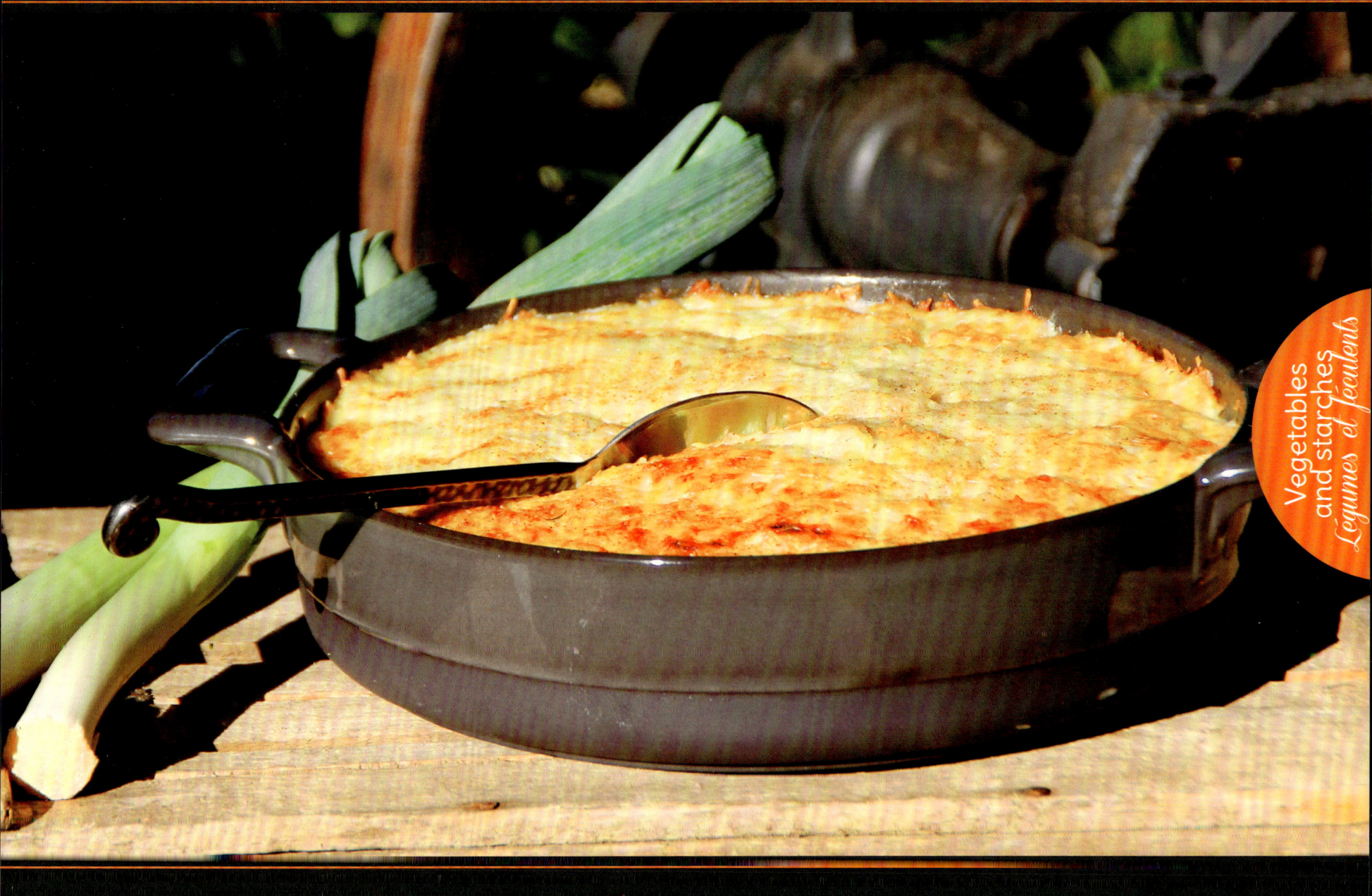

A satisfying, tasty dish which complements any meat or fish.

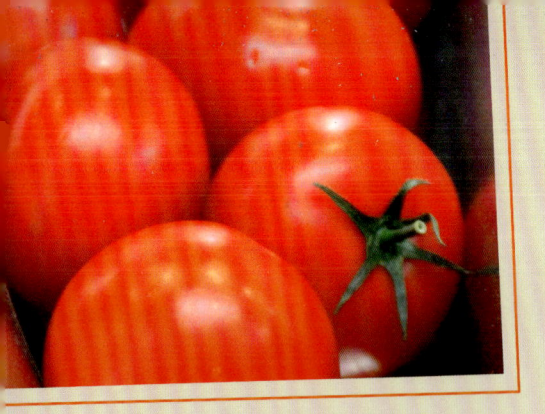

Potato and tomato bake
Gratin de pommes de terre aux tomates

Finely slice the potatoes. *Do not rinse them after they have been sliced as the starch found in the potatoes helps to thicken the gratin.*

Dissolve the stock cube in the boiling water then add it to the cream.

Layer half the potatoes into a well-greased ovenproof dish (21 x 27 x 6 cm or 27 cm diameter).

Sprinkle over the chopped garlic cloves. Season with salt and pepper.

Layer over the rest of the potatoes. Pour over the cream and season with a little more salt and pepper.

Cook for 40 minutes. *Take care during cooking that the potatoes do not turn black. If you notice they are beginning to darken, press them down with a slotted spoon to allow the cream to cover them.*

Arrange the slices of tomatoes on top, season with salt and pepper and sprinkle with *herbes de Provence* and parsley. Cook for a further 40 minutes.

Arrange the *raclette* slices on top and cook for another 15 minutes.

This bake can be made one or two days in advance omitting the final stage of adding the raclette slices. Allow to cool and place in the fridge. For serving, heat until warmed through before adding the raclette and cook for a further 15 minutes.

Serves approx. 10 - 12 persons

Oven: 180°C

- 1 kg potatoes, peeled*
- 700 g tomatoes, sliced
- 2 garlic cloves, crushed
- Salt and pepper
- 250 ml boiling water
- 1 vegetable stock cube
- 250 ml double cream
- 300 g *raclette* cheese
- 2 bunches fresh parsley, chopped
- 1 teaspoon *herbes de Provence*

*Choose potatoes that are suitable for baking (such as Agatha in France).

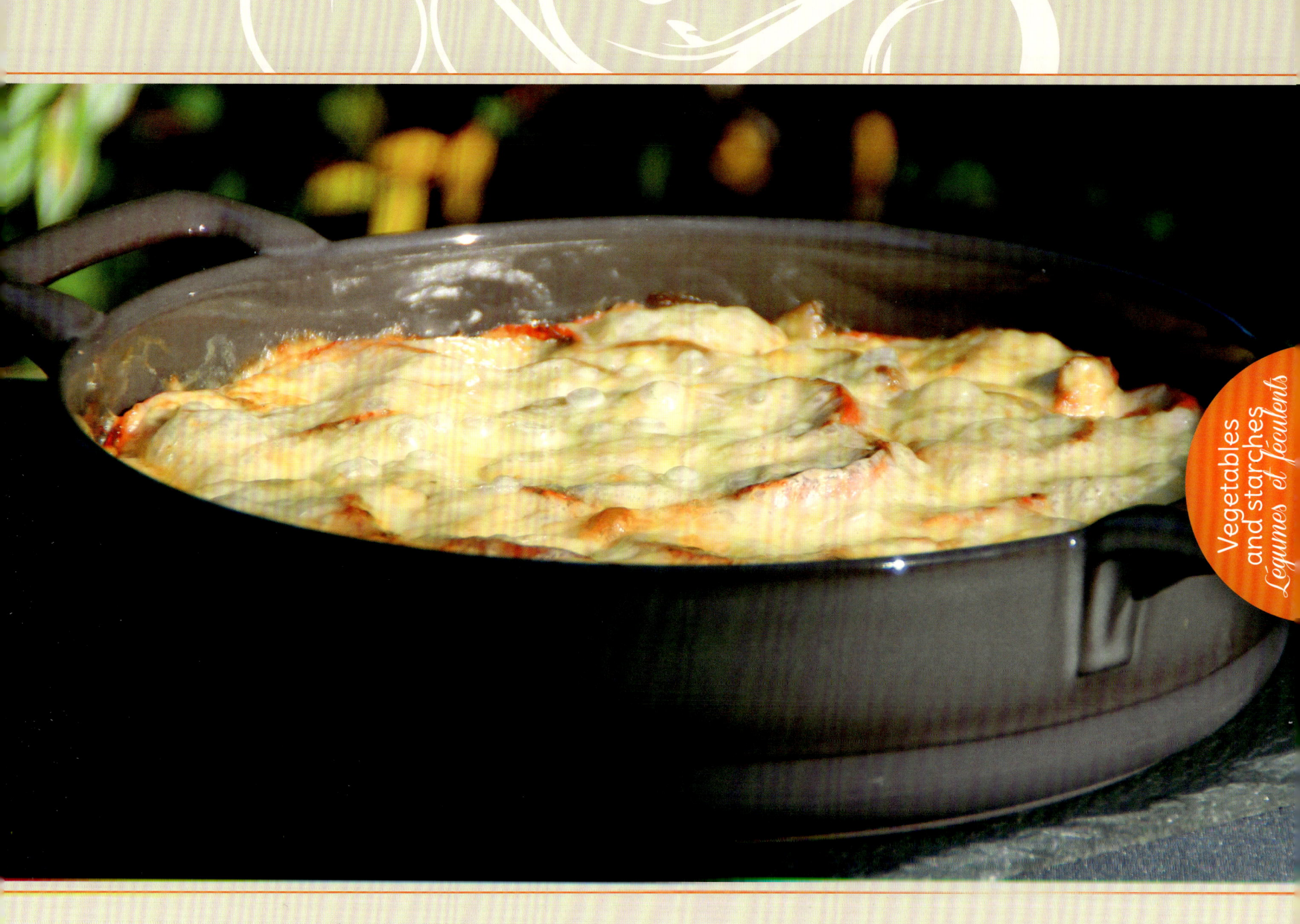

The addition of juicy tomatoes adds a delightful flavour and colour to this tasty, substantial potato dish.

Vegetables and starches
Légumes et féculents

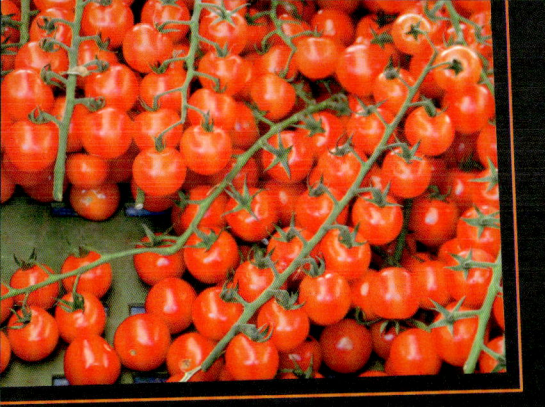

French beans with cherry tomatoes
Haricots verts aux tomates cerises

Cook the beans for about 10 - 15 minutes in salted water until tender. Drain. *The best way to cook beans without losing their colour is to cook them uncovered in plenty of boiling water. As soon as they are cooked, plunge them quickly into iced water. (The thermal shock helps to fix the chlorophyll in the beans.)*

Heat the olive oil in a frying pan. Add the garlic, onion and tomatoes. Cook until the tomatoes and garlic are beginning to soften.

Add the cooked beans and toss them in the tomatoes, onion and garlic.

Season well with salt and pepper.

Serve hot.

Serves 8 – 10 persons

- 800 g French beans
- 40 ml olive oil
- 1 onion, chopped
- 2 garlic cloves, crushed
- 225 g small cherry tomatoes
- Salt and pepper

VARIATION:
French beans with tomatoes
Haricots verts aux tomates

Fry the garlic and onion in the saucepan with the olive oil then add 500 g of ripe tomatoes or 6 tablespoons of tinned, chopped tomatoes. Add the cooked beans and mix together. Roast the cherry tomatoes in the oven (180°C) for about 10 minutes then serve them on top of the beans.

Vegetables and starches
Légumes et féculents

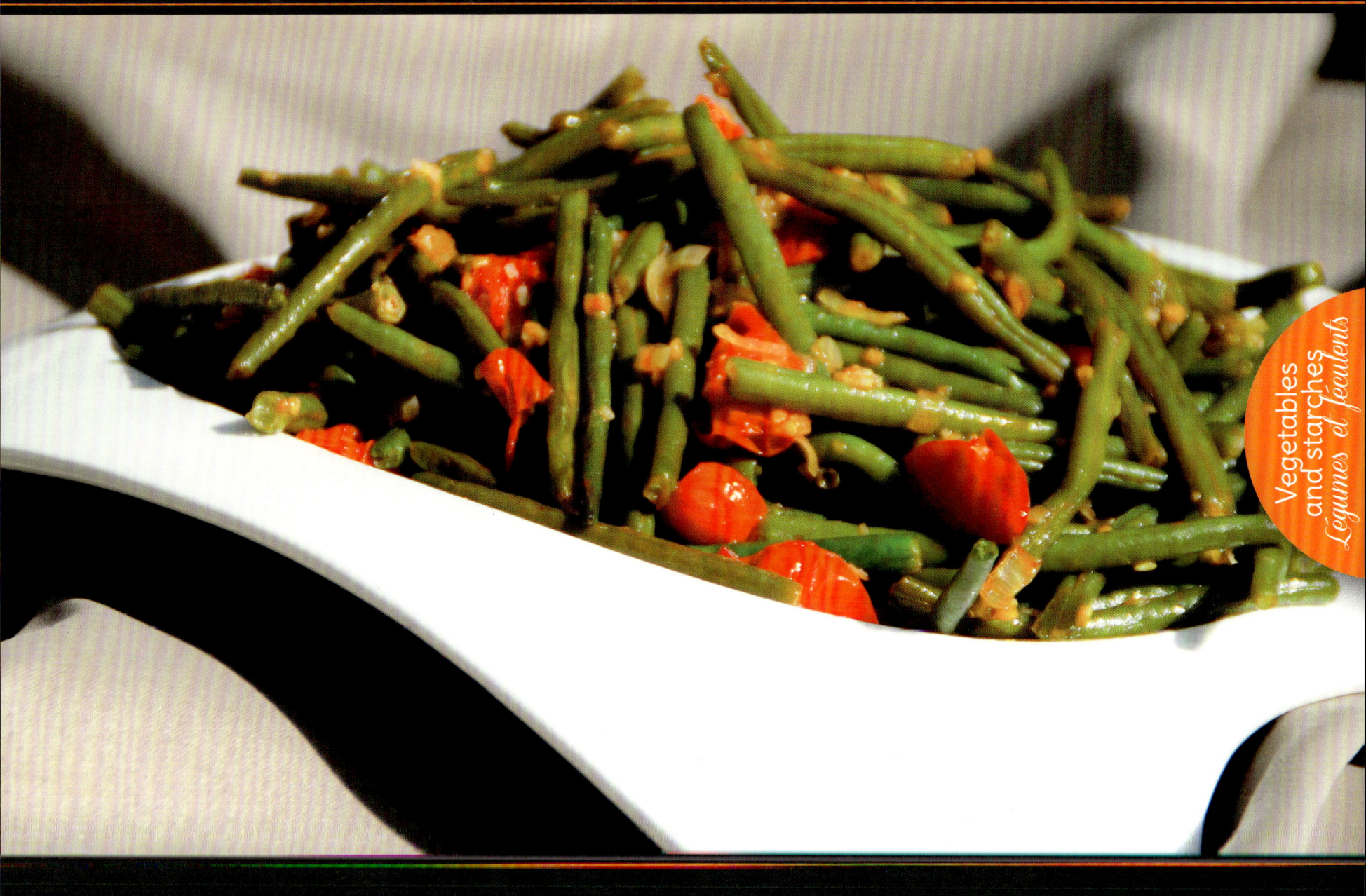

Originating from America, fresh beans have become very popular in France where the thin, green varieties are customary.
Yellow or green beans are full of vitamins, minerals and fibres and are low in calories.
The best time to eat fresh beans in France is from June to October, when they are young and tender.

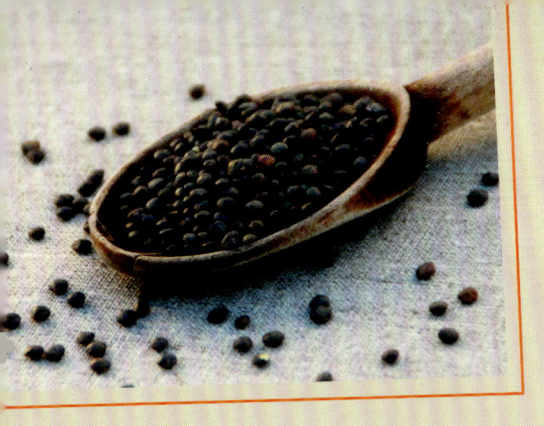

Lentils with sausages
Lentilles aux saucisses

PREPARE THE LENTILS: Place the lentils in a saucepan with 500 ml unsalted water. Cover and bring to the boil. Leave to simmer for about 20 minutes. Drain and reserve the cooking juice.

MAKE THE *SAUCE ROUSSE*: Measure the reserved cooking juice and add a little water, if necessary, to make it up to 400 ml. Heat approximately 3 tablespoons of the cooking juice and add the stock cube. Stir to dissolve. Add to the rest of the cooking juice. Heat the olive oil in a saucepan. Add the shallot and bacon and sauté until golden. Add the flour and mix together on the heat until the mixture becomes dry then gradually add the stock, mixing thoroughly between each addition. Bring to the boil, stirring until the sauce thickens.

Cut each sausage into four pieces. *If using large sausages, they should be pre-cooked.*

Cover the bottom of an ovenproof dish with some of the sauce. Pour the lentils over the sauce. Put the sausages on top of the lentils, and then cover with the remaining sauce. Sprinkle over with breadcrumbs (optional).

Cook for 30 minutes.

Serves approx. 3 persons

Oven: 180°C

- 150 g lentils
- 140 g pork sausages

Sauce Rousse:
- 1/3 stock cube
- 1 tablespoon olive oil
- 1 shallot, chopped finely
- 20 g plain flour
- 75 g chopped bacon
- Breadcrumbs (optional)

Vegetables and starches
Légumes et féculents

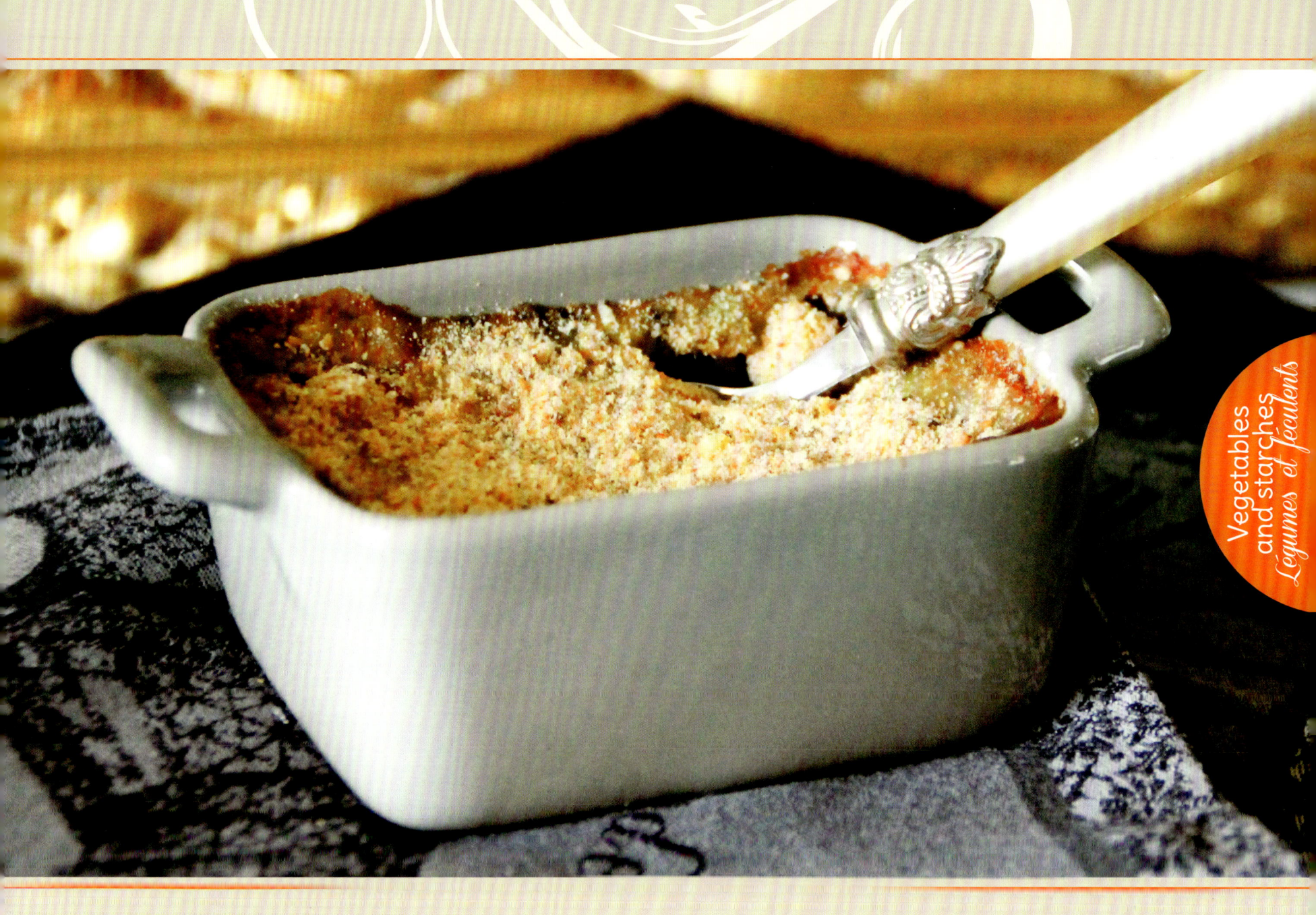

Pulses should be eaten weekly: they are vegetable proteins, with no excess of saturated fat, and a source of fibre and minerals (iron and magnesium in particular)

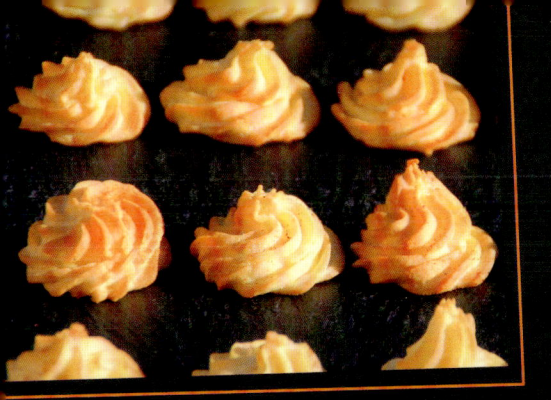

Sautéed potatoes
Pommes de terre sautées

Peel and cut the potatoes into small cubes.

Heat the oil in a large frying pan. Add the potatoes and sauté on a medium heat for about 10 minutes.

Cover and cook for about 5 minutes on a lower heat, stirring from time to time to avoid them burning. *Covering the pan enables the steam to cook the potatoes.*

Add the onion and garlic clove and continue to cook for another 5 minutes. *The cooking time will depend on the type of potatoes used. Vary accordingly.*

Sprinkle with salt and pepper and *herbes de Provence*. Cover and leave to stand for several minutes before serving.

Serve hot.

Serves approx. 4 persons

- 800 g potatoes*
- 50 - 60 ml olive oil
- 1 medium onion, chopped
- 1 garlic clove, finely chopped
- 1 teaspoon *herbes de Provence*
- Salt and pepper

*Choose potatoes that are suitable for steaming.

Duchess potatoes
Pommes duchesses

Boil or steam the potatoes until soft. Drain well.

Mash (using a potato masher or a vegetable mill). Add the butter and mix to make a smooth purée. *The purée should be fairly dry. If it appears too liquid, heat slightly in a saucepan to help dry out.*

Add the egg yolks, one by one, and continue mixing. Season with salt, pepper and grated nutmeg.

Using a piping bag with a star nozzle, pipe small rosettes onto a well greased baking tray. Chill for about 1 hour.

Cook for 30 minutes.

Makes approx. 40 - 50

Oven : 180°C

- 1 kg peeled potatoes*
- 100 g butter, softened
- 4 egg yolks
- Salt and pepper
- Grated nutmeg

*Choose potatoes that are suitable for mashing.

Vegetables and starches
Légumes et féculents

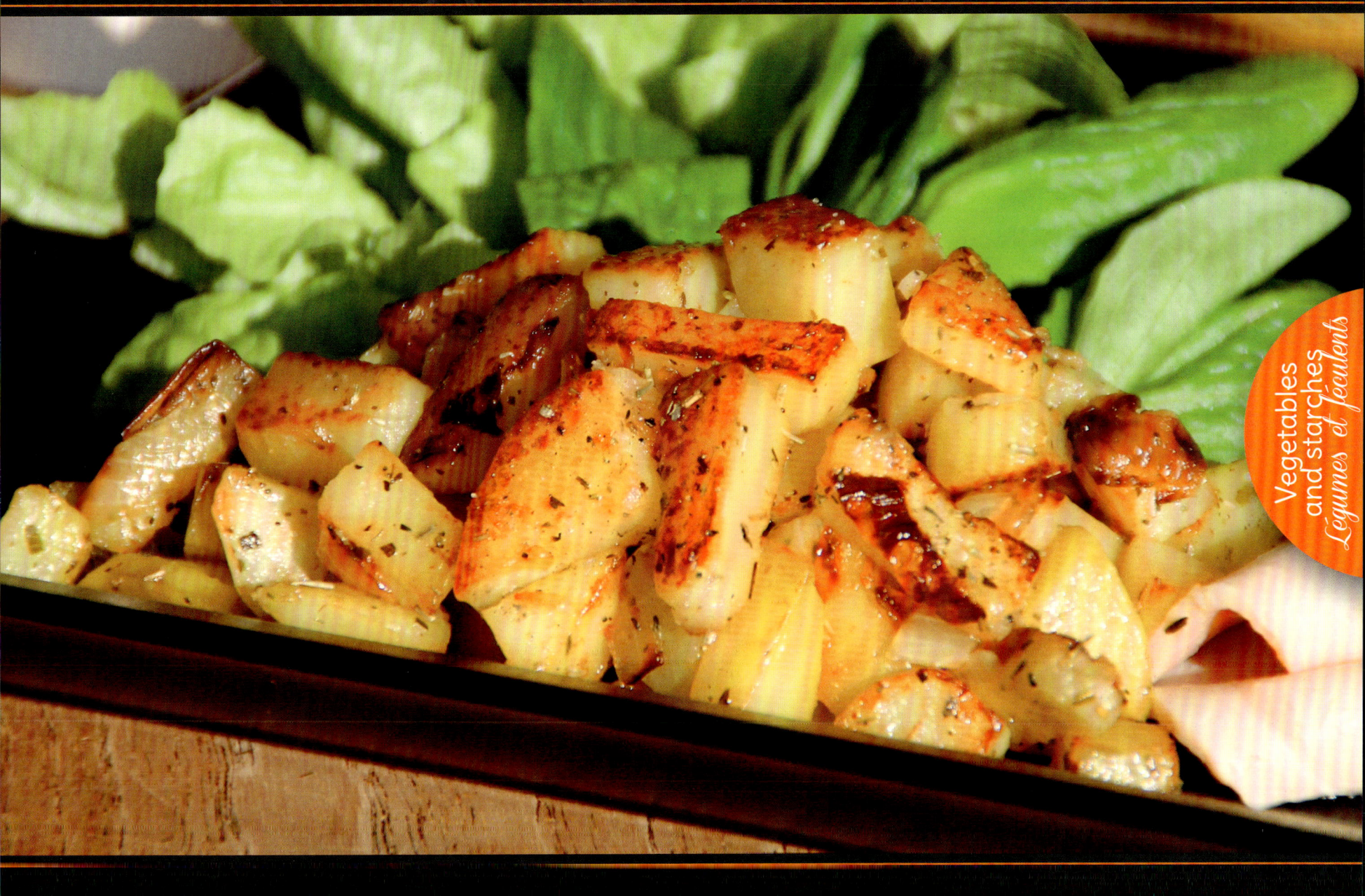

Potatoes contain more starch than any other vegetable and should be regarded in the same category as bread and pastas, although they do contain a variety of vitamins and minerals.
Those with blue, purple, yellow or red flesh contain more antioxidants than the white varieties.

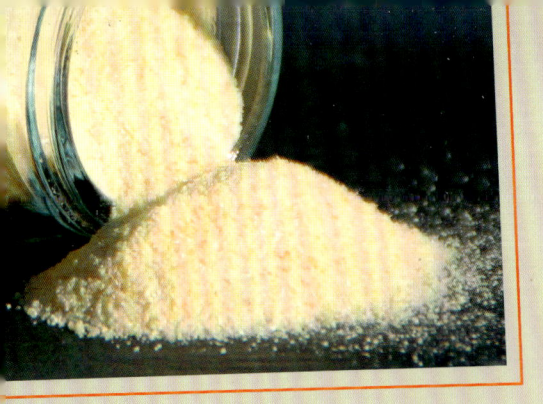

Semolina quenelles
Quenelles à la semoule

PREPARE THE QUENELLES: Place the milk, butter, salt, pepper and nutmeg in a saucepan and bring to the boil.

Mix together the semolina and flour and add to the milk all at once. Stir with a wooden spoon until the mixture comes off the sides of the saucepan. Place back on the heat and cook for about 2 minutes, stirring, to dry the mixture and until it makes a compact ball.

Leave to cool for about 10 minutes and add the eggs, one by one, stirring well between each addition. *Use the 'K' beater if using an electric beater.* Add the grated cheese.

Leave to cool.

Turn onto a floured surface, and with floured hands, roll into a cylinder shape of about 3 cm diameter. *If preferred use a piping bag with a plain 3 cm diameter nozzle.* Cut into lengths of about 10 cm. Shape each *quenelle* by rolling onto the surface and between floured hands.

Bring a large saucepan of salted water to the boil and plunge the *quenelles* (only 5 or 6 at a time) into the water. Cook until they rise to the surface. Carefully remove and place in a bowl of cold water.

Drain well and place them, well-spaced apart, into an ovenproof gratin dish. *Allow plenty of space in between each quenelle for them to rise.*

MAKE THE SAUCE FINANCIÈRE according to the recipe.

Cover the *quenelles* with the *sauce financière*.

Cook in the oven for about 45 minutes to 1 hour. *Cover with foil during cooking if the top begins to burn.*

Makes approx. 12 *quenelles*

Oven: 180°C

- 450 ml milk
- 90 g butter
- Salt and pepper
- A pinch of nutmeg
- 150 g fine semolina
- 100 g plain flour
- 3 eggs
- 150 g grated cheese

- 1 quantity *sauce financière* (see *recettes de base*)

Vegetables and starches
Légumes et féculents

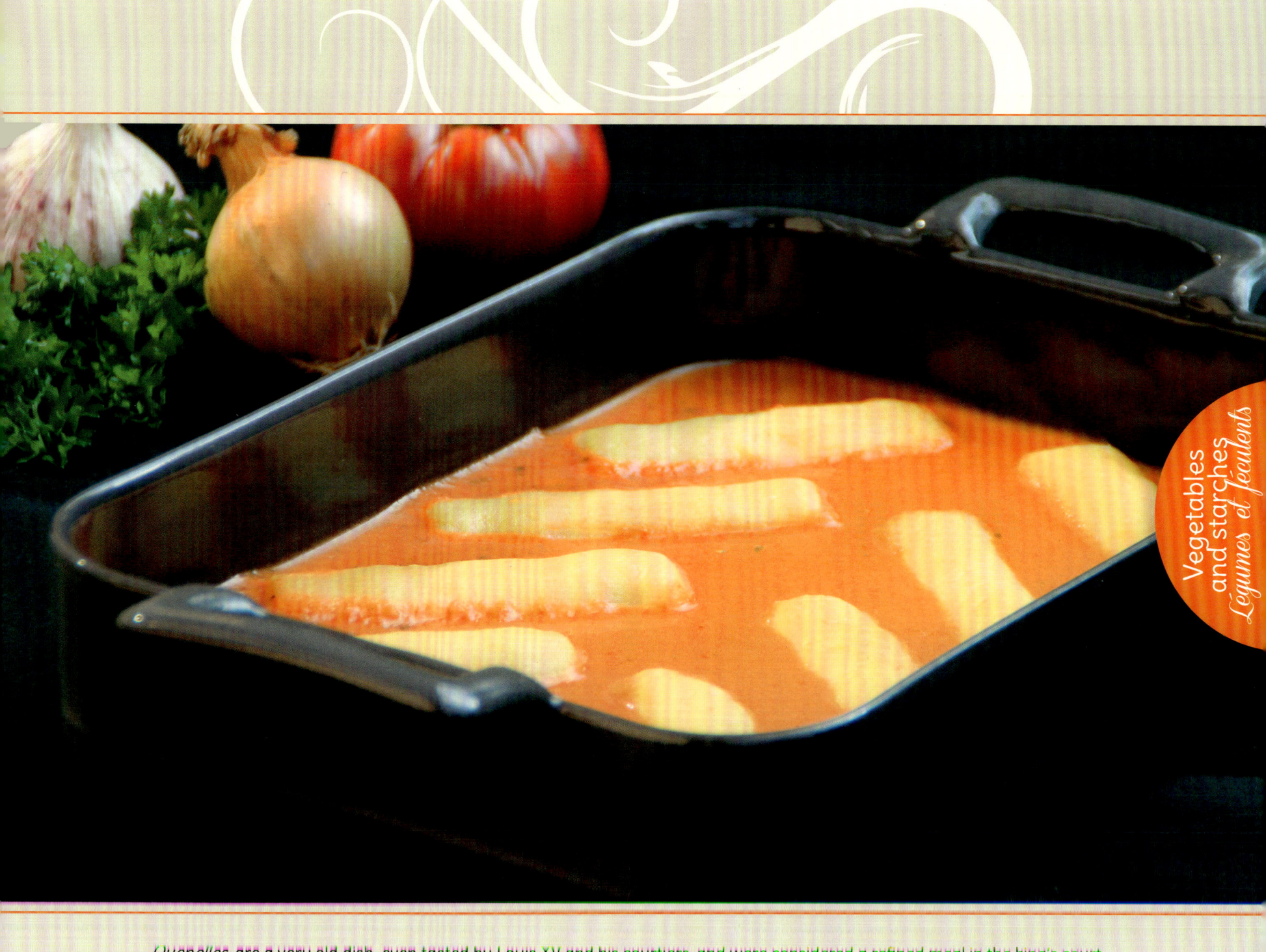

Quenelles are a very old dish, even tasted by Louis XV and his courtiers, and were considered a refined meal in the king's court. Over the years the recipe has altered tremendously. According to some, *quenelles lyonnaises* first appeared in about 1830. During this time the River *Saône* was teeming with pikes and a master cook decided to create a recipe using the flesh of this fish and mixing it with choux pastry. Later the recipe changed, substituting pike for poultry or rabbit. During the Second World War, due to the rationing of fish and meat, *quenelles* were cooked plain with no added meat. Today, *quenelles* are part of Lyon's gastronomic heritage. Manufacturers produce many different flavours: freshwater crayfish, *truffes*, *foie gras*, *morilles* (type of mushroom) etc. and can be bought from delicatessens and other specialists.

211

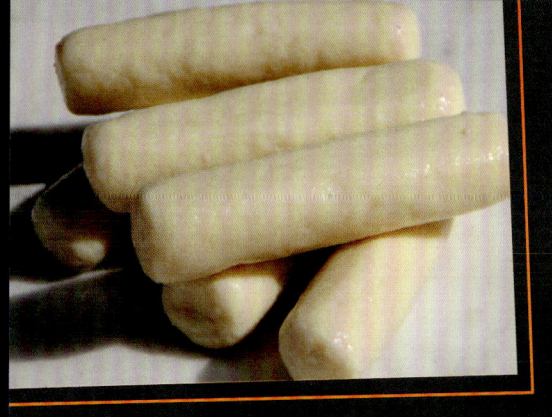

Flour quenelles
Quenelles à la farine

PREPARE THE *QUENELLES*: Place the water, milk, butter and some salt into a saucepan and bring to the boil.

Remove from the heat and add the flour in one addition. Stir vigorously with a wooden spoon. Place back on a low heat and cook for about 5 minutes, stirring, to dry the mixture.

Remove from the heat and add the eggs, one at a time, stirring well between each addition. *Use the 'K' beater if using an electric beater.*

Turn onto a floured surface, and with floured hands, roll into a cylinder shape of about 3 cm diameter. Cut into lengths of about 10 cm. Shape each *quenelle* by rolling on the surface with your hands.

Bring a large saucepan of salted water to the boil and plunge the *quenelles* (only 5 or 6 at a time) into the water. Cook until they rise to the surface. Carefully remove and drain them.

Place the *quenelles* well-spaced apart into an ovenproof gratin dish. *Allow plenty of space in between each quenelle for them to rise.*

MAKE THE *SAUCE FINANCIÈRE* according to the recipe.

Cover the *quenelles* with the *sauce financière*.

Cook for about 45 minutes. *Cover with foil during cooking, if the top begins to burn.*

Makes approx. 12 *quenelles*

Oven: 180°C

- 200 ml water
- 200 ml milk
- 60 g butter
- 260 g plain flour
- 4 eggs
- Salt

- 1 quantity *sauce financière* (see *recettes de base*)

Vegetables and starches
Légumes et féculents

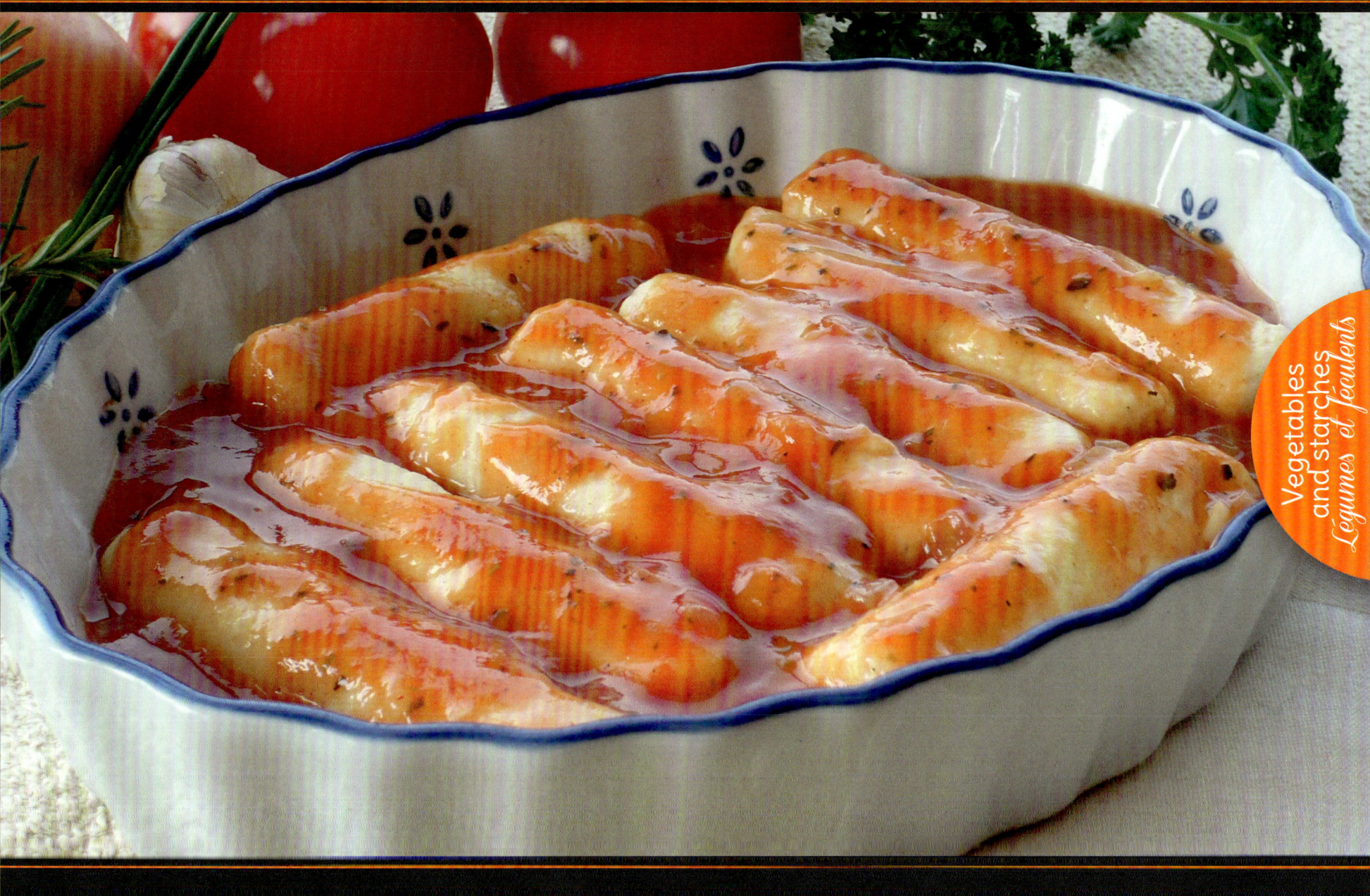

A great Lyon speciality, the *quenelle* is a beige, smooth roll with a slightly rough apperance and rounded ends, composed of semolina or flour, butter, milk (or water) and seasonings. More traditionally, it can be made with pike, veal or poultry. Prepared in several ways, simply fried in butter or sliced in rounds and used to stuff *vol-au-vents* with chicken livers, *quenelles* are best placed in a dish and cooked in the oven where they inflate up to triple in volume, and topped with a sauce (tomato, béchamel, etc.) and sprinkled with cheese. It is an ideal dish to serve as a main meal or as an accompaniment.

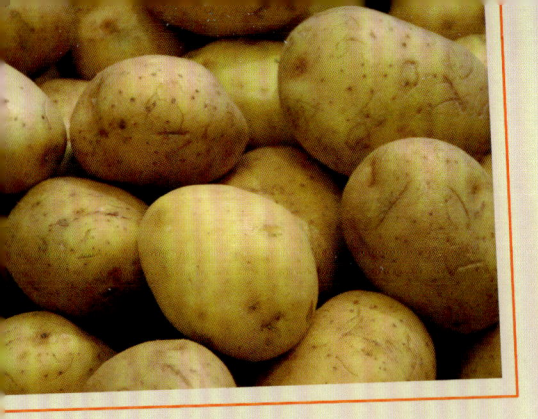

Grated potato cakes
Râpée de pommes de terre

Peel and finely grate the potatoes.

Add the eggs, salt, pepper, garlic and chives. Mix together well.

Heat the oil in a large frying pan. Once it is really hot, pour in the potato mixture. Cover and cook on a medium heat. Once the base begins to golden, carefully turn the *râpée* over, adding a little more oil if necessary.

Turn it regularly during cooking to prevent it from burning. The total cooking time should be about 20 minutes. *It should be soft in the middle and crispy on the edges.*

Serve warm with a fresh green salad.

Serves 4 persons

- 1 kg potatoes*
- 2 eggs, beaten
- Salt and pepper
- Pinch garlic powder
- 2 teaspoons chopped chives
- 4 tablespoons oil

*Choose a type of potato that is suitable for mashing.

For a variation, divide the mixture into 4 and make individual *rapées*. Fry them separately in a small frying pan. These are even nicer and crispier!

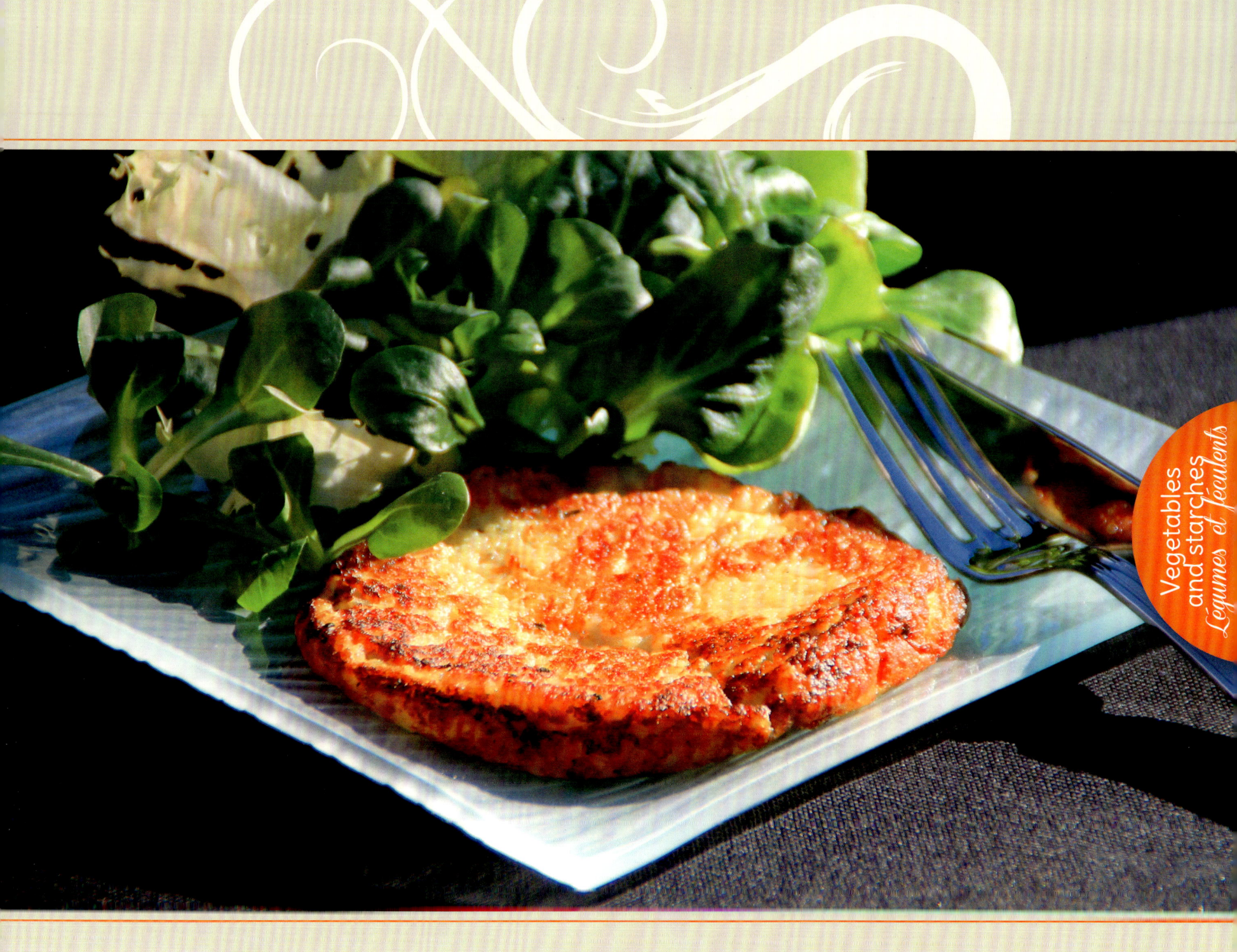

Râpée de pommes de terre are often known as *râpée stéphanoise* as they originate from St Etienne. Principally a mixture of potatoes with beaten eggs, it is similar to the *Ardèche* (or Lyon) *crique*. Authentic recipes have originated from peasants who used their own farm produce to provide cheap and hearty dishes.

Vegetables and starches
Légumes et féculents

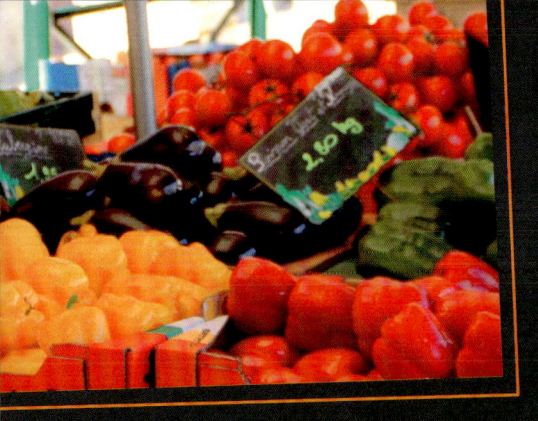

Ratatouille
Ratatouille

Peel the tomatoes. *Make a cross on the bottom of each one, plunge into boiling water for about 10 seconds (or a little longer if the tomatoes are not very ripe). Remove and peel.*

Cut the peeled tomatoes into quarters. Slice the aubergines, onions and courgettes. Remove the seeds from the peppers and discard. Slice into strips.

Heat 3 tablespoons of olive oil in a large saucepan and lightly fry the onions and peppers until they are soft. Add the tomatoes, garlic, *herbes de Provence* and the bay leaf.

Season with salt and pepper, and leave to simmer uncovered for 45 minutes. *Do not cover as the water from the tomatoes needs to evaporate.* Remove the bay leaf.

Meanwhile heat some oil in a frying pan and fry the aubergines and courgettes separately for about 15 minutes. *Use approximately 5 tablespoons of olive oil to fry the aubergines, adding more if necessary, and only 2 tablespoons of olive oil to fry the courgettes.*

Once they are cooked, add to the tomato mixture and continue cooking on a low heat for about 10 minutes.

Season with more salt and pepper if necessary.

Vegetables and starches
Légumes et féculents

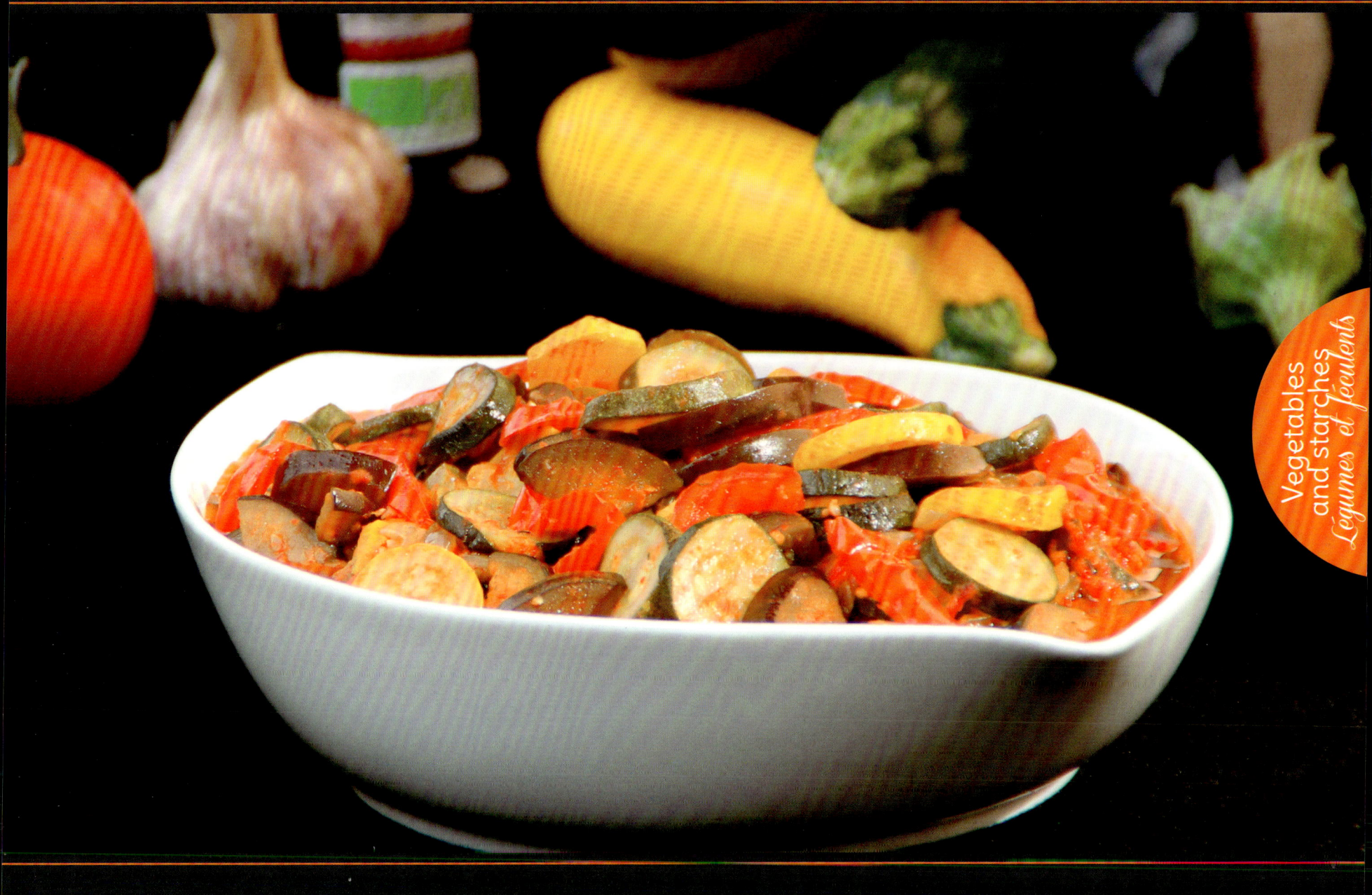

This is a delicious dish to prepare in the height of summer, when vegetables ripen to their peak and are found in abundance in the garden or at the market.
The flavour improves if it is made the day before.

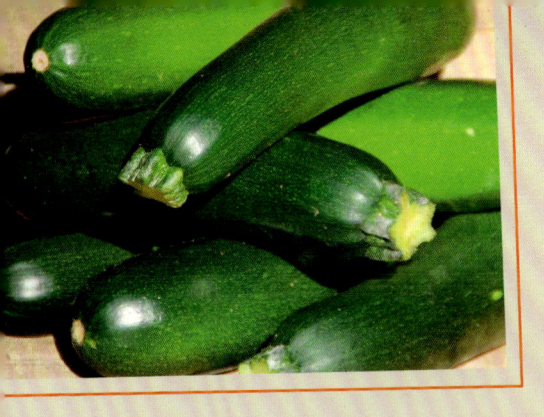

Courgette soufflé
Soufflé à la courgette

Cook the courgettes for 8 minutes in boiling water or until they are soft. Drain and liquidise with the milk until it becomes a smooth purée.

Melt the butter in a heavy-based saucepan and add the flour. Mix thoroughly. Cook on a low heat for two minutes, stirring continuously. Do not allow it to brown. Remove from the heat and add the courgette purée. Mix together until smooth. Return to the heat and bring to the boil. Leave to simmer for 3 minutes, stirring. Remove from the heat and pour into a mixing bowl with the cheese. Season with the salt and pepper. Leave to cool.

Add the egg yolks one by one and mix thoroughly.

Brush the inside of a 1.5 litre soufflé dish with the melted butter, and then sprinkle with the breadcrumbs (or the flour). Turn and shake the dish to coat the surface evenly.

Whisk the egg whites with a pinch of salt until stiff. Carefully fold a quarter of the whisked egg whites into the courgette mixture. Carefully fold in the rest. Pour into the prepared dish filling it about 2/3 full. Chill for about 2 hours.

Cook for about 45 minutes. The soufflé must be well risen, but still soft to touch. Insert a metal skewer into the soufflé—it should come out dry or slightly damp.

Serve immediately.

VARIATION :
Broccoli soufflé
Soufflé au brocoli

Replace the courgettes with the same quantity of broccoli. Boil the broccoli florets for 10 minutes or until soft.

The courgette or broccoli mixture can be made a day in advance and left in the fridge.

Serves 4 persons

Oven: 180°C

- 15 g melted butter
- 1½ tablespoons breadcrumbs (or plain flour)
- 350 g courgettes, grated *(zucchini)*
- 120 ml milk
- 30 g butter
- 40 g plain flour
- 75 g cheese, grated
- 4 eggs, separated
- Salt and pepper

Vegetables and starches
Légumes et féculents

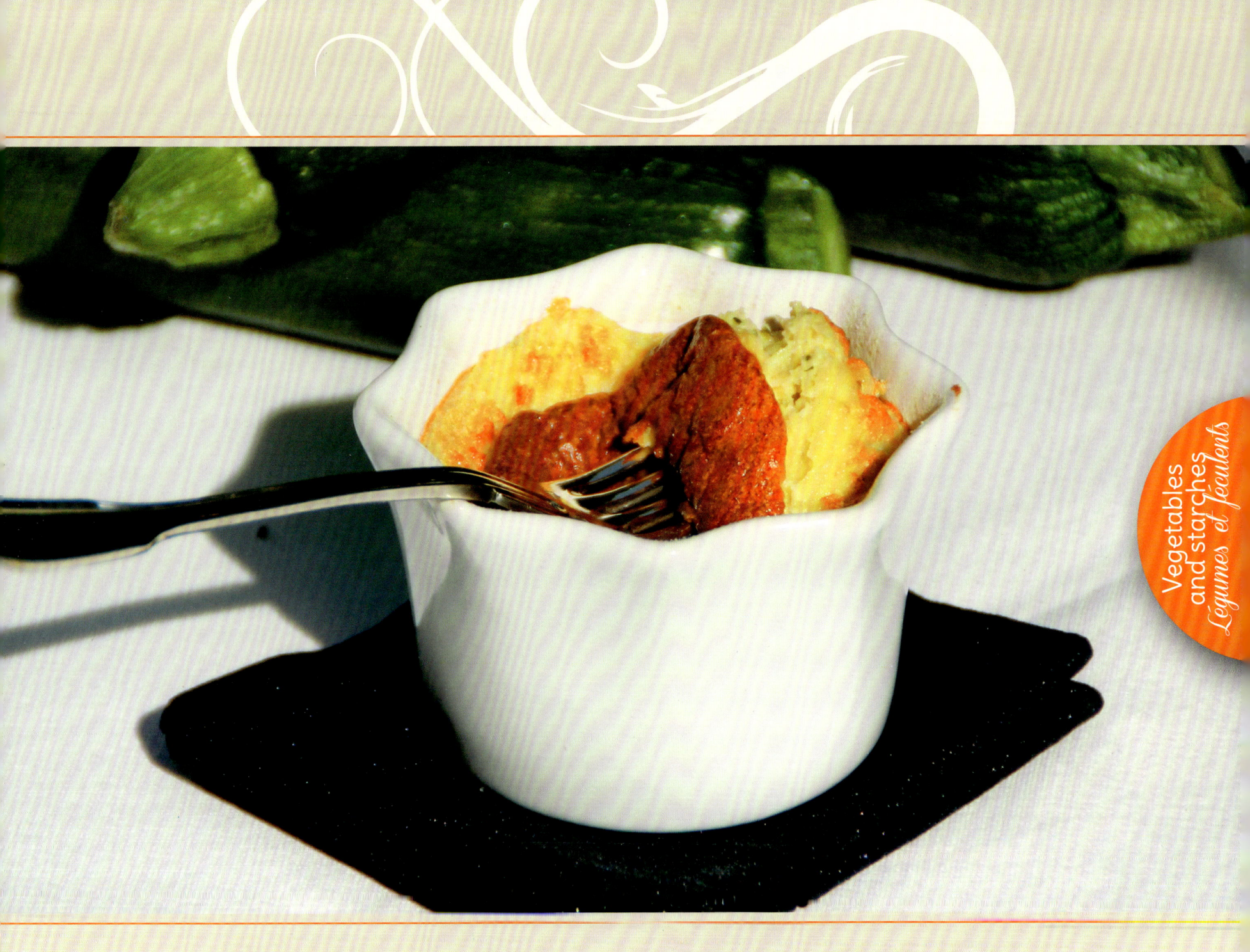

One of the secrets of a successful soufflé is to ensure the egg whites are beaten until really stiff. Another is to serve the dish immediately: "Soufflés don't wait for the visitors—visitors must wait for the soufflés!"

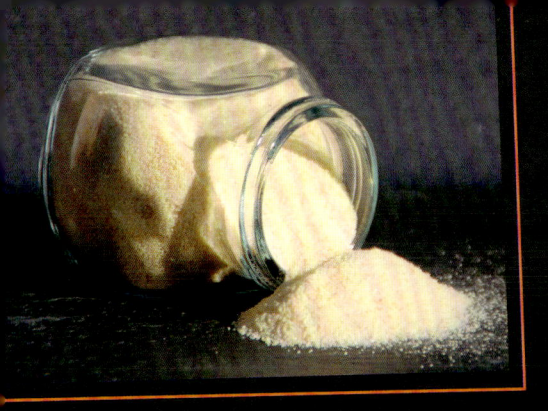

Semolina soufflé
Soufflé de semoule

Bring the milk to the boil with the salt, pepper and nutmeg.

Pour in the semolina. Cook over a low heat, stirring, for about 10 minutes, or until the mixture no longer sticks to the side of the saucepan.

Take off the heat and mix in the butter, cream, eggs and cheese.

MAKE THE *SAUCE TOMATE* according to the recipe and pour into an ovenproof dish. Pour over the semolina mixture, cover with the rest of the *sauce tomate* and sprinkle with some cheese.

Cook for about 1 hour.

Serves approx. 6 persons

Oven: 180°C

- 750 ml milk
- Salt and pepper
- Nutmeg
- 150 g fine semolina
- 60 g butter
- 2 eggs
- 100 g cheese, grated
- 250 ml double cream
- Grated cheese for topping

- 1 quantity of *sauce tomate* (see *recettes de base*)

Vegetables and starches
Légumes et féculents

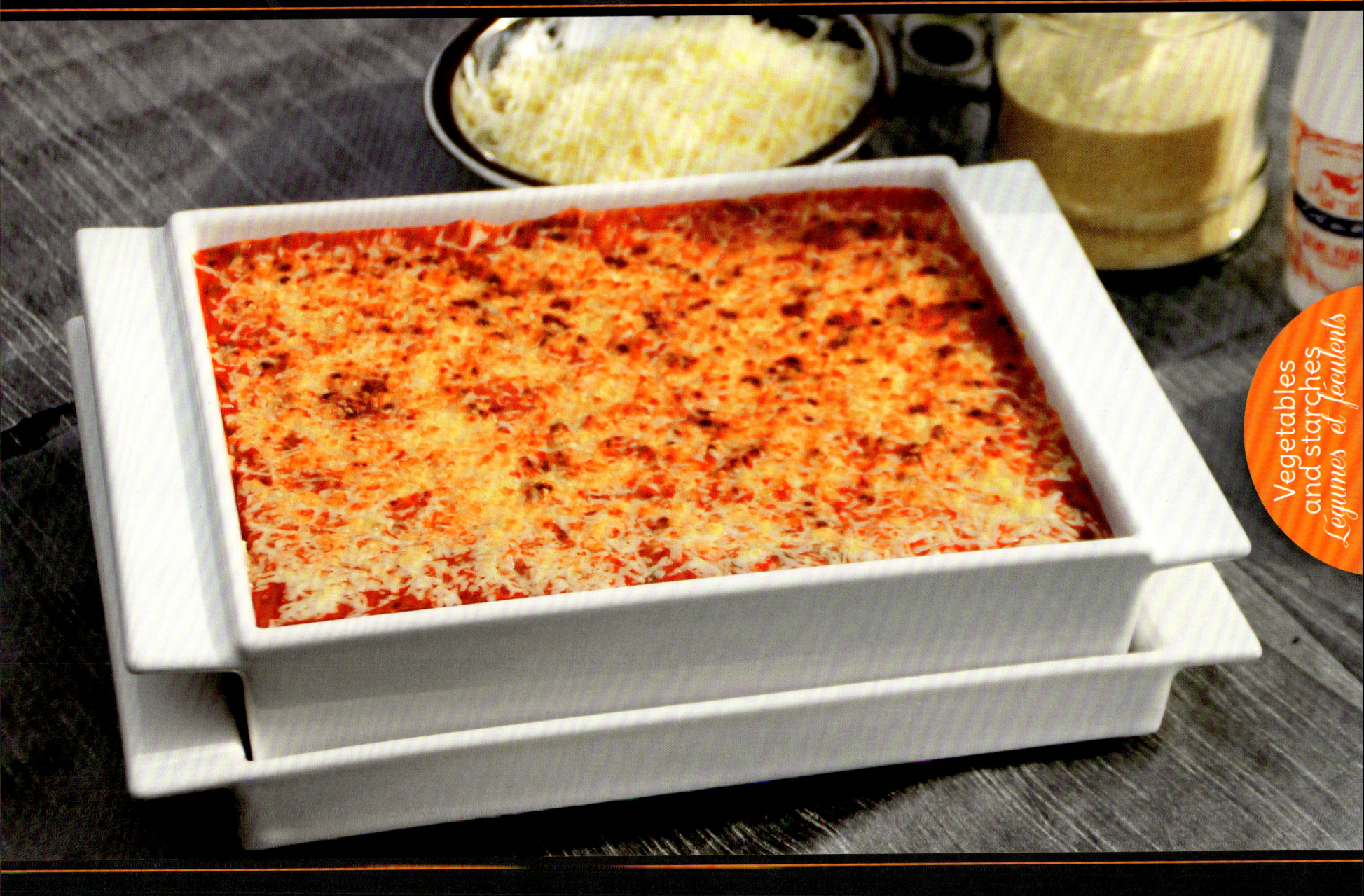

A very economical and tasty dish, which is simple to prepare and an excellent standby.

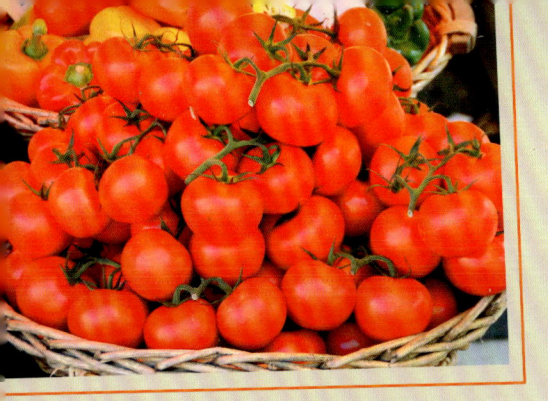

Provençale-style tomatoes
Tomates à la provençale

Wash the tomatoes and cut in half. Place cut sides up in an ovenproof dish. Season with salt and pepper.

Blend the bread or breadcrumbs with the garlic clove and parsley. Sprinkle over each tomato. Drizzle with olive oil and sprinkle with *herbes de Provence* (optional).

Place in the oven. Cook for about 50 minutes. *They are much tastier overcooked than undercooked!*

Serve warm.

Serves 8 persons

Oven: 200°C

- 8 medium tomatoes
- 1 - 2 garlic cloves
- 40 - 50 g dry bread, or breadcrumbs
- 2 tablespoons fresh parsley, chopped
- Olive oil
- Coarse grain salt and pepper
- *Herbes de Provence* (optional)

Vegetables and starches
Légumes et féculents

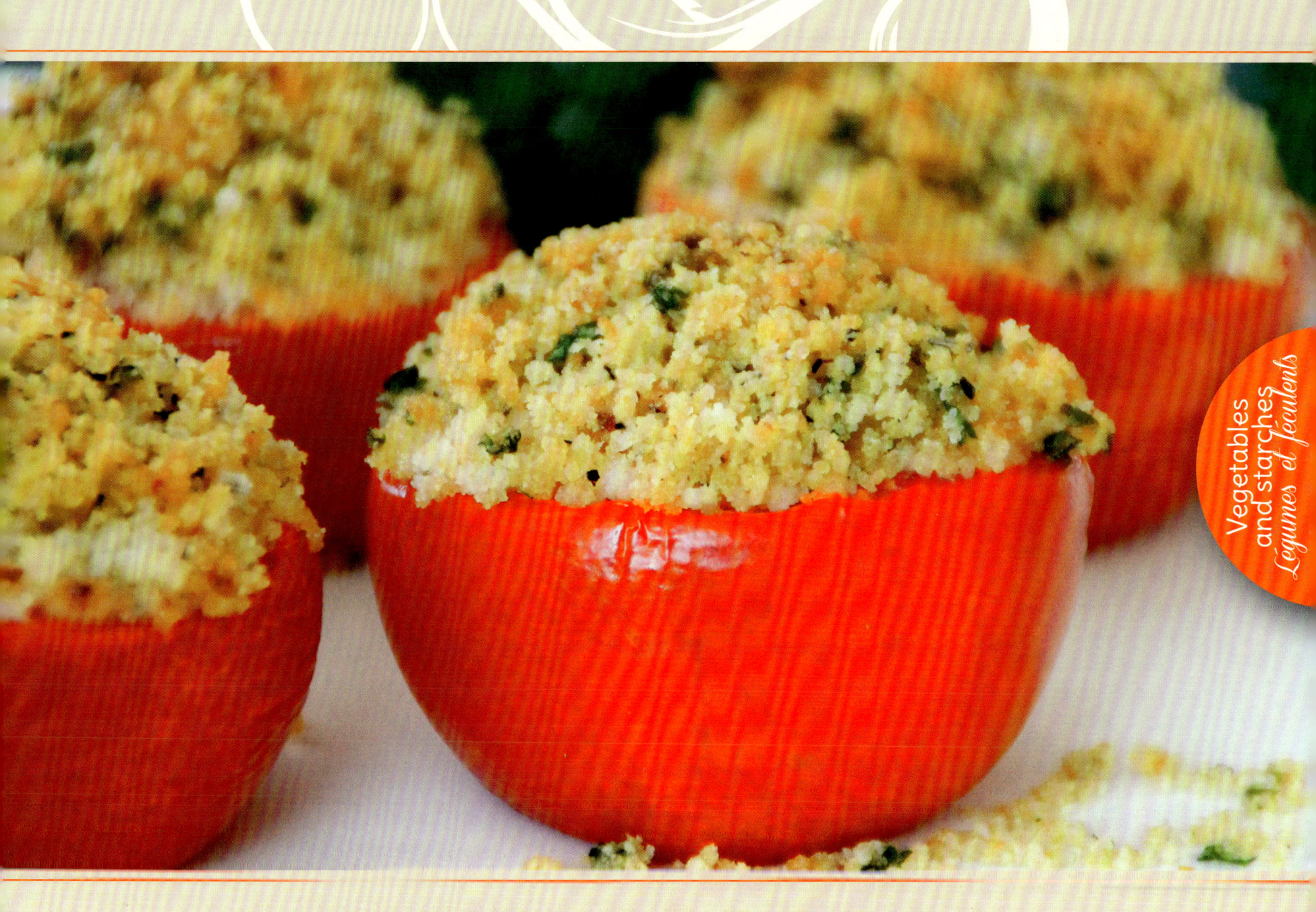

A delicious, yet simple and light accompaniment to grilled meats or fish dishes.
Les tomates à la provençale are a great classic in the South of France and are best prepared in summer to enjoy the incomparable flavour of sun-ripened tomatoes.

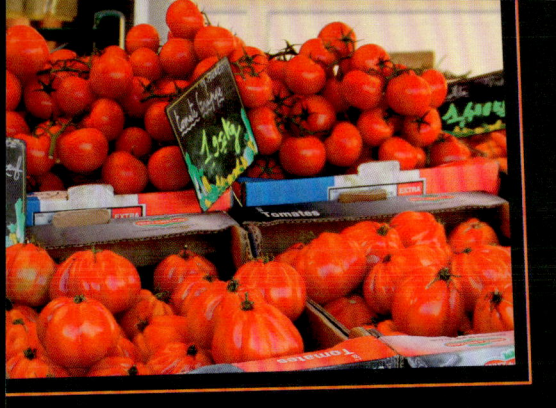

Stuffed tomatoes
Tomates farcies

Cut the tops off the tomatoes, reserve. Scoop out the pulp with the seeds, reserving enough flesh to hold the tomatoes together. Reserve the pulp and seeds of 6 tomatoes and cut into small pieces. *More pulp may be used, depending on the size of the tomatoes: alter the quantity as desired.*

Heat the oil in a frying pan and cook the onion until soft.

Add the garlic and continue cooking for a few minutes.

Add the minced meat with the parsley, tomato flesh, and salt and pepper and cook for about 10-15 minutes, or until the liquid has evaporated, stirring from time to time.

Put the milk and the breadcrumbs into a saucepan. Heat gently until the milk is absorbed.

Add the soaked breadcrumbs to the meat mixture with the egg and grated cheese.

Fill the tomatoes with the mixture and place the tops back on.

Cook for about 50 - 60 minutes.

Serve warm.

Oven: 170°C

- 8-10 large ripe tomatoes
- 400 g minced meat (a mixture of beef, veal and sausagemeat)
- 1 onion
- 3 tablespoons olive oil
- 1-2 garlic cloves, chopped finely
- 40 g breadcrumbs
- 60 ml milk
- 1 egg
- 1 tablespoon fresh parsley
- Salt and pepper
- 50 g grated cheese

For a variation, use the filling to stuff courgettes or marrows.

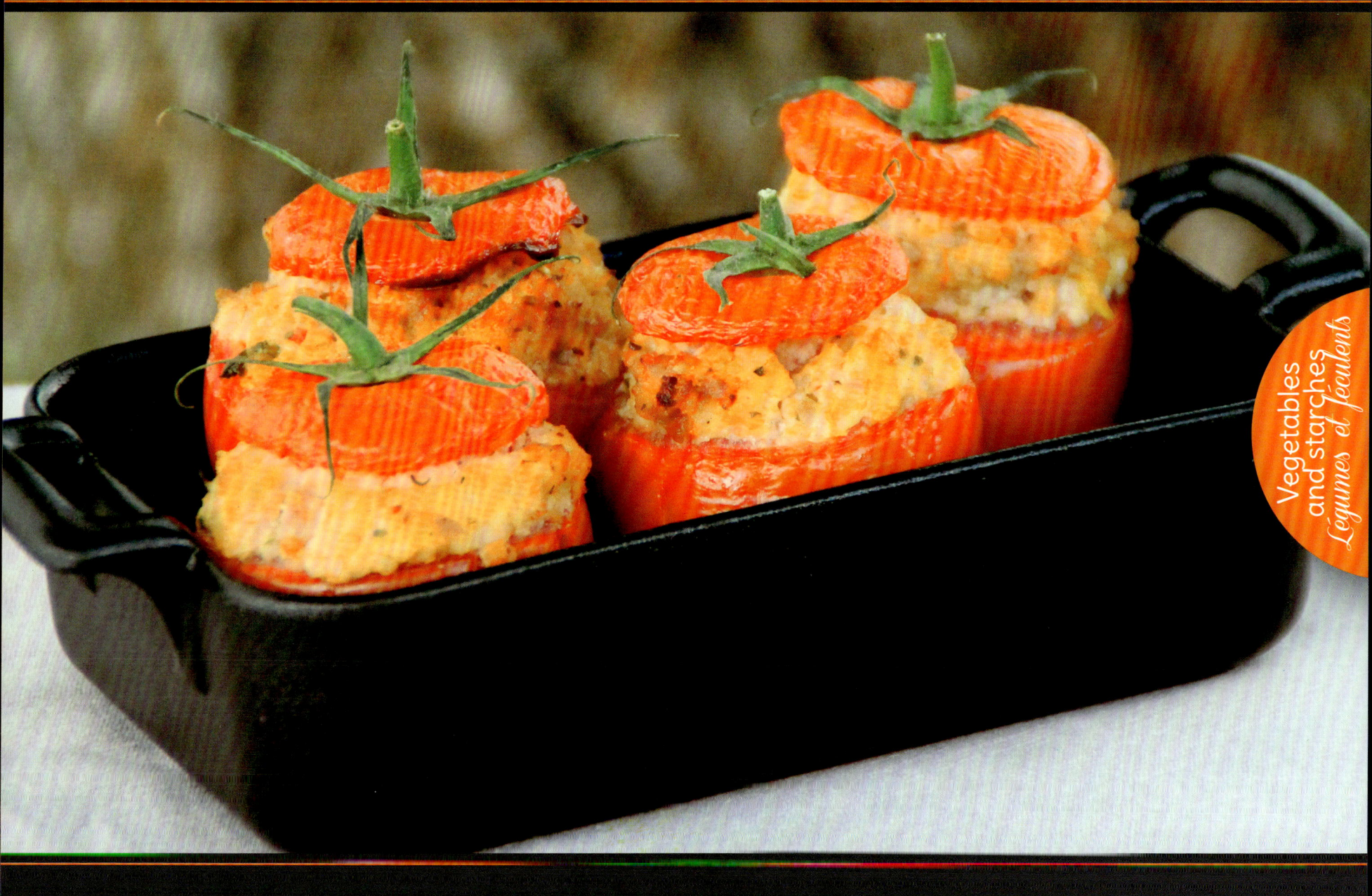

A delicious way of using an over-abundance of homegrown vegetables.
This can be made using cooked or uncooked meat and is an excellent way of using up leftover, cooked meat without having that reheated taste!

Vegetables and starches
Légumes et féculents

Cheese favourites
Autour du fromage

230 *Savoie*-style fondue
Fondue savoyarde

232 Tips for a successful cheese fondue
Astuces pour une bonne fondue

234 *Savoie*-style potatoes
Pommes de terre savoyardes

236 The origin of *raclette*
L'origine de la raclette

238 *Savoie*-style *raclette*
Raclette savoyarde

240 *Tartiflette*
Tartiflette

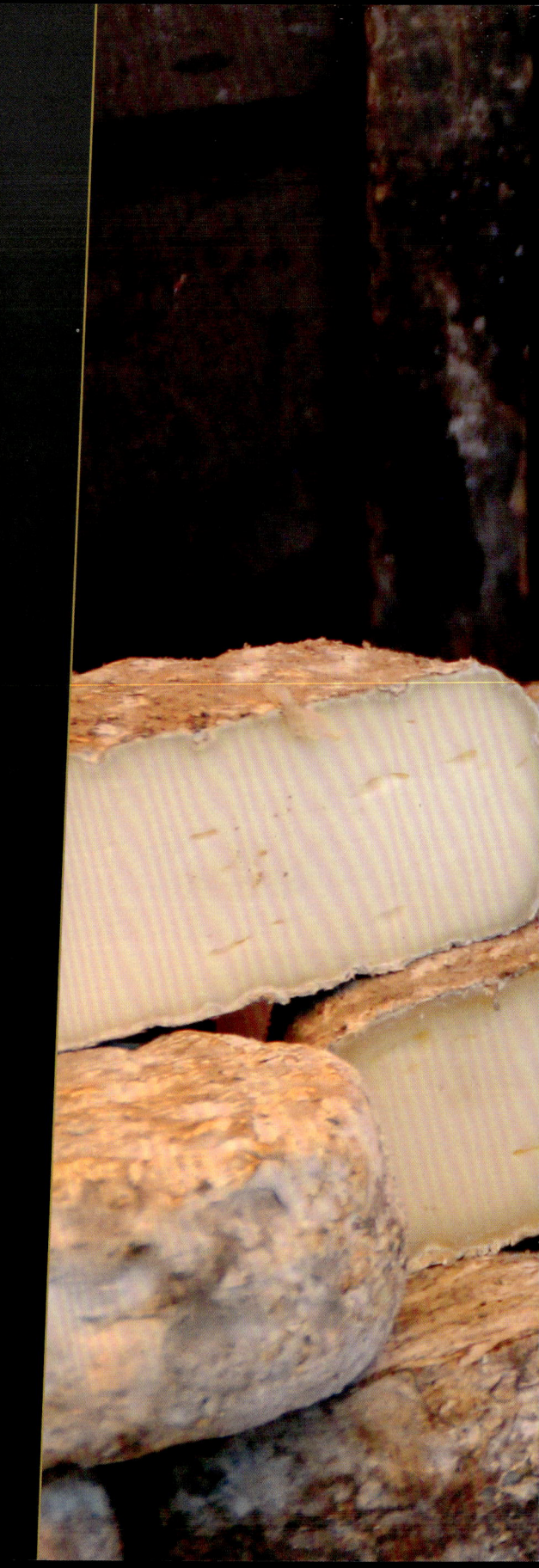

Warning !
Some recipes contain alcohol.

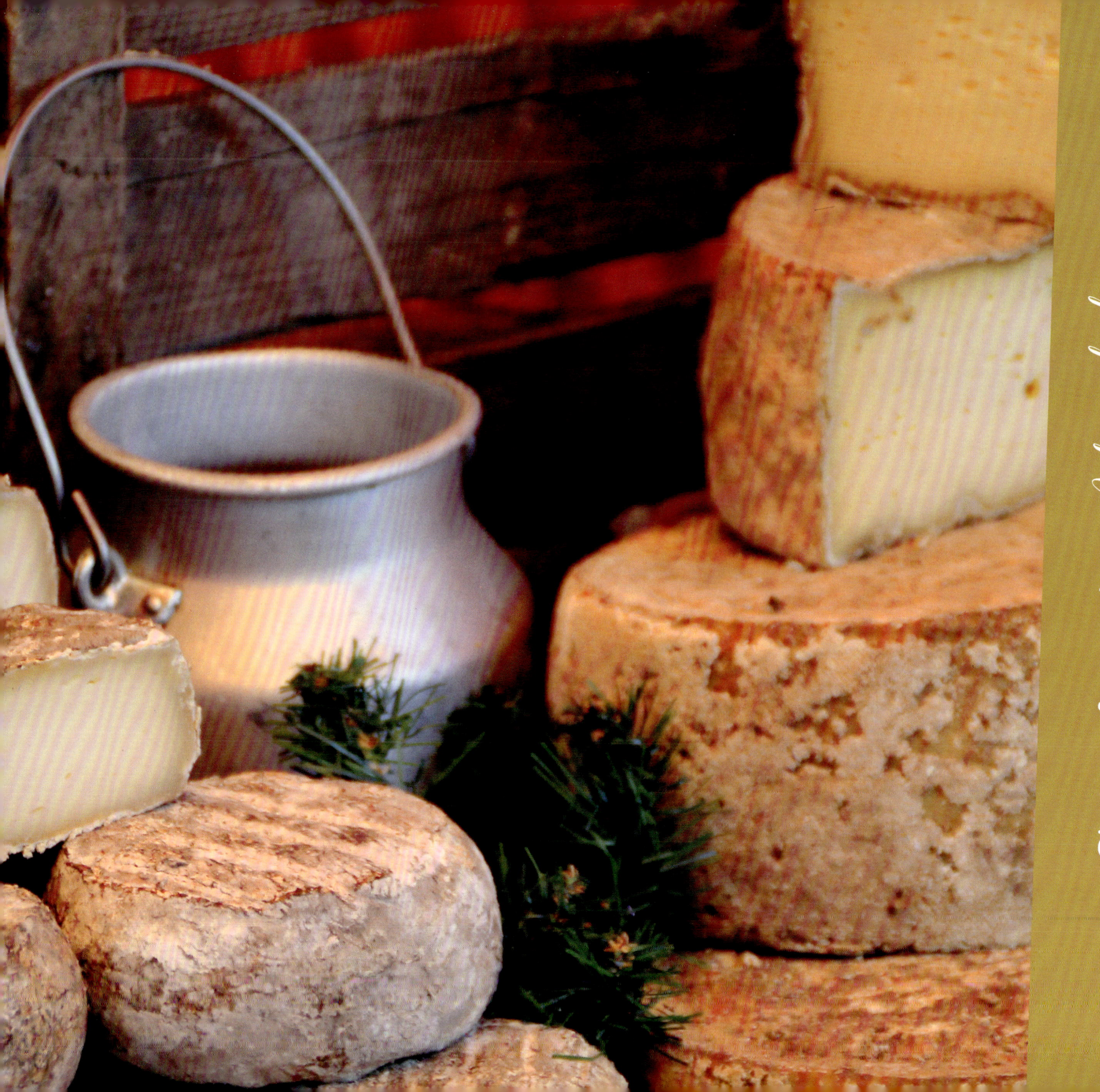

Cheese favourites *Autour du fromage*

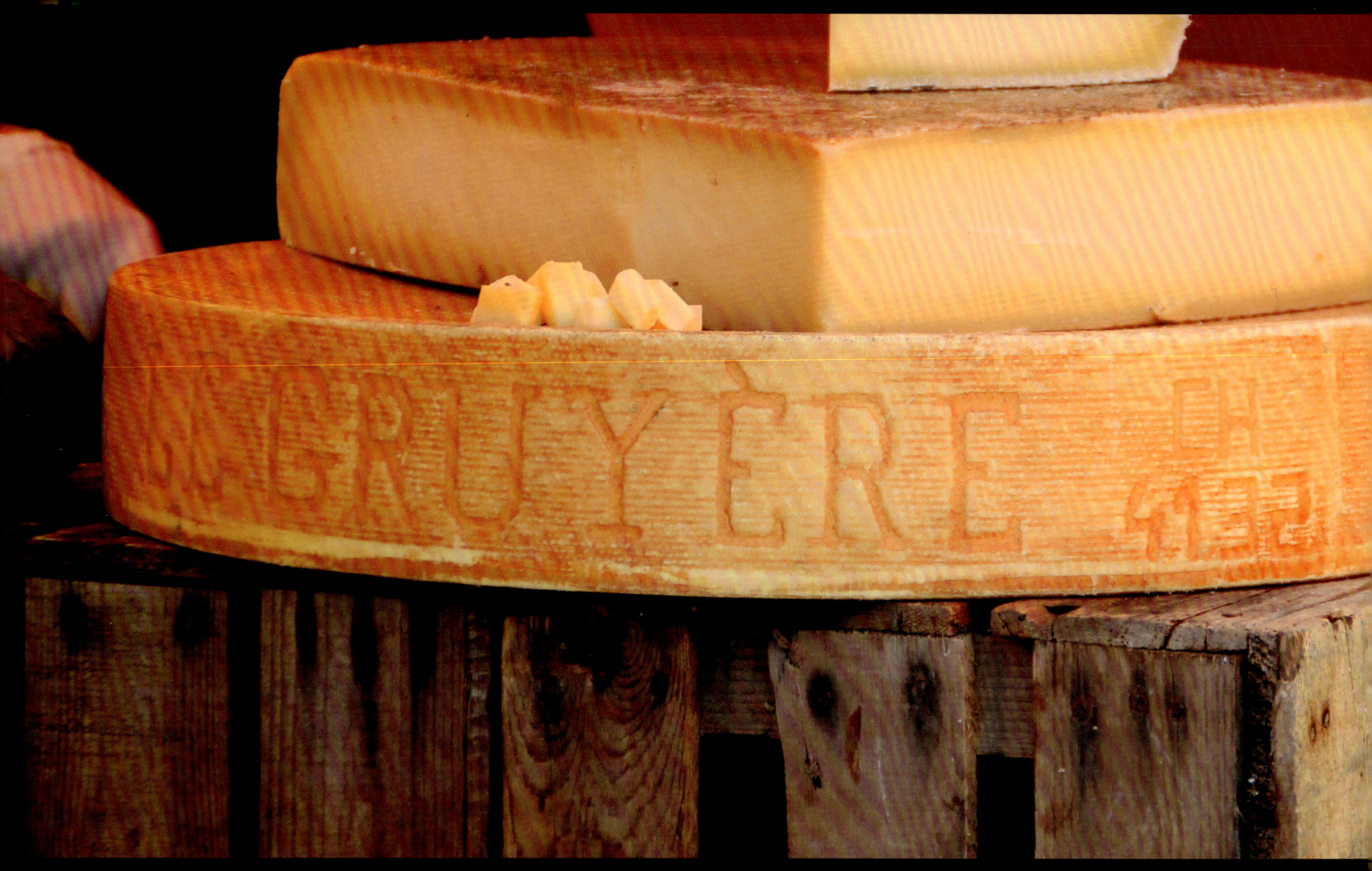

France's inviting traditions...

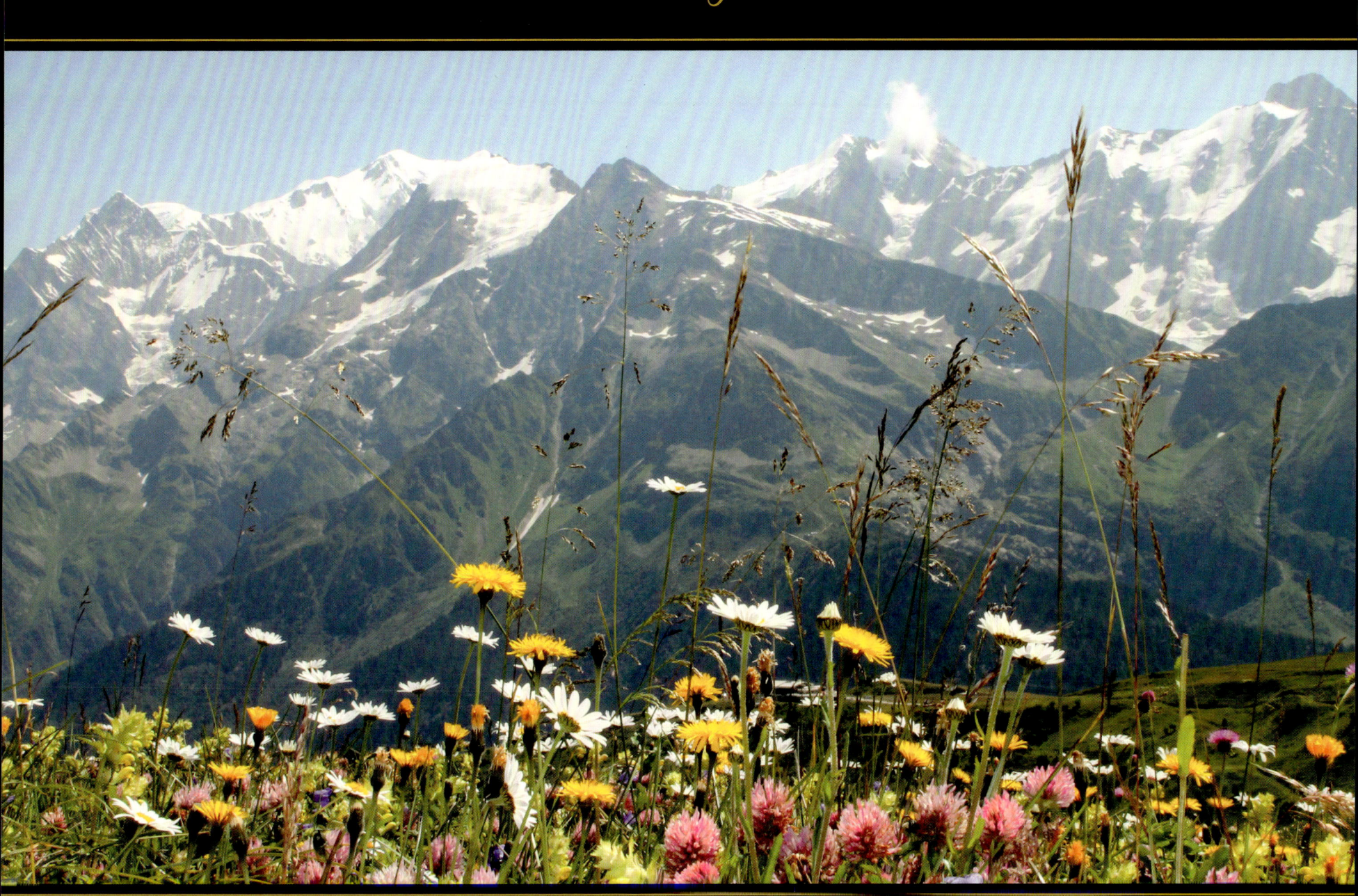

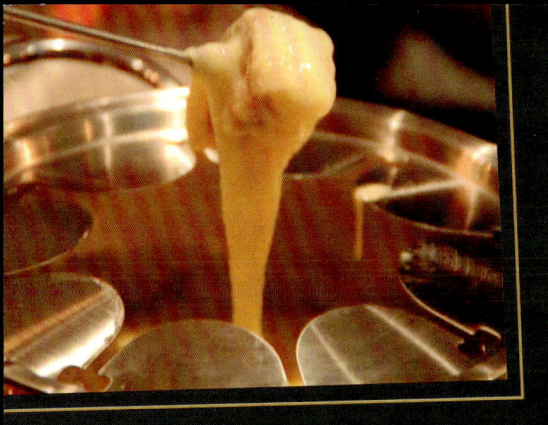

Savoie-style fondue
Fondue savoyarde

Remove and discard the rind from the cheeses then cut into slices, strips or cubes and place in a bowl.

Pour the cornflour over the cheeses and mix together well.

Rub the inside of the fondue bowl with the garlic clove, cut in half. Add the wine and heat.

Add the cheese and heat gently or moderately, stirring constantly with a wooden spoon, making figures of 8. *This action is important to stop the cheese becoming stringy. (Always stir in the same direction.)* Continue stirring until the wine is completely mixed into the cheese.

Add the Kirsch. *This is what gives the fondue its unique flavour!*

Place the fondue bowl in the centre of the table over a lit tabletop burner.

To serve, allow your guests to spear pieces of bread on the long-handled fondue forks and plunge them into the smooth, bubbling, cheesy mixture. Allow the bread to soak long enough to cover it with the melted cheese. Keep the fondue over a low heat to allow it to simmer throughout the meal.

Serve with a strong, dry white wine (preferably from Savoie), some *savoyard charcuterie* (thin slices of dried meat, ham and cured ham) and accompanied with gherkins, pickled onions and a crisp green salad or *salade aux noix* (walnut salad).

Serves 4 persons

- 200 g *Emmental* cheese
- 100 g *Comté* cheese
- 100 g *Beaufort* cheese
- 2 tablespoons cornflour
- 1 garlic clove
- 300 ml white wine
- 2 tablespoons Kirsch

- 1 large country loaf

See tips for a successful *Savoie*-style fondue on the following page.

Cheese favourites
Autour du fromage

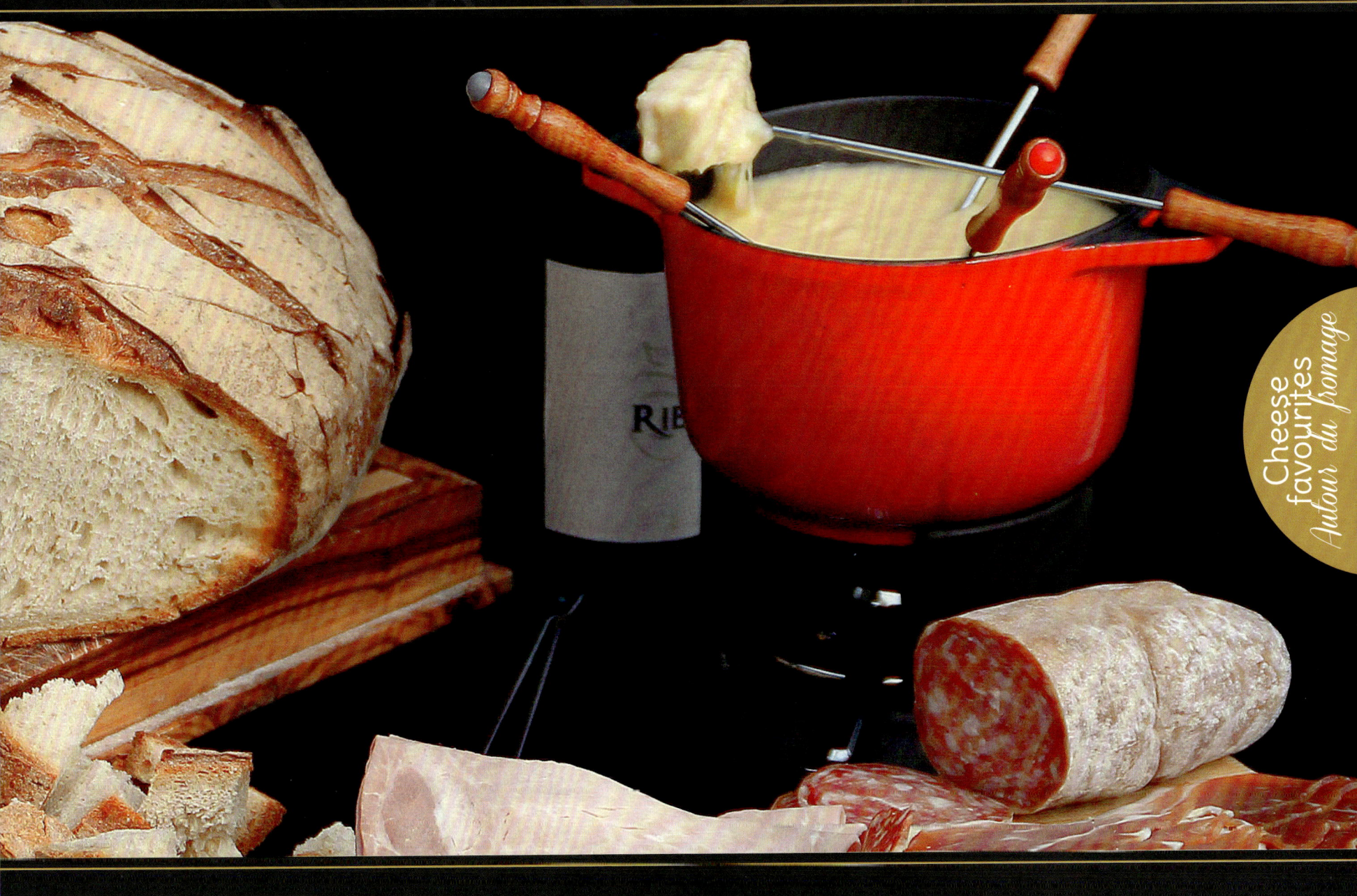

Fondue is a speciality from the Alps and is one of the most tempting *rendez-vous* for all cheese amateurs! A real classic for winter evenings in the mountains, it has emerged from a rustic-style cuisine with cheese being the key ingredient, which changes from region to region (*Comté, Cantal, Emmental* and others). Mostly, mature cheeses are used to give a rich flavour. The *Savoie*-style recipe consists of mature *Beaufort*, mild fruitier-flavoured *Beaufort*, dry white wine and Kirsch.
To follow, a light dessert is recommended such as a fresh fruit salad with a sorbet.

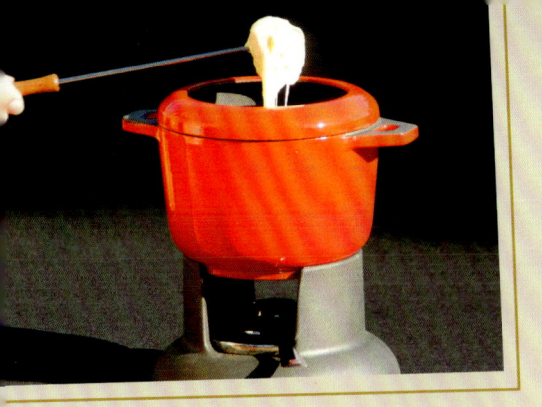

Tips for a successful cheese fondue
Astuces pour une bonne fondue

Easy to prepare and one of the most welcoming and convivial meals on a cold winter's day—follow a few helpful tips to guarantee a successful fondue.

Allow about 120 g to 200 g of cheese per person and 150 g to 200 g of bread per person. (Choose bread that is not too fresh and with a good crust).

Ensure that the temperature remains gentle and constant with the cheese barely simmering during the meal. If it is too hot, it can curdle—too cool, it will thicken and begin to set.

Adding the cornflour should prevent it from curdling as the grains of starch hold the cheese in suspension and help to keep the mixture stable.
Although other cheese can be experimented, the cheeses suggested in the recipe are recommended as melting well.

If preparing for a large company, ensure there are enough fondue bowls and forks for everyone to reach. Don't double the recipe—make several batches.
Continue to stir the fondue during the meal, always in the same direction, to prevent it sticking to the base.

Avoid drinking cold water or fruit juices with a fondue as the melted cheese will coagulate in the stomach and produce indigestion—instead a dry white wine or herb tea is recommended.

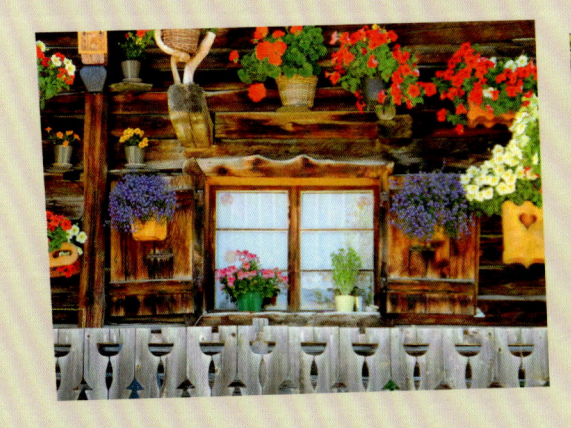

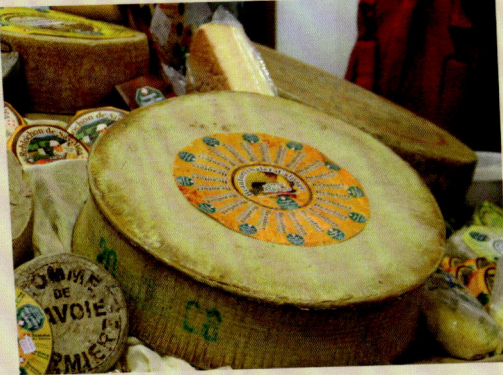

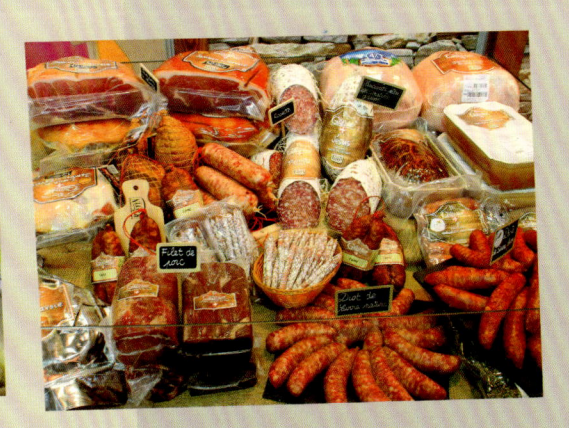

Cheese favourites
Autour du fromage

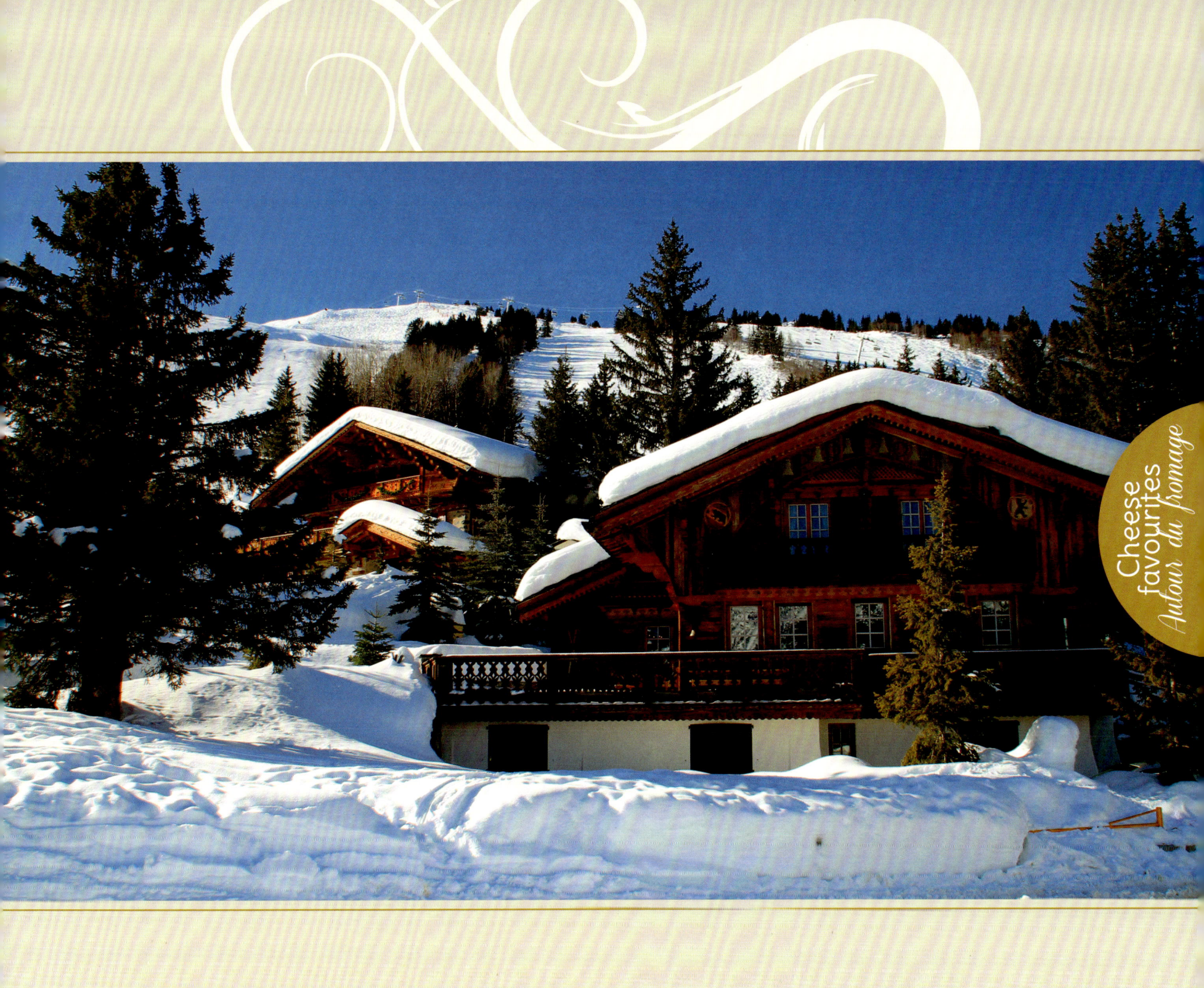

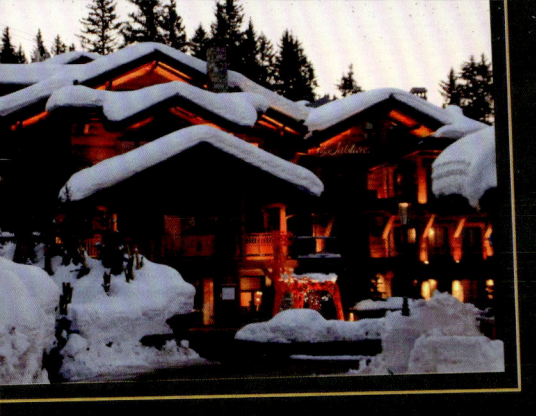

Savoie-style potatoes
Pommes de terre savoyardes

Cook the potatoes in boiling, salted water for about 20 minutes or until soft. *The cooking time will vary according to the type and size of the potatoes.*

Drain them and leave until just warm. Peel them and then leave aside until cold. Cut each potato into 3 horizontally. Insert a piece of *raclette* cheese in between each slice of potato.

Wrap a rasher of streaky bacon around each potato joining underneath, and then another rasher joining on top. Fix with a cocktail stick.

Season with salt and pepper, dot with butter and sprinkle with dried, chopped thyme.

Put in the oven and cook for about 15 minutes or until the cheese is melted and the potatoes crisp and golden.

Decorate with a sprig of fresh thyme.

Serves approx. 4 persons

Oven: 220°C

- 4 medium firm potatoes
- 6 slices of *raclette* cheese (140 g)
- 8 rashers streaky bacon
- 2 teaspoons dried thyme
- Butter
- Salt and pepper
- A bunch of fresh thyme to decorate

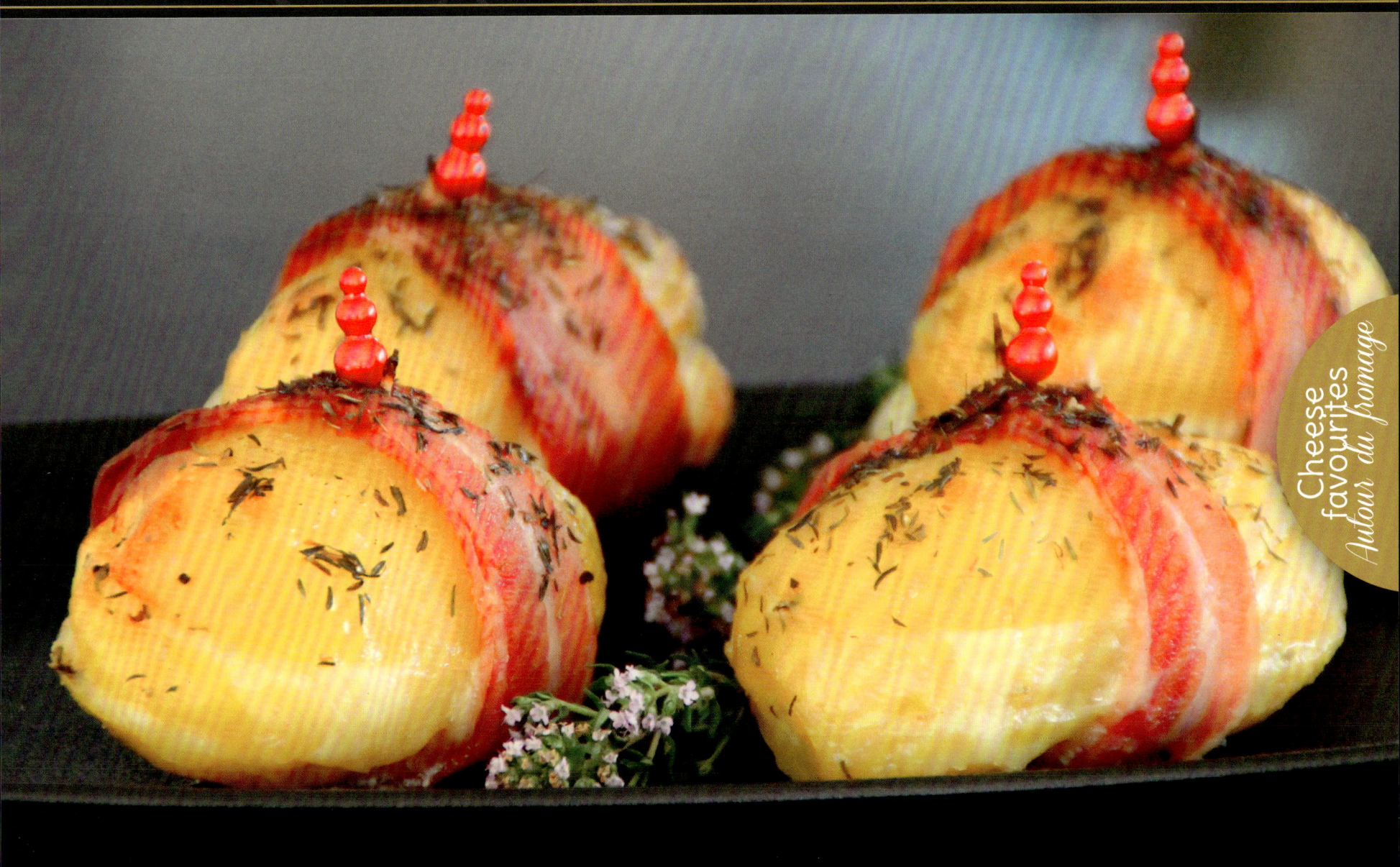

This recipe can be enjoyed as a main course if served with white meat and a green salad.

Cheese favourites — Autour du fromage

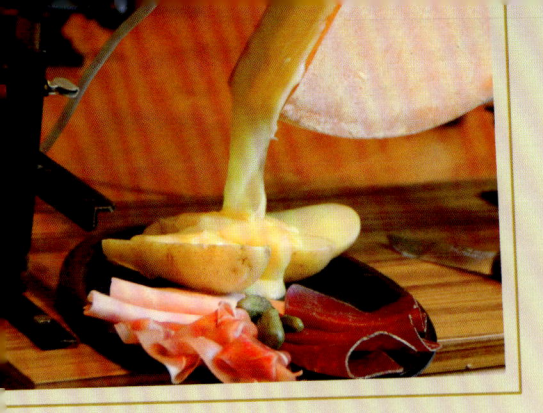

The origin of raclette
L'origine de la raclette

In the days when whole flocks of sheep were taken to the Alps to graze in summertime, the shepherds lived in almost total isolation for over three months. Having only very limited provisions, they had the idea of roasting a piece of cheese over the open fire, and scraping it onto their bread as it melted.

This led to an electric grill being designed to replace the rustic wood fire, to heat a half round of *raclette* cheese. The melted cheese was scraped off with a knife and poured over hot potatoes rather than bread.

Modern *raclette* grills have individual metal pans for melting slices of *raclette* cheese, and are safer and quicker to use as well as being more convivial.

A choice of *charcuterie* are traditional accompaniments such as *Bayonne*—a cured ham, and *saucisson*—a mixture of uncooked meats, seasoned with either spices, peppers, hazlenuts, cheese, etc. then salted and dried to preserve it. Gherkins and pickled onions are normally served with *raclette* also.

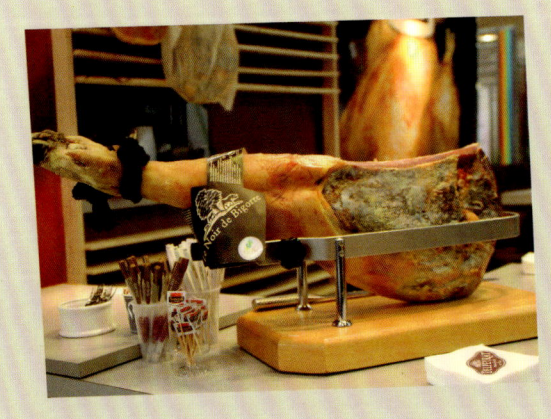

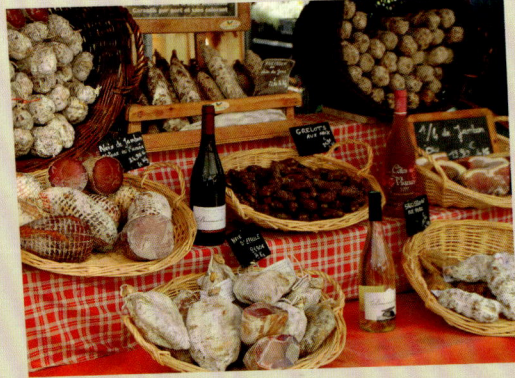

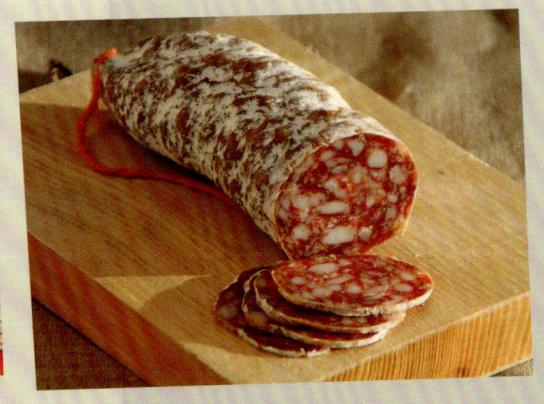

Bayonne

Saucisson

Cheese favourites
Autour du fromage

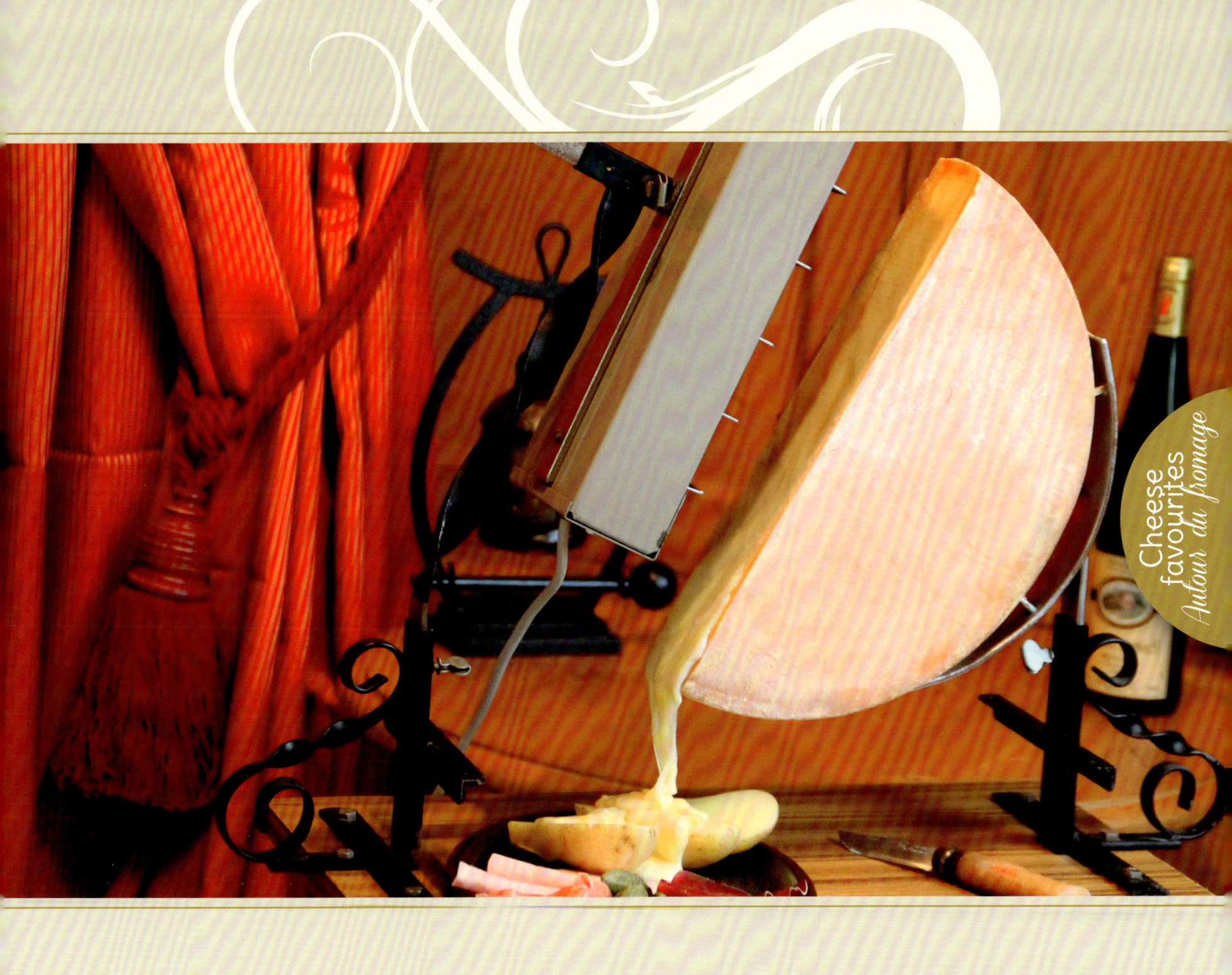

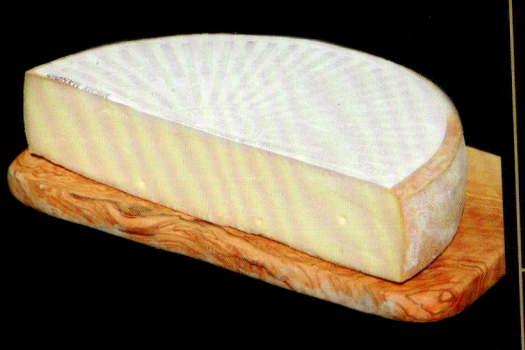

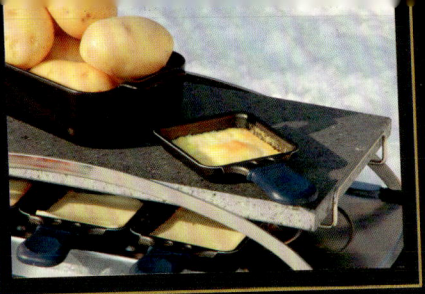

Savoie-style raclette
Raclette savoyarde

Scrub the potatoes and cook either in a steamer or in a large saucepan of boiling, salted water. Keep warm.

Arrange the *charcuterie* on a serving plate.

Cut the cheese into 5 mm slices (if not already sliced) and arrange on a plate.

Heat the *raclette* grill and start melting the cheese, when everyone is at the table.

Serve with the hot potatoes, *charcuterie*, gherkins and pickled onions.

IDEAS TO ACCOMPANY A *SAVOIE*-STYLE RACLETTE

- Button mushrooms
- Finely chopped onions mixed with parsley
- Slices of salted tomatoes
- Stoned prunes soaked in white wine
- Mini corn on the cobs
- A green salad with a vinaigrette sauce

Serves approx. 8 persons

- 800 g *raclette* cheese

- 1 kg new potatoes

Charcuterie:
- 8 slices ham
- 8 slices *Bayonne* ham
- 8 slices dried beef
- 16 slices bacon
- 24 slices *saucisson*

- Gherkins
- Pickled onions

Cheese favourites
Autour du fromage

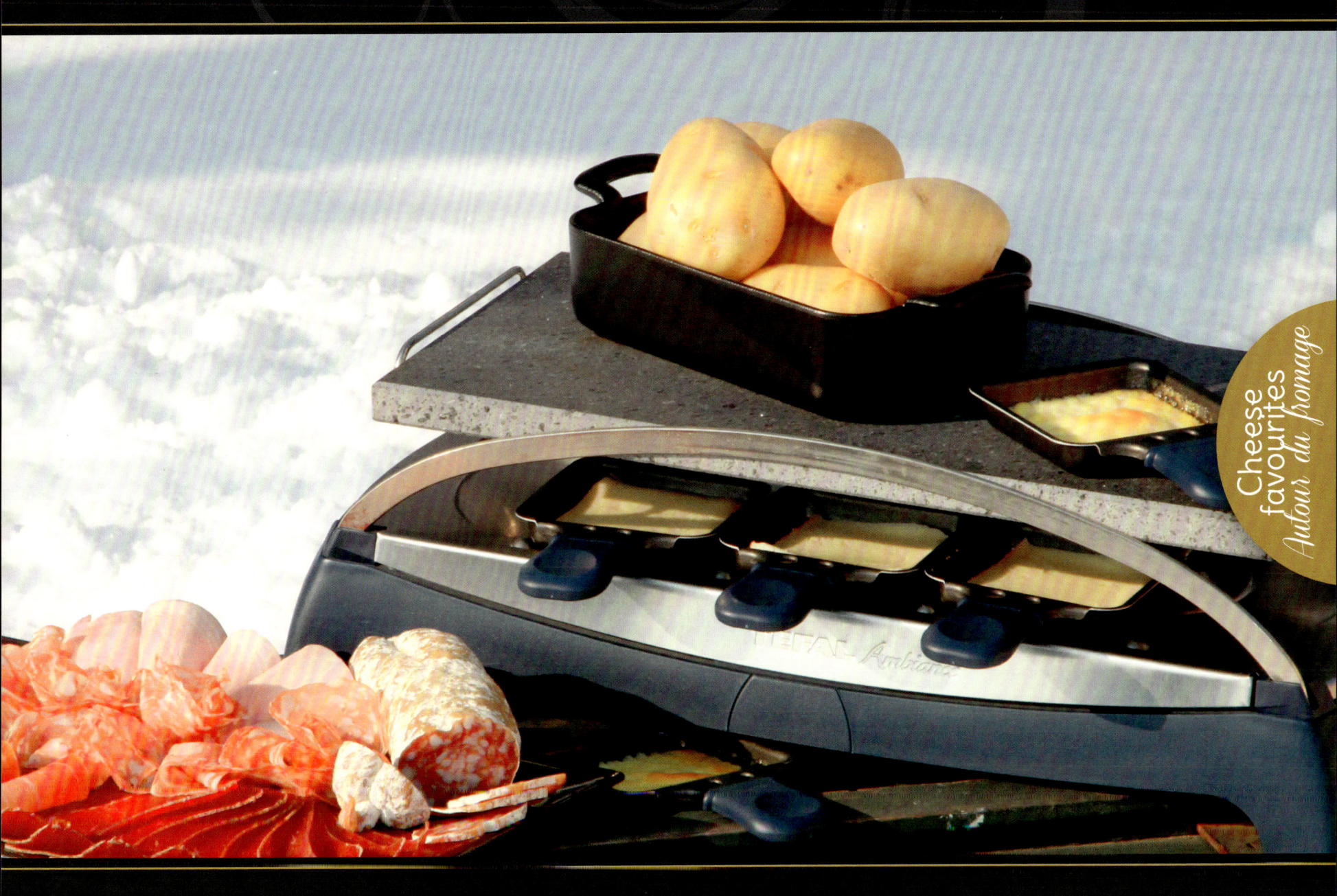

This is a very warming and satisfying meal in the cold winter months, especially after a day spent outside in the snow. Quick to prepare, it does not need a starter or the traditional cheese course. However, a fruit salad or a light mousse is always appreciated as a dessert.

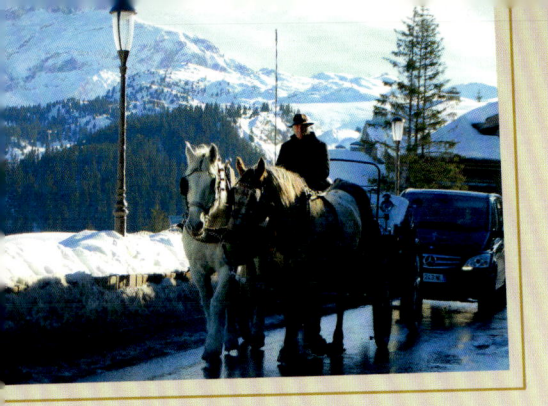

Tartiflette
Tartiflette

Cook the potatoes in boiling, salted water for about 20 minutes or until just soft. Peel and cut into thin slices.

Chop the onions finely and fry in olive oil until transparent. Add the bacon and cook on a low heat for about 10 minutes, stirring from time to time.

Rub the garlic over the base and sides of an ovenproof dish (approx. 26 x 22 cm, 6 - 7 cm deep).

Place half the potatoes in the dish, and then sprinkle with the onions and bacon. Cover with the rest of the potatoes.

Pour over the wine and the cream. Season generously with pepper and lightly with salt.

Cut the cheese in half, and place the 2 rounds (outer side up) on top of the potatoes. *For a slightly milder flavour, scrape the surface of the cheese before cutting in half.*

Cook for about 30 minutes.

This can be prepared 1 or 2 days in advance and kept in the fridge. Leave the final oven cooking until just before serving.

Serves approx. 6 - 8 persons

Oven: 210°C

- 1.5 kg medium, firm potatoes
- 1 whole *tartiflette* cheese (*Reblochon*)
- 4 onions
- 1 garlic clove, halved
- 100 ml white wine
- 180 ml double cream
- 300 g smoked bacon, chopped
- Salt and pepper

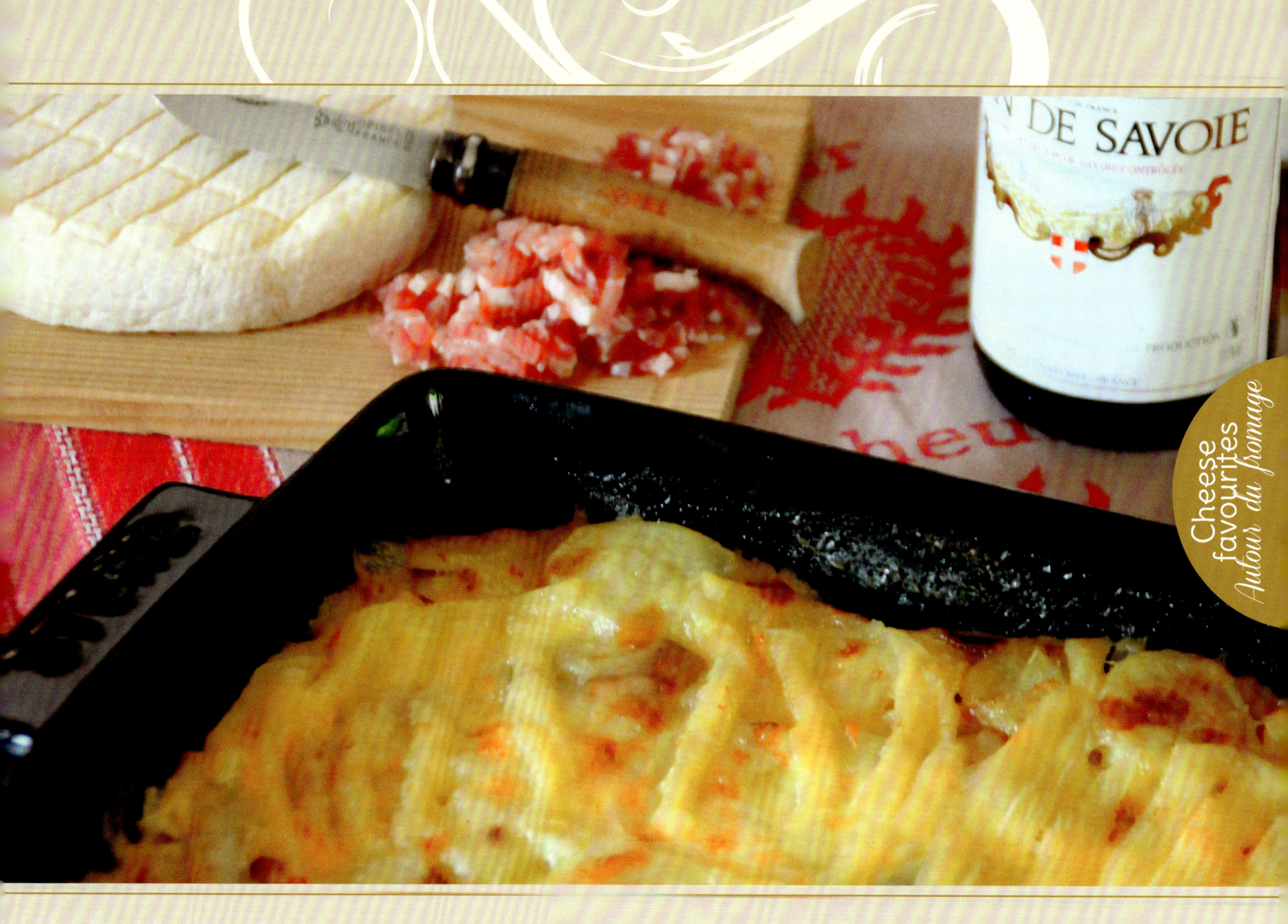

This ancient recipe from *Haute-Savoie*, originally named *Pêla des Aravis* was made using cheese remnants and cooked in a frying pan. In more recent years, it has been modernised and renamed *Tartiflette* using *Reblochon* cheese, bacon and white wine, and baked in the oven. *Reblochon* is a soft cheese, produced in *Savoie* and *Haute Savoie*, about 14 cm in diameter and 3.5 cm thick, weighs about 450 g – 550 g, and is covered with an orange-yellow coating which is then covered again with a thin white mousse.

Cheese favourites
Autour du fromage

Basic recipes
Recettes de base

244 *Vinaigrette* sauce
Vinaigrette

245 Mayonnaise
Mayonnaise

246 Hollandaise sauce
Sauce hollandaise

247 Cocktail sauce
Sauce cocktail

248 Tomato coulis
Coulis de tomates

249 Tomato sauce
Sauce tomate

250 Bechamel sauce
Sauce béchamel

250 Bechamel sauce with cheese
Sauce béchamel au fromage

251 *Financière* sauce
Sauce financière

252 Pizza dough
Pâte à pizza

253 Shortcrust pastry
Pâte brisée

Warning!
Some recipes contain alcohol.

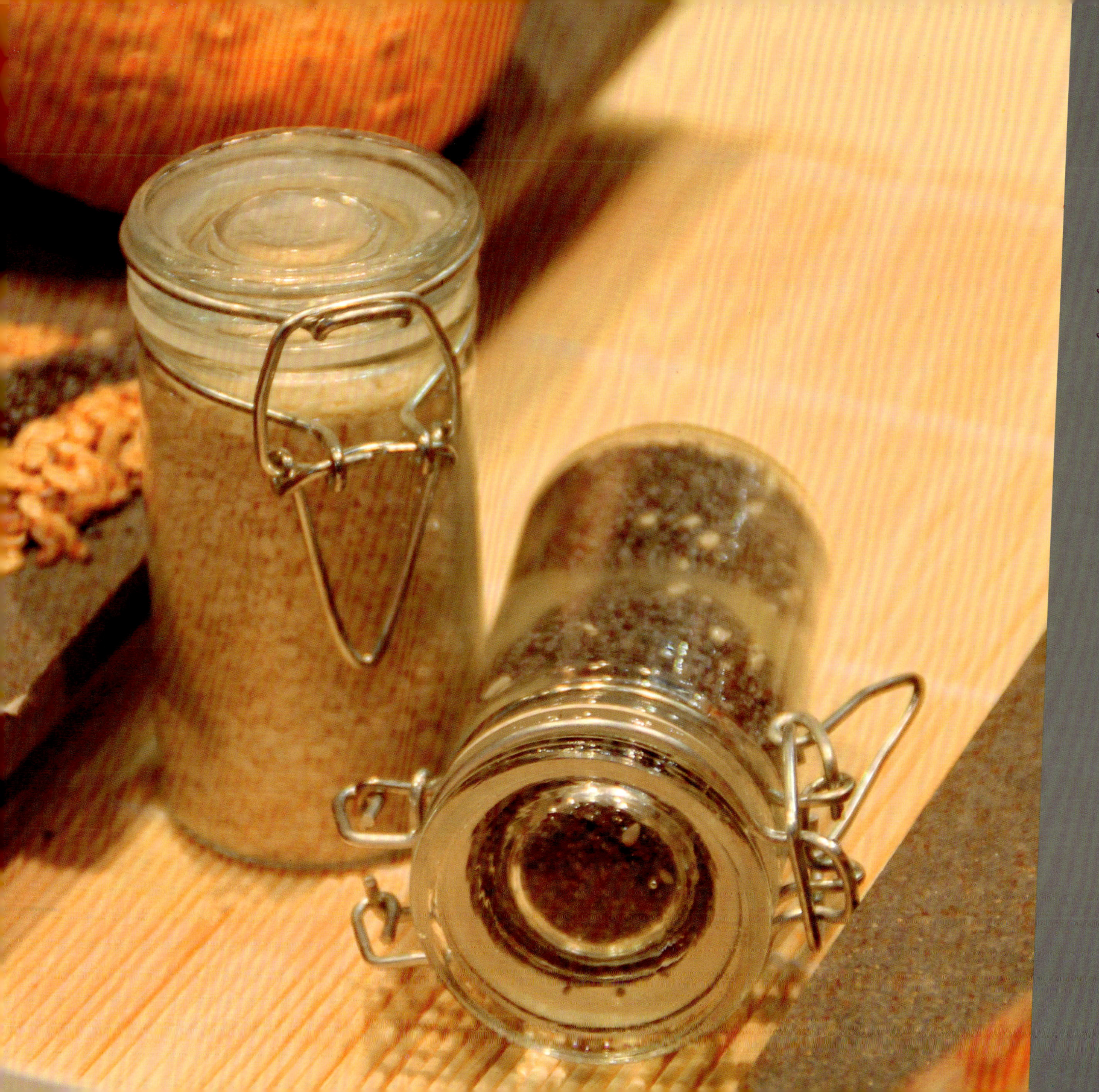

Basic recipes *Recettes de base*

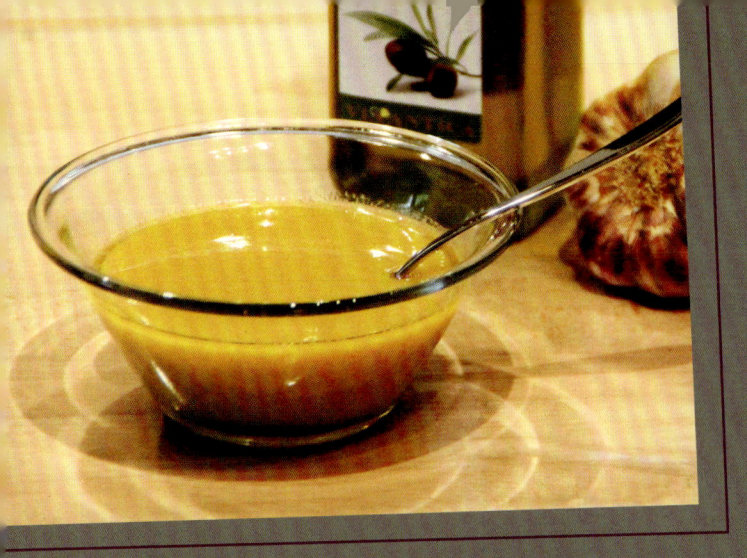

Vinaigrette sauce
Vinaigrette

Put the mustard with the salt into a small bowl and mix in the vinegar and a few drops of liquid seasoning with a spoon until smooth. Slowly pour in the oil steadily, stirring all the time until the vinaigrette turns thick. Add the pepper to taste.

Experiment by adding a little chopped shallot. Make in advance and leave a garlic clove in the mixture. Remove before serving.

- 1 level tablespoon Dijon mustard
- 3 tablespoons cider vinegar or red wine vinegar
- A few drops of liquid seasoning (e.g. *arome Maggi®**)
- 6 tablespoons vegetable oil
- 3 tablespoons olive oil
- Salt and pepper

**Arome Maggi® is a liquid seasoning used frequently in France for flavouring salad dressings, soups, sauces, vegetables dishes or simply sprinkled over rice or pasta. If unavailable, use soya sauce.*

Note: The flavours of *vinaigrettes* vary tremendously just by changing the few ingredients—oil, vinegar or mustard. For example: using red wine vinegar with shallots gives a slight onion flavour, replacing one or two tablespoons of vegetable oil with walnut oil gives the salad a nutty flavour. For a lighter *vinaigrette*, replace a little of the oil with water, adding a little extra mustard.

Vinaigrettes are an essential part of the whole dish. Freshly made vinaigrettes are much tastier than any bottle you can buy from a supermarket. Everyone has their own way of making them.

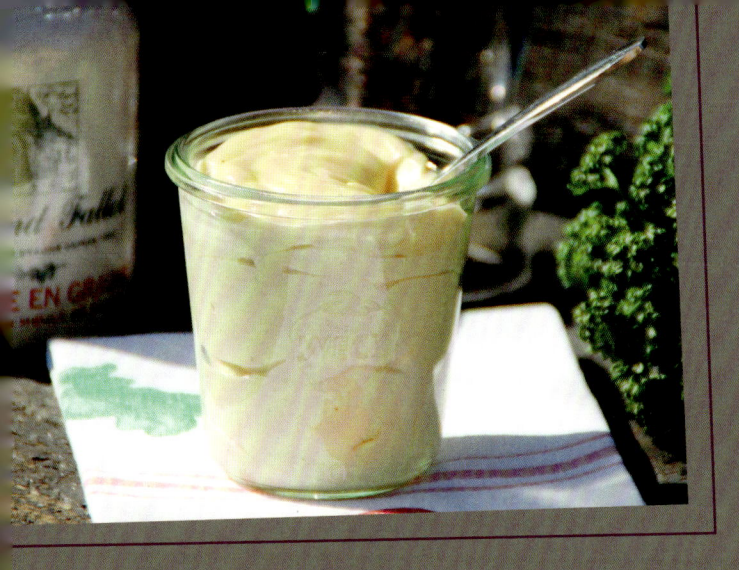

Mayonnaise
Mayonnaise

All ingredients <u>must</u> be at room temperature.

This recipe can be made using an electric whisk or electric mixer.

Measure the oil into a jug with a very fine pouring spout, so that only a few drops of oil can be poured out at a time. *This is very important for a successful mayonnaise.*

Beat together the egg yolk and mustard with the salt and pepper.

Once they are completely mixed, begin adding a few drops of oil, whisking all the time (on medium speed). *Do not rush this process.*

Once the emulsion has 'taken' and thickened, mix a little vinegar or lemon juice with some oil then add to the mayonnaise in a slow stream, whisking constantly.

- 1 egg yolk
- 2 teaspoons strong Dijon mustard
- 250 ml oil (sunflower, rapeseed or corn)
- Salt and pepper
- A drop of vinegar or lemon juice

Room temperature should not be too warm or the mayonnaise will be difficult to set and will collapse quickly.
If the mayonnaise does not 'take', blend in a hard-boiled egg.

A favourite accompaniment for cold meats, fish, crudités, asparagus, hard-boiled eggs, chips or sandwiches. Mix with a *vinaigrette* to make a dressing for a mixed salad.

Basic recipes *Recettes de base*

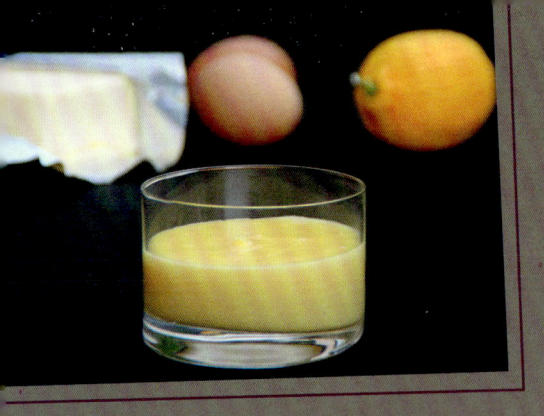

Hollandaise sauce
Sauce hollandaise

Clarify the butter by slowly melting it in a small saucepan over a very low heat. Skim the froth from the surface once it has totally melted.

Pour the butter very slowly into another bowl leaving the milky whey which is left on the base of the pan. *This butter must be kept warm, but not hot, either over another bowl of hot water or on a hob kept at a very low temperature.*

Place the egg yolks in a bowl over a saucepan of hot, but not boiling water. *Ensure that the base of the bowl does not touch the water.* Season with salt and a pinch of *Espelette* chilli. Add 7 tablespoons of water.

Whisk the egg yolks well over a low heat until the mixture starts to thicken and turns frothy (approx. 65°C). Remove from the heat.

Slowly and carefully add the melted butter, whisking continuously to emulsify the sauce. *The butter must be added only a few drops at a time whisking well in between each addition. Hollandaise sauce will separate if the butter is added too quickly.*

Add the lemon juice and adjust the seasoning if necessary. Keep warm in a bain-marie, off the heat. *If the sauce is too thick, add some warm water, several drops at a time (as for the butter), until the desired consistency is reached.*

For a richer sauce, replace the water with the same quantity of dry white wine. It can be seasoned with fresh, cut herbs as well as the lemon juice.

If the sauce separates:

- Whisk an egg yolk in a small bowl and gradually whisk in the curdled sauce.

or

- Pour 15 ml water into a medium-sized bowl and whisk in a little of the curdled sauce until it becomes creamy. Slowly add the rest of the sauce, whisking vigorously all the time.

Hollandaise sauce is the perfect accompaniment to fish, seafood, eggs and vegetables such as asparagus and broccoli.

- 300 g butter, good quality
- 5 egg yolks
- Juice of ½ a lemon
- Salt
- A pinch of *Espelette* chilli

If making in advance, keep in the fridge and reheat very slowly in a bain-marie making sure that the water does not boil or come in contact with the bowl.

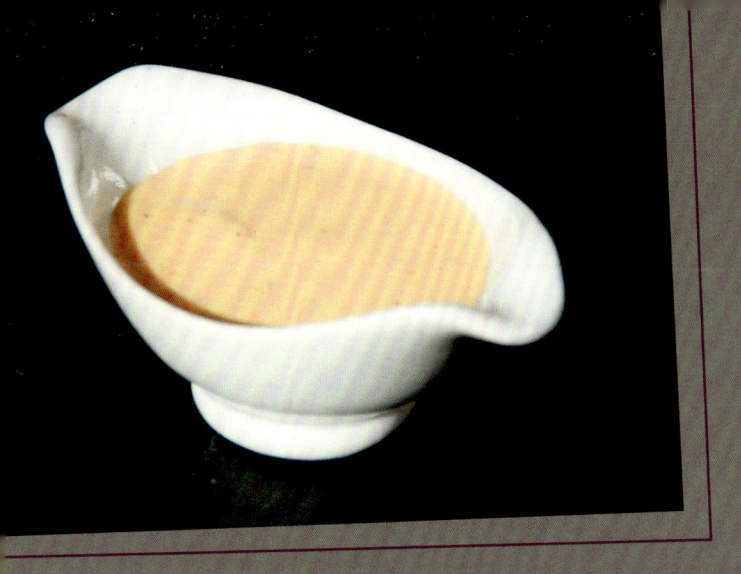

Cocktail sauce
Sauce cocktail

Finely chop the shallot. Heat the wine in a small saucepan. Add the chopped shallot and simmer gently until all the liquid has evaporated. Leave aside to cool.

Mix together the mayonnaise with the mustard, ketchup, Tabasco®, vinegar, Cognac and lemon juice until smooth.

Add the chopped shallot and season with the salt, pepper and paprika.

- 150 g mayonnaise
- 1 shallot
- 100 ml dry white or rosé wine
- 1 tablespoon cider vinegar
- 1 teaspoon Dijon mustard
- 1 - 2 tablespoons tomato ketchup
- 2 teaspoons Cognac
- Juice of 1 lemon
- 4 drops Tabasco®
- Salt and pepper
- Paprika

Basic recipes
Recettes de base

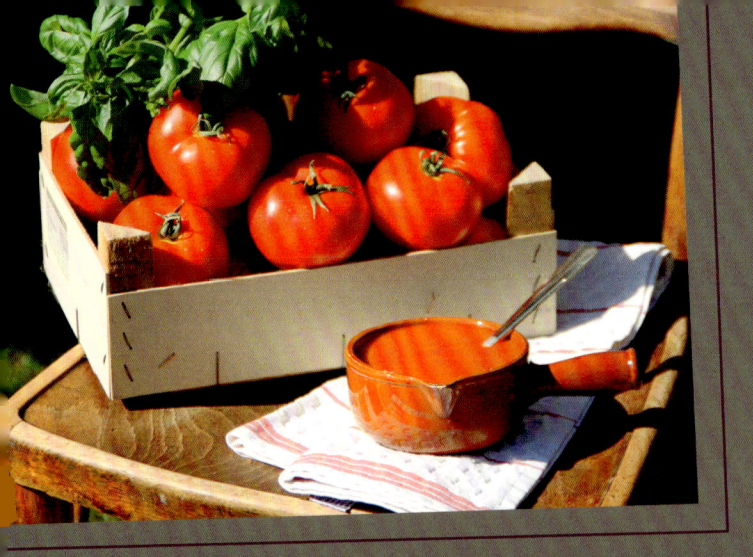

Tomato coulis
Coulis de tomates

Wash the tomatoes then score a cross in the bottom of each one, using a sharp knife. Place into a saucepan full of boiling water. Boil for about 2 minutes. Take off the heat and plunge the tomatoes immediately into cold water to remove the skins.

Cut the peeled tomatoes into small pieces.

Peel and finely cut the onion. Heat the olive oil in a saucepan and add the onion and garlic. Cook until onions begin to turn transparent. Add the chopped tomatoes, parsley, thyme and bay leaf.

Heat uncovered on a medium heat, stirring occasionally until the water has evaporated and the sauce thickened. Add a pinch of sugar to take away the acidity of the tomatoes. Season with salt and pepper. Remove the bay leaf and sprig of thyme.

Leave to cool slightly before blending until smooth.

- 500 g tomatoes
- 1 onion
- 1 garlic clove, crushed
- 3 tablespoons olive oil
- 1 tablespoon chopped fresh parsley
- 1 sprig fresh thyme
- 1 bay leaf
- Pinch of sugar
- Salt and pepper

This sauce can be kept in the fridge for at least one week. Alternatively, pour while still very hot into clean, warmed glass jars and close immediately. This will preserve it for several months.

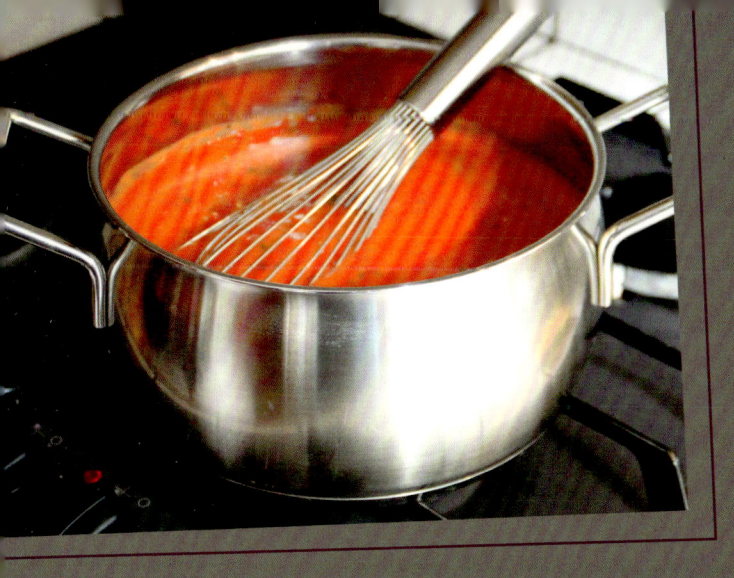

Tomato sauce
Sauce tomate

Heat the oil in a large saucepan and fry the onion and garlic until transparent.

Stir in the flour and cook until foaming.

Gradually add the tomato purée and the water, whisking constantly until the mixture thickens.

Add the *herbes de Provence*. Season to taste with salt and pepper.

Reduce the heat and simmer for a few minutes.

- 6 tablespoons olive oil
- 1 onion, finely chopped
- 70 g plain flour
- 600 g tomato purée
- 600 ml water
- 2 teaspoons *herbes de Provence*
- 1 garlic clove, crushed
- Salt and pepper

Basic recipes
Recettes de base

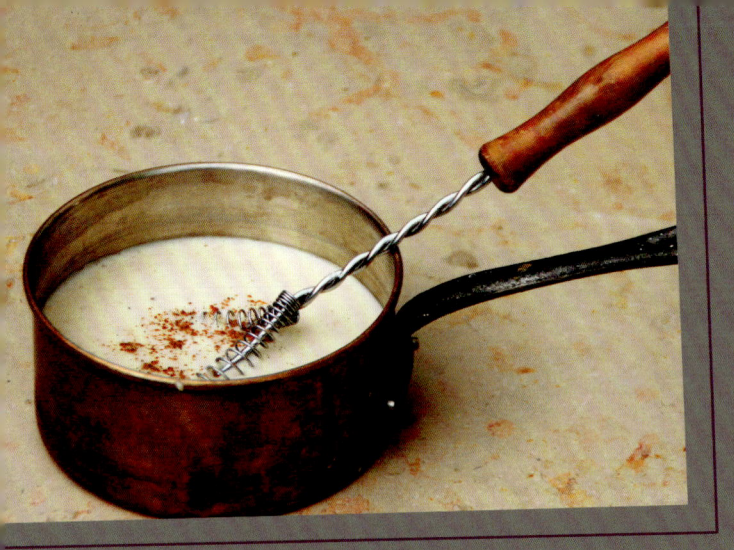

Bechamel sauce
Sauce béchamel

Melt the butter or the oil over a low heat. Stir in the flour and cook until foaming (1 - 2 minutes). Remove from the heat.

Add the milk, a little at a time, whisking until smooth. Place back on a moderate heat and cook until thick, stirring continuously. Allow to boil for 1 - 2 minutes, still stirring. Remove from the heat and season with salt, pepper and nutmeg according to taste.

- 30 g butter or oil
- 30 g plain flour
- 500 ml milk
- Salt, pepper and nutmeg

Bechamel sauce with cheese
Sauce béchamel au fromage

Add grated cheese to the hot sauce and stir until it melts.

Use to accompany vegetables.

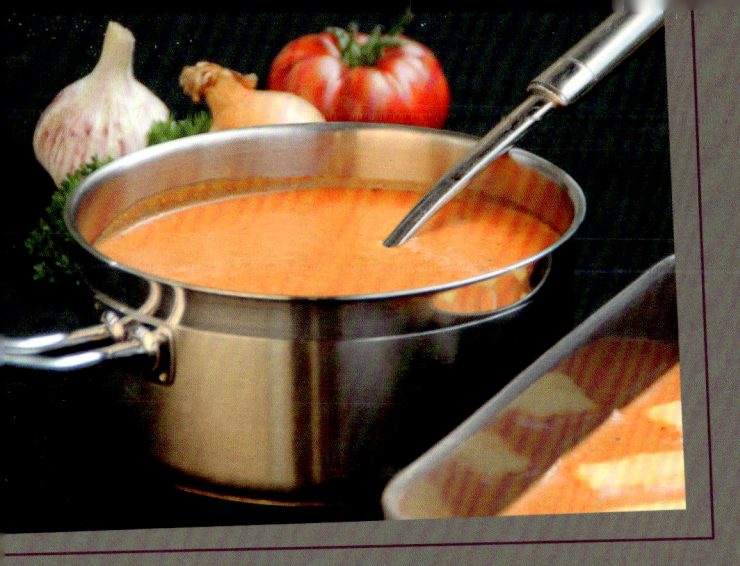

Financière sauce
Sauce financière

Heat the oil and cook the onions and garlic until transparent. Add the flour and mix well with a whisk. Cook for about 3 minutes, stirring from time to time to prevent it burning. Remove from the heat.

Slowly add the milk and stock, stirring well to remove any lumps.

Add the chopped tomatoes, concentrated tomato paste and wine. Put back on the heat and allow to simmer, covered, for about 30 minutes.

Blend. Season with the salt, pepper, *herbes de Provence* and basil. Add the olives and mushrooms.

Add the bicarbonate of soda to correct the acidity.

- 60 ml olive oil
- 2 large onions (or 4 medium), chopped
- 4 garlic cloves, crushed
- 40 g plain flour
- 500 ml milk
- 500 ml chicken stock (made with 1 stock cube)
- 2 tins of 400 g chopped tomatoes
- 2 teaspoons concentrated tomato paste
- 100 ml white wine
- Salt and pepper
- 2 teaspoons *herbes de Provence*
- A few fresh basil leaves
- A few stoned green olives, chopped
- A few tinned button mushrooms, sliced
- ½ teaspoon bicarbonate of soda

Basic recipes
Recettes de base

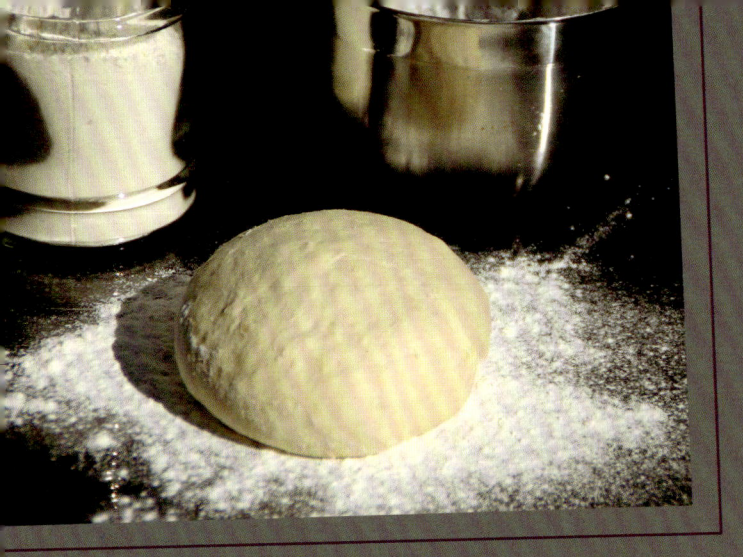

Pizza dough
Pâte à pizza

Crumble the yeast with the sugar into the warm water. Leave aside in a warm place until the yeast froths.

Put the flour in a large bowl and make a well in the centre. Add the salt and olive oil. Pour in the yeast liquid and knead together until smooth and the sides of the bowl clean. Leave covered in a warm place until double in size.

- 10 g fresh yeast
- 1 teaspoon sugar
- 150 ml warm water
- 250 g strong white flour
- 1 teaspoon salt
- 2 tablespoons olive oil

The quantity of liquid may have to be altered depending on the type of flour used.

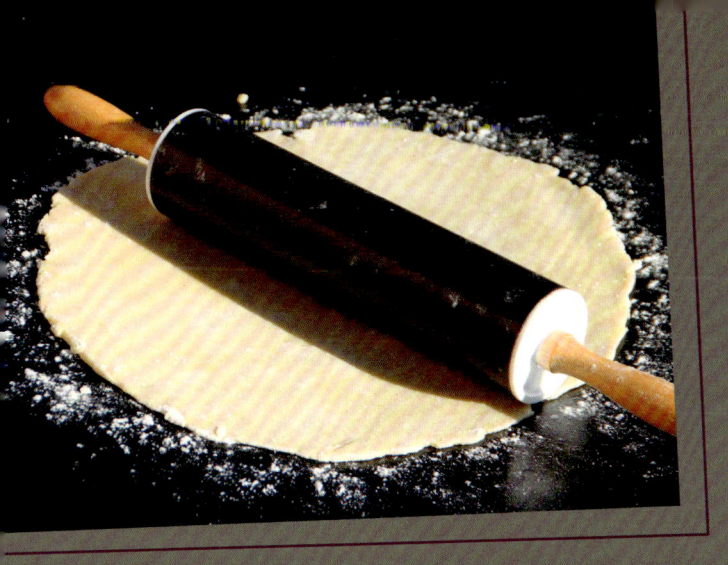

Shortcrust pastry
Pâte brisée

Place all the ingredients in a large bowl in the order shown in the list of ingredients.

Mix together quickly and lightly with a wooden spoon.

Make into a ball and roll out on a lightly floured surface.

- 50 g butter, melted
- A generous pinch of salt
- 2 tablespoons olive oil
- 70 ml water
- 200 g plain flour

Basic recipes / Recettes de base

Although very quick and easy to make, this pastry is not a dough that should be kneaded. It must be handled lightly or the final result will be hard and tough.

This was *Grand-mère's* recipe before the days of ready-made pastry. It is very easy to make and can be rolled out straight away without leaving it to rest.

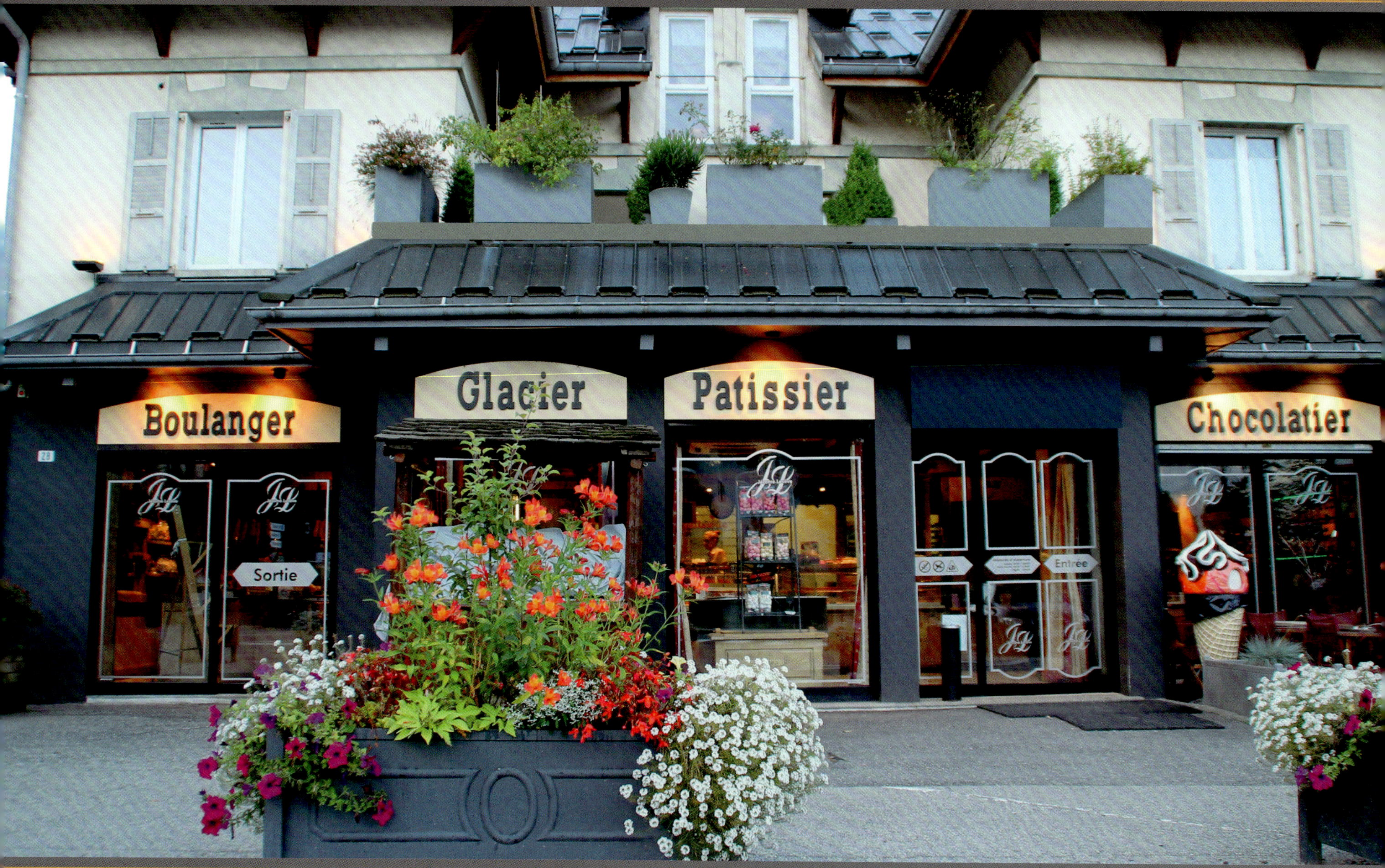
Boulanger
Glacier
Patissier
Chocolatier
Sortie
Entree

Speciality breads from France

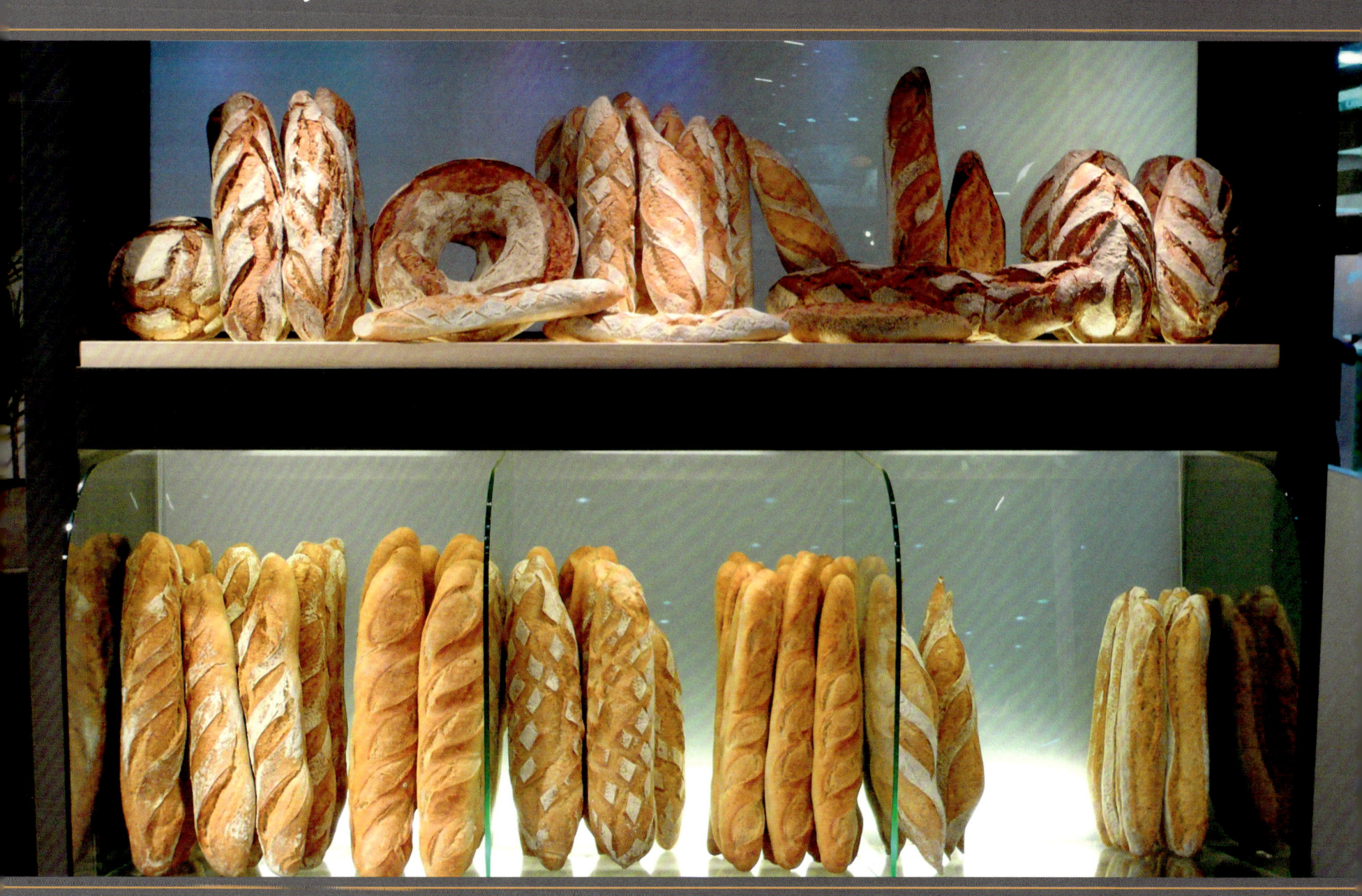

Bread
Le pain

Fresh bread is very important to the French and is normally served at each meal. A visit to the *boulangerie* (baker) every day, to buy fresh bread, has become part of French culture and tradition. Thanks to a 19th century law, every town and village has to have at least one *boulangerie*.

Mostly family owned, *boulangers* (bakers) are artisans who have passed their skills down the generations and reflect a heritage craft. Every stage of bread making is critical; from the type of flour and yeast to the methods of proving and cooking and every *boulanger* practices their own techniques to succeed in producing such exceptional results.

From early in the morning the *boulanger* works to continue this tradition and offers an impressive selection of breads, brioches, cakes and pastries. Batches of bread are cooked throughout the day allowing the population to have fresh supplies any time of the day.

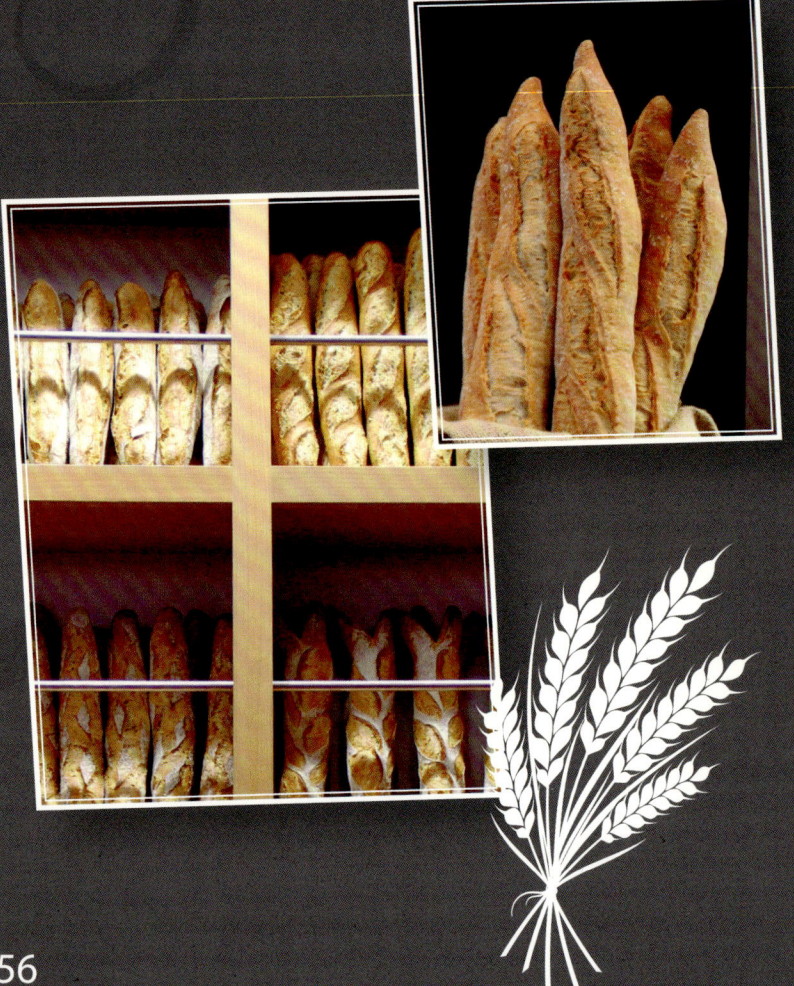

Baguette Parisienne

Renowned all over the world for its delicious golden, crunchy crust and soft, airy inside, the *baguette* is customarily present at every French meal. It first appeared during the reign of King Louis XIV and is now a national pride as it represents about 80% of bread purchased in France.

Baguettes are made of only simple ingredients: wheat flour, water, yeast or leaven and salt. The preparation is fairly long and requires kneading, fermentation, dividing the dough into pieces, resting time then shaping and finally, the famous incisions by the artisan before cooking. The elongated shape reduces the time needed for rising and cooking.

Delicious spread with jam or made into a crisp sandwich, bakers compete in creativity to offer varied and original alternatives such as using wholemeal or organic flour, adding dried seeds or even spices. It doesn't keep well, however, and is at its best only when freshly baked.

Each year a competition is held in Paris to award the best baker of *baguettes* and the winner is awarded the right to deliver the President his *baguette* at the *Elysée* palace every day for one year!

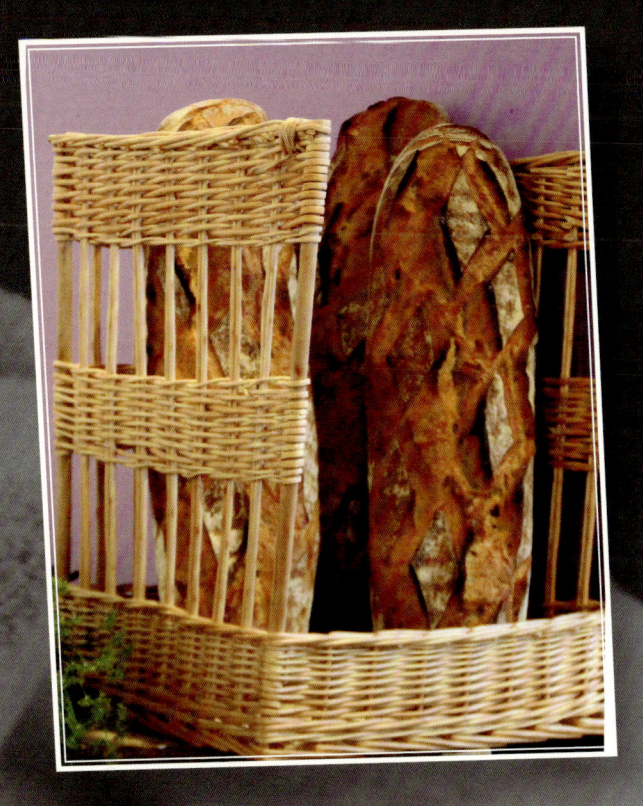

Pain de campagne

A very rustic type of bread, which was the staple diet of the poor in the days when only the rich could afford white bread. Although their form varies from one area to another, they all have a hard, rich brown crust, dusted with flour. The bread stays fresh for up to a week, and the flavour actually improves with keeping.

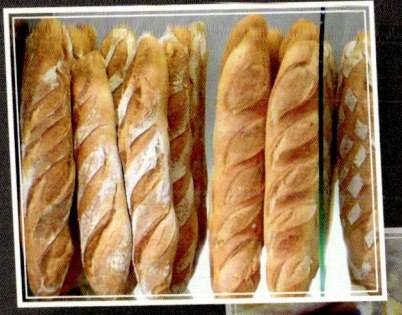

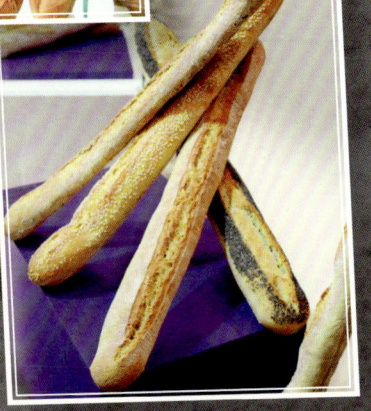

Flûte and ficelle

Although a *flûte* is larger than a *baguette* and a *ficelle* smaller, they are both baked in the same way.

Pain de seigle

This rye bread originates from mountain areas such as the *Vosges* and the *Pyrennées*. It is particularly good when thinly sliced, generously buttered and served with oysters. Rye bread normally contains about two thirds of rye flour and one third of wheat flour.

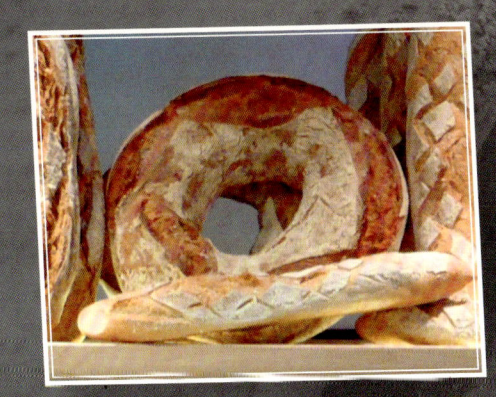

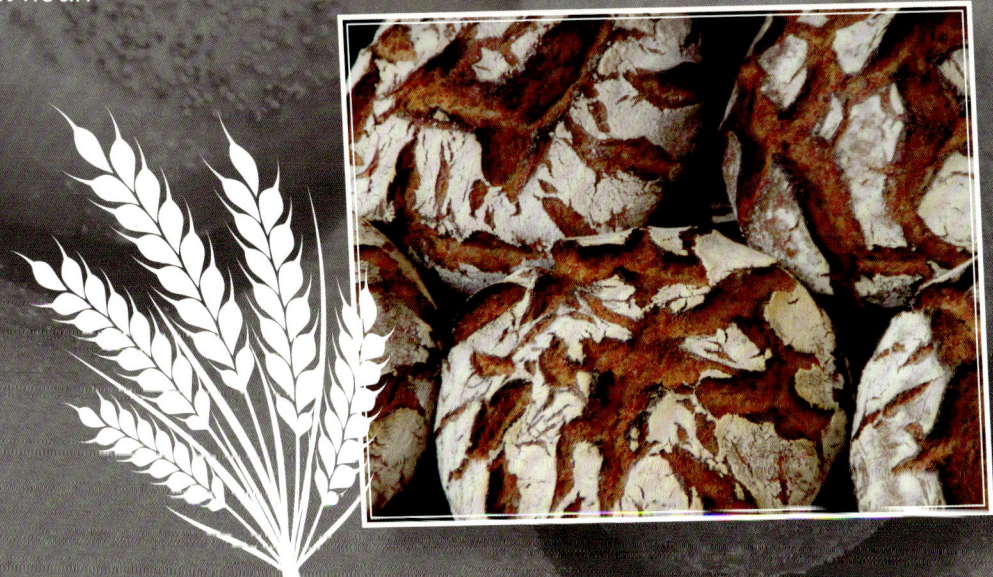

Couronne

This crown-shaped loaf is especially appreciated for its generous crust and is designed to be transported by hanging from your arms or even the handlebars of a bike!

Bread
Le pain

257

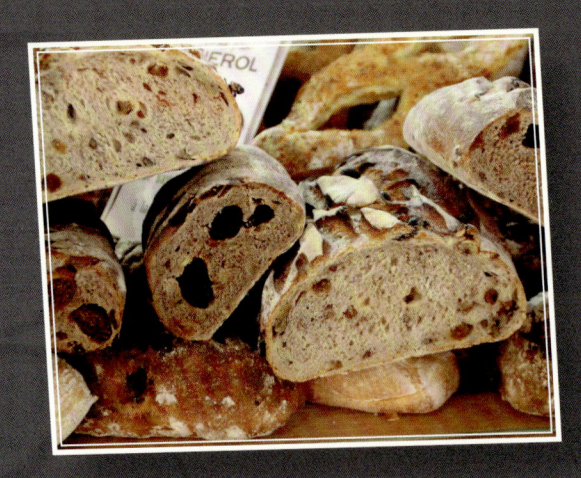

Pains aux céréales

These are breads made from wheat flour but have added cereals (spelt, corn, millet, oats etc.) and/or seeds (linseed, poppy seeds, sunflower etc).

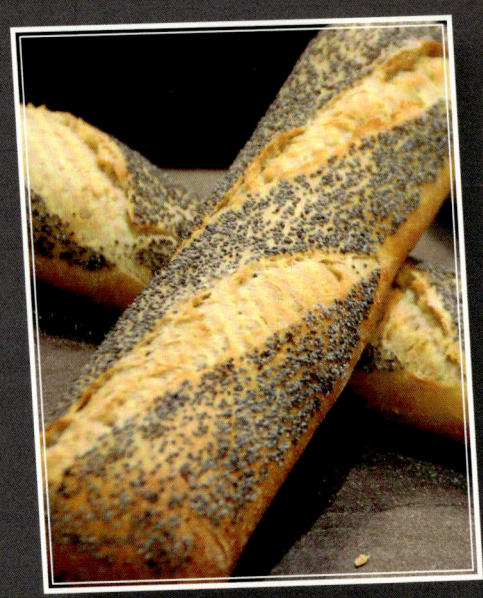

Pains spéciaux

Special breads contain supplementary ingredients such as walnuts, bacon, cheese, raisins, figs etc. Walnut bread is an excellent accompaniment to seafood as well as goats' and sheep cheeses, such as *Roquefort* and *bleu des Causses*.

Sweet bread and pastries
Viennoiseries

Boulangeries also offer a delicious range of *viennoiseries*. These are baked delicacies made from yeast-leavened dough as in bread, but with added ingredients such as eggs, butter, milk, cream and sugar, giving them a richer, sweeter composition, tempting for the youngest to the eldest! From the crack of dawn right through to the evening, there is something there for every gourmand!

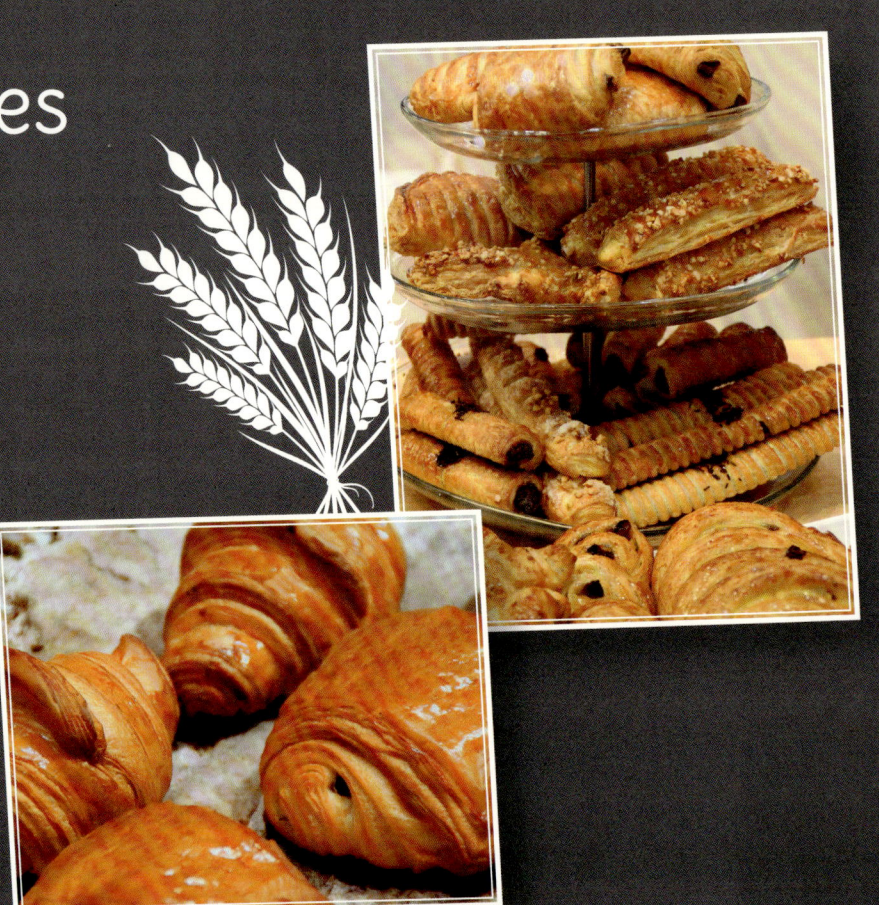

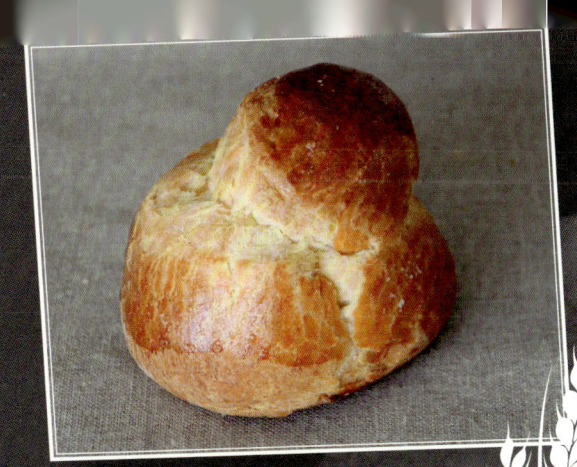

Brioche

This is the richest of all yeast breads, containing large quantities of butter and eggs in the ingredients and comes in many different forms, the most classic being the *Brioche Parisienne* with its characteristic fluted base and rounded hat.

Pain au chocolat

These incomparable flaky pastries conceal a band of melted chocolate—a firm favourite for the children.

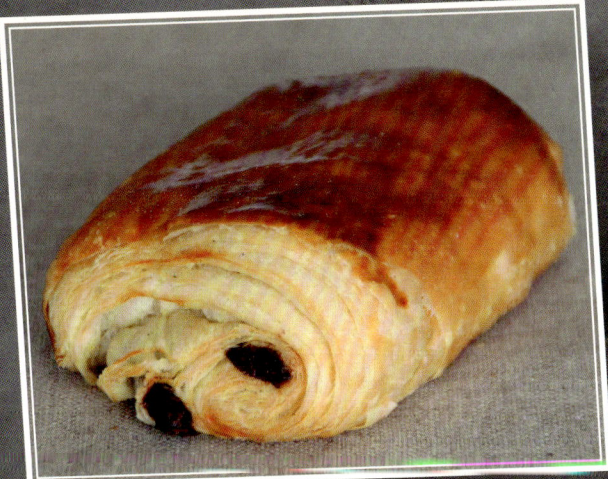

Croissants

One of the essential components of French breakfast! In fact, no breakfast *à la française* would be complete without the renowned buttery croissant. Deliciously rich, these crispy, flaky delicacies require no additional butter or jam—they are tasty just as they are!

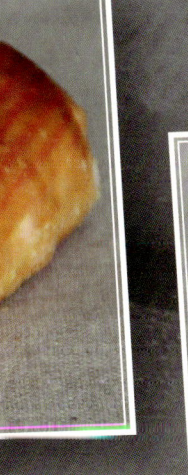

Pain aux raisins

A brioche spiral generously filled with vanilla cream and raisins.

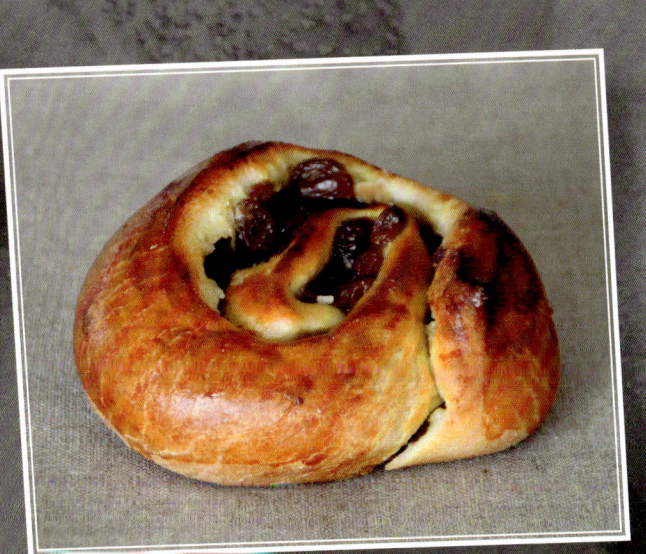

Bread / *Le pain*

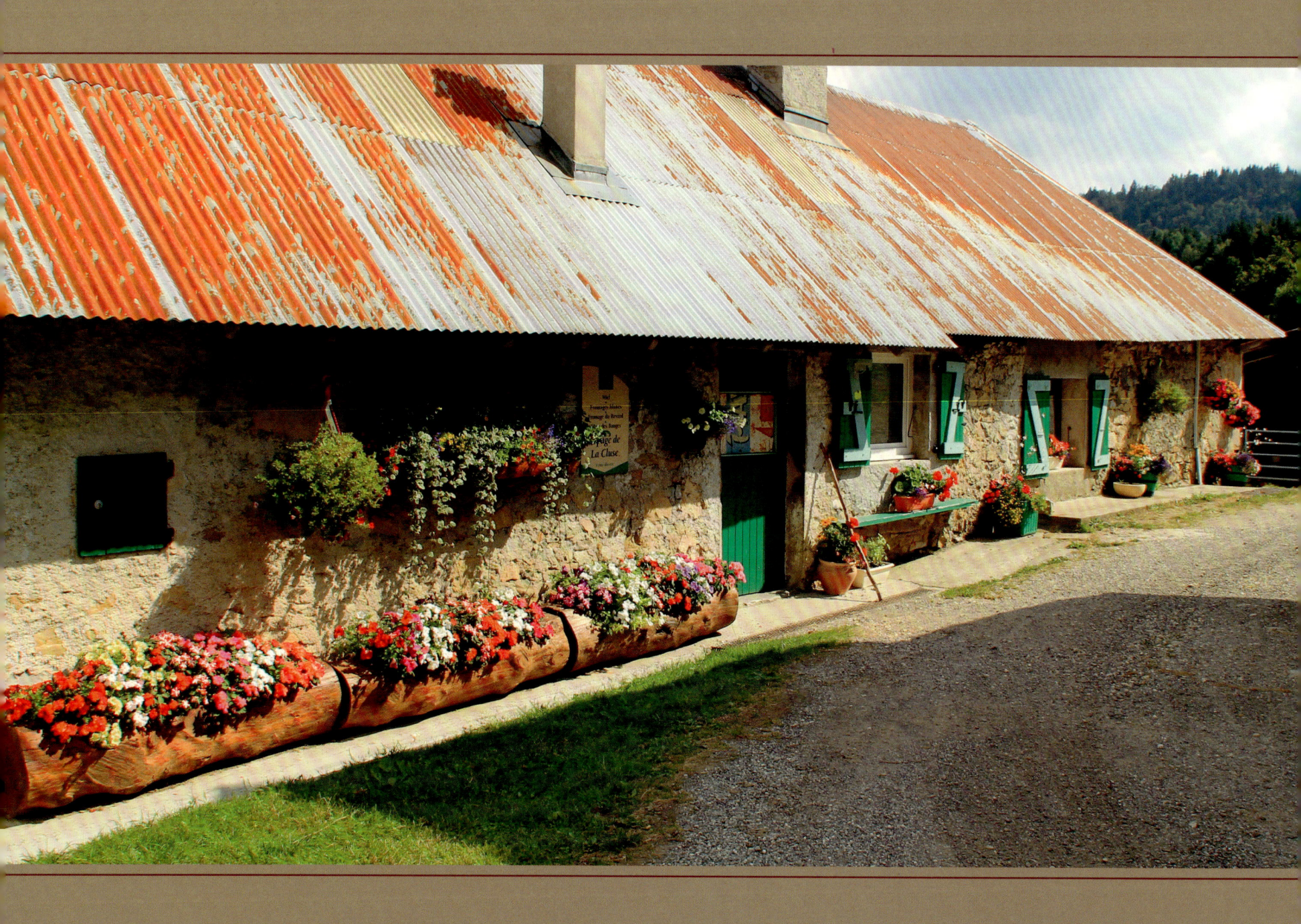

French cheeses

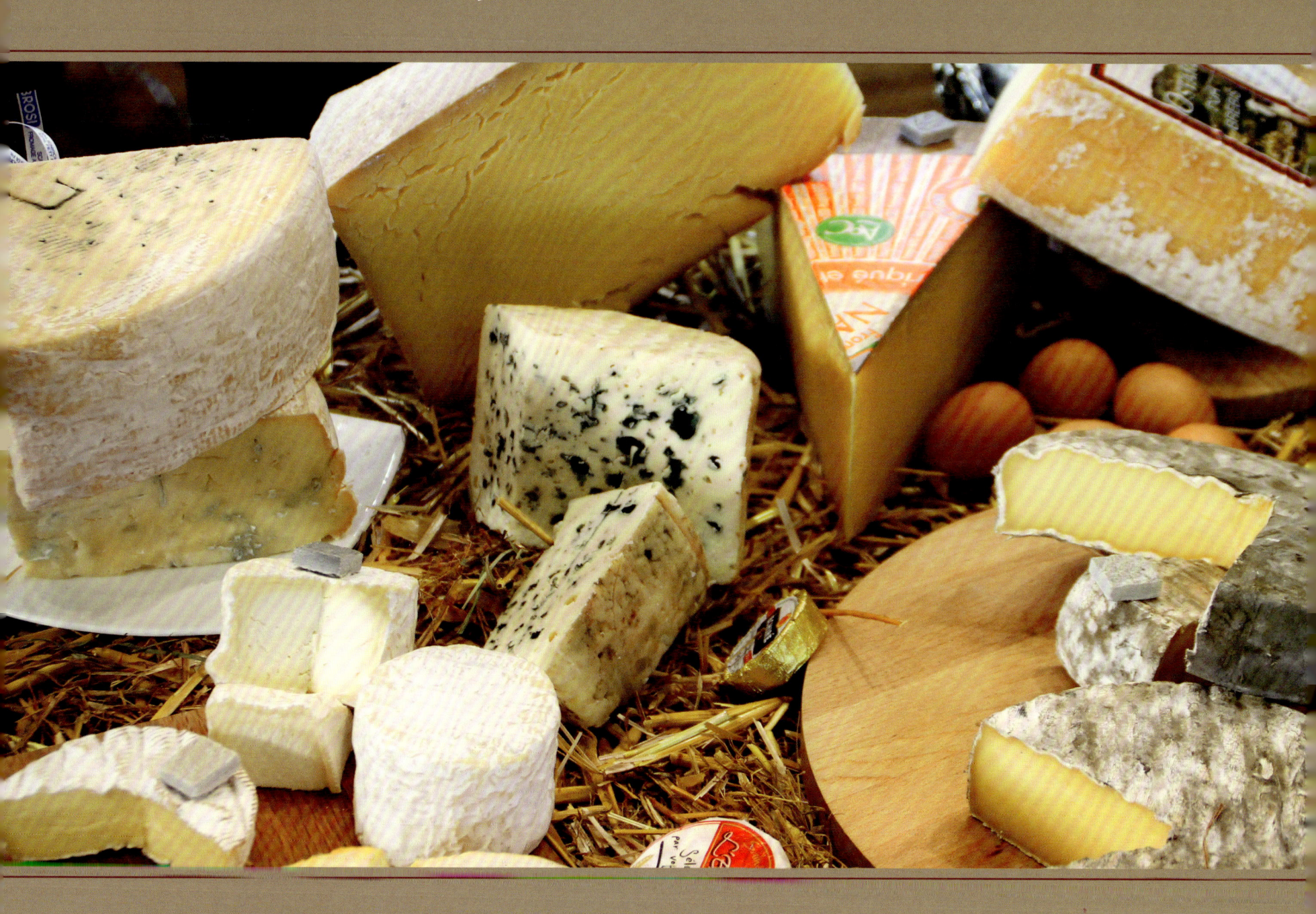

Cheese
Le fromage

France produces **more than 500 varieties of cheeses**, with every region and province having its own unique methods of production. Many towns and villages have their own speciality, offering a huge choice of flavours and textures.

Although the methods of producing cheese have changed over the years, one thing hasn't changed—France is by far the biggest consumer of cheese in the world!

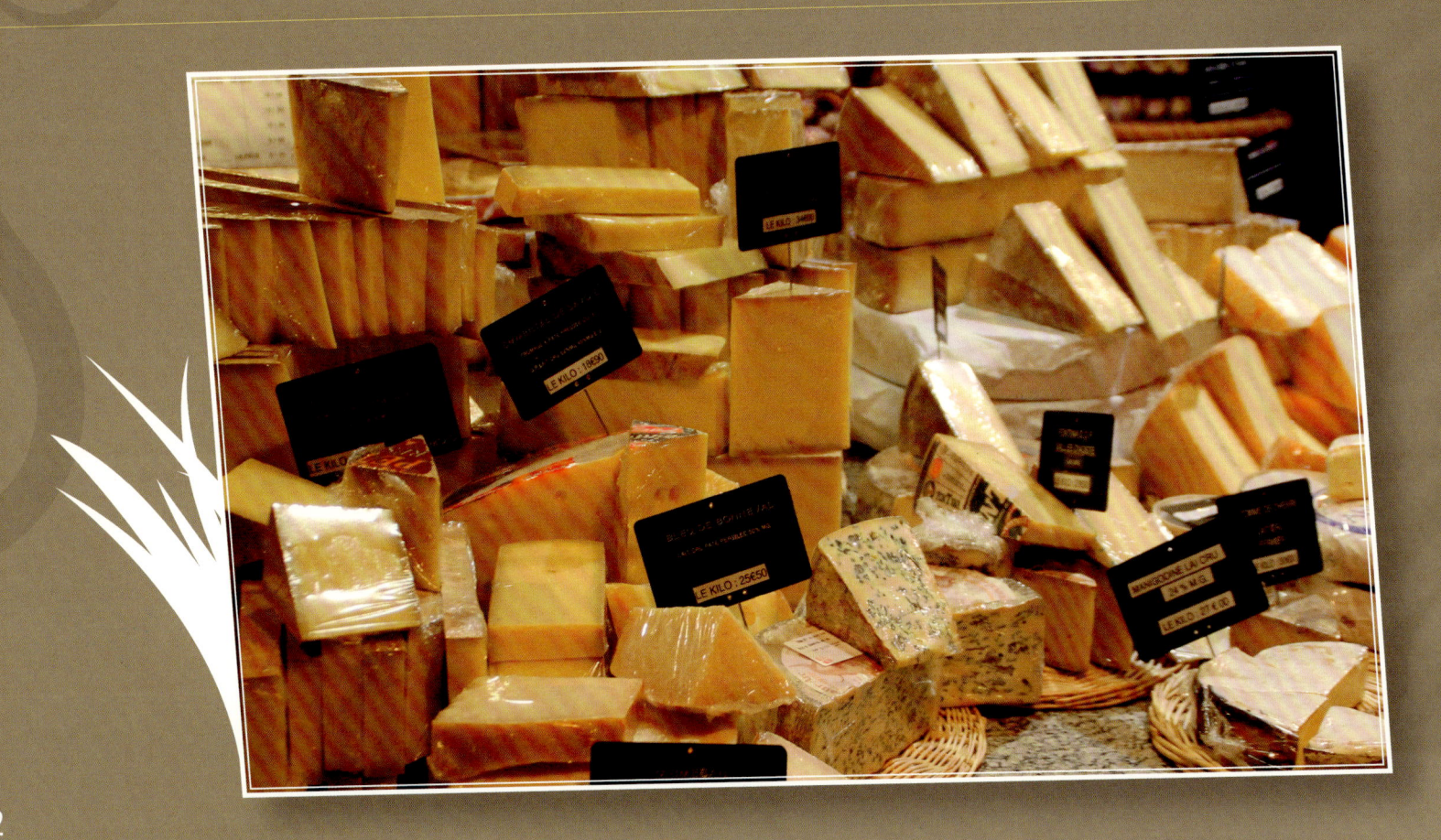

Cheese is produced in four main stages

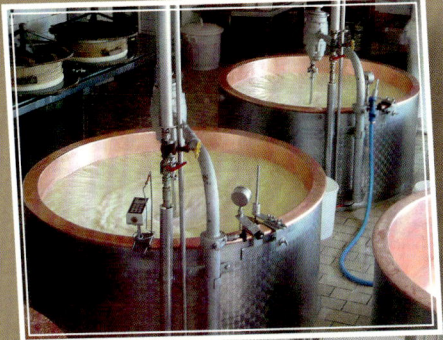

Curdling
In the first stage, a fermenting agent is added to the milk or cream to curdle it, although in some cases this is a natural process caused by the production of lactic acid.

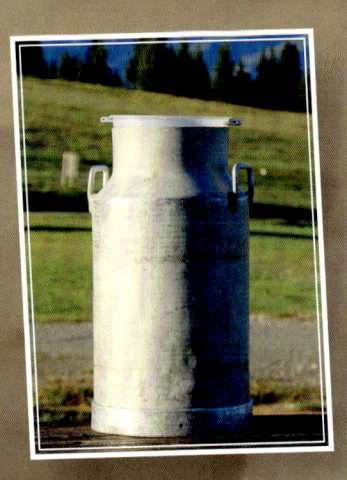

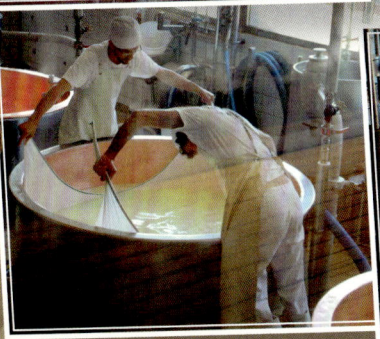

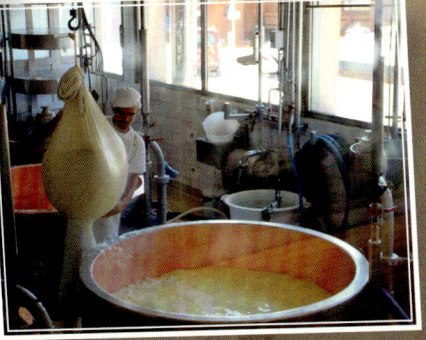

Straining
Whey is strained from the curd. This can be done by using a press or by leaving the curd in a cloth to drain naturally. It will depend on the type of cheese required as to how much it is strained.

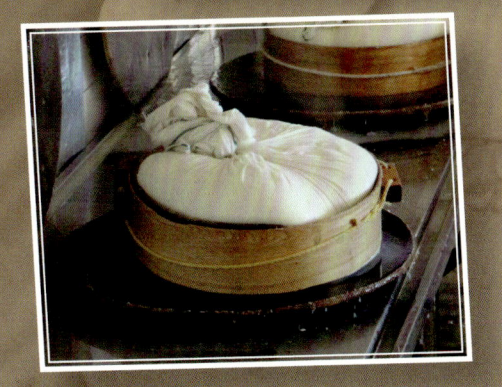

Salting and moulding
Adding salt, which can be done by soaking it in a brine bath, is an integral part of manufacturing. This not only preserves the cheese but has an impact on the flavour and texture, and also forms the outer crust. The curd is then placed in different moulds depending on the required shape.

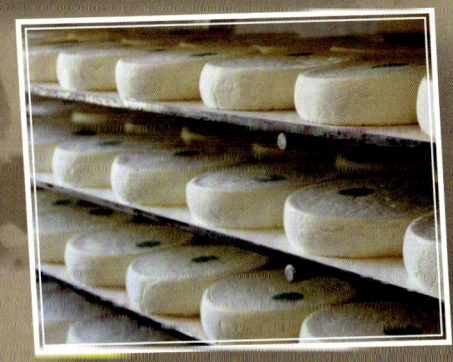

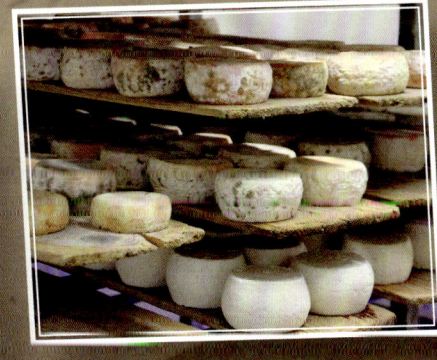

Maturing
Depending on the type of cheese, it is then matured in a cellar for several days, months, or years. With time, the cheese becomes harder and fuller in flavour.

Cheese
Le fromage

The types of cheeses

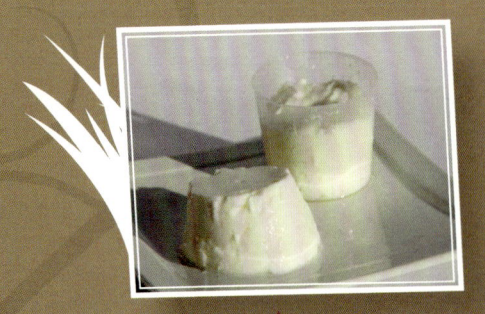

SPECIAL CHEESES:

Fresh cheeses | *Fromages frais*
(*Fromage blanc, Faisselles, Petit Suisse*, etc.)
Fresh cheeses are not left to mature. They are curdled naturally and only briefly strained, hence their refreshing taste and light texture.

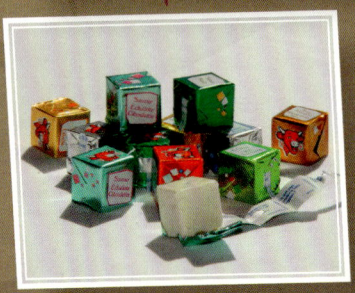

Processed cheese | *Fromages à pâte fondue*
(*Apéricube®, La vache qui rit®*, etc.)
Processed cheeses are a combination of soft and hard cheeses mixed with other milk products (such as butter, etc.)

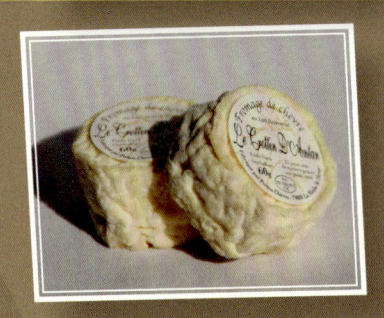

Goat's cheeses | *Fromages de chèvre*
(*Chabichou, Crottin de Chavignol, Picodon, Pélardon, Rocamadour*, etc.)
Unlike other cheeses, they can be eaten at four or five stages of maturity.
When fresh, they are soft and creamy but they become chalky and bitter as they mature. They are whiter than cows' cheeses and the flavour is more pronounced. Shapes and sizes vary; pyramid, brick, log ...

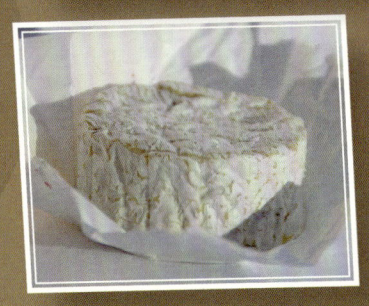

SOFT CHEESES:

Cheeses with a fluffy white coating | *Fromages à croûte fleurie*
(*Brie, Camembert, Coulommiers, Neufchâtel*, etc.)
These soft and creamy cheeses are easily recognisable by their edible, velvety white coating. They are often made with pasteurised milk and soften as they mature.

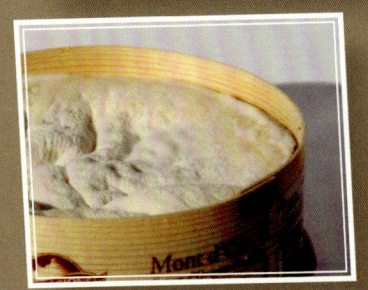

Cheeses with a washed rind | *Fromages à croûte lavée*
(*Epoisses, Munster, Livarot, Maroilles, Mont d'Or, Reblochon*, etc.)
These soft cheeses are regularly washed or brushed with brine and sometimes beer or wine during the maturing process. The rind is smooth and often orange coloured. They have a delicate to strong flavour with a pronounced perfume.

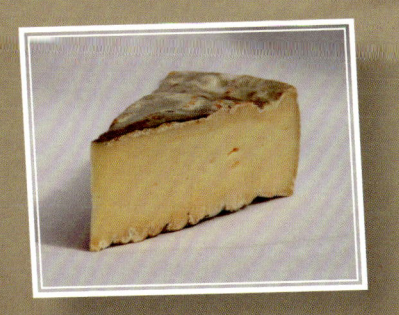

SEMI-SOFT CHEESES:

Uncooked cheeses / *Fromages à pâte non-cuite*

(*Cantal, Morbier, Raclette, Tome de Savoie, Saint Nectaire*, etc.)
These cheeses are matured for a fairly long period of time, in a cool, very damp atmosphere (7 – 10°C with 90% humidity). They have a dense texture, a pale yellow colour and a fruity, sweet flavour.

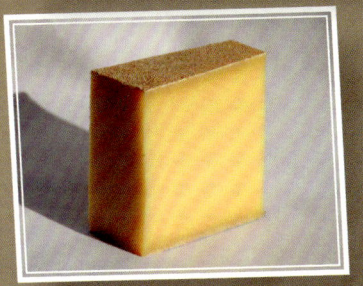

Cooked cheeses / *Fromages à pâte cuite*

(*Abondance, Beaufort, Comté, Emmental, Gruyère*, etc.)
These are 'cooked' cheeses in that the curd has been heated to make a firmer and more compact cheese. The maturing process lasts from 4 – 18 months and a whole round can weigh up to 130 kg.

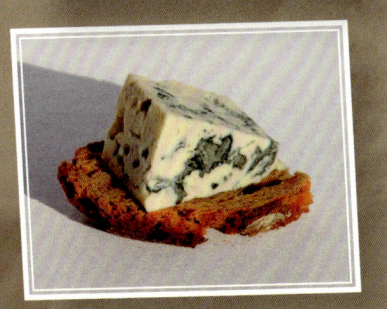

Blue cheeses / *Fromages à pâte persillée*

(*Bleu d'Auvergne, Bleu de Bresse, Fourme d'Ambert, Roquefort*, etc.)
Blue cheeses are made by injecting starter bacteria into the cheese with long needles. The bacterial growth results in blue-green veins which run along the natural grain of the cheese. Whether creamy or crumbly, dry or firm, blue cheeses, although very different, have the same piquant, almost peppery flavour.

HARD CHEESES:

These are strong, dry cheeses mostly made by craftsmen in rural areas. They can be stored easily and are consumed by shepherds and people working outdoors.

Serving cheese

Cheese is always served at the end of the main course before the dessert, with red wine-which is said to counteract the cholesterol found in cheese-and is very much part of French tradition and culture. Ideally they should be removed from their packaging and left at cool room temperature for about an hour before serving.

The perfect cheese plate should include one semi-soft, one blue and one or two soft cheeses and served with a basket of fresh, crusty bread.

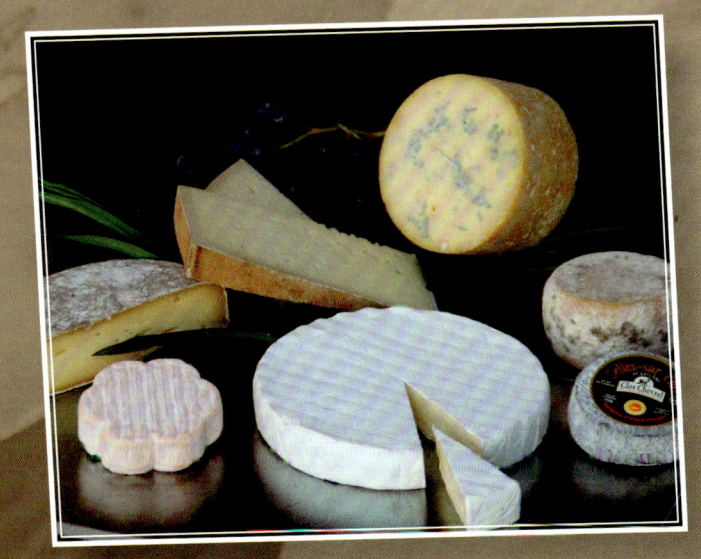

Cheese / *Le fromage*

Production of a semi-soft cheese Beaufort

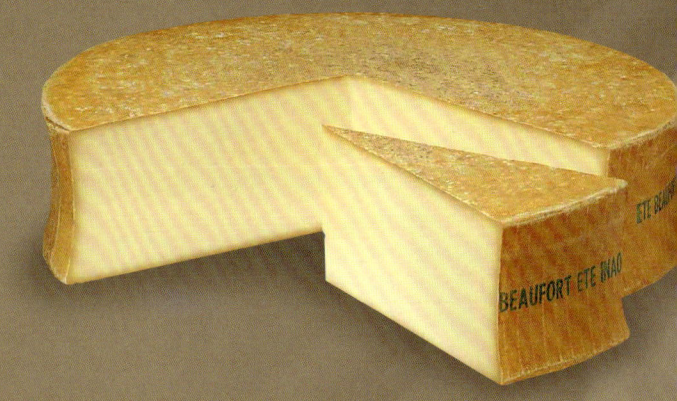

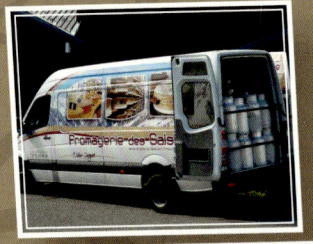

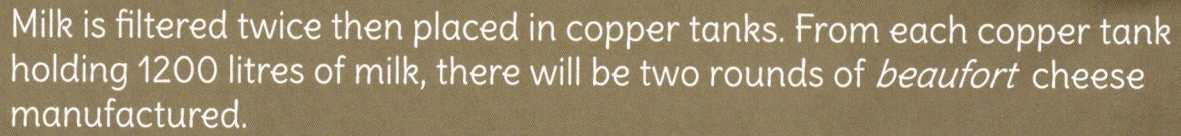

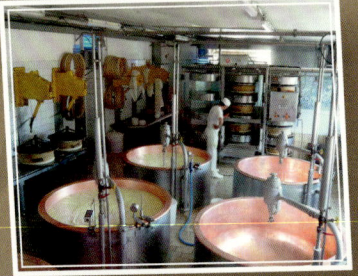

Milk is filtered twice then placed in copper tanks. From each copper tank holding 1200 litres of milk, there will be two rounds of *beaufort* cheese manufactured.

Milk is heated to 32°-34°C and rennet is added to help the milk coagulate. The curds are cut with a curd slice and then is heated up to a temperature of 52°-55°C in only 30-40 minutes. This process separates the curd and whey.

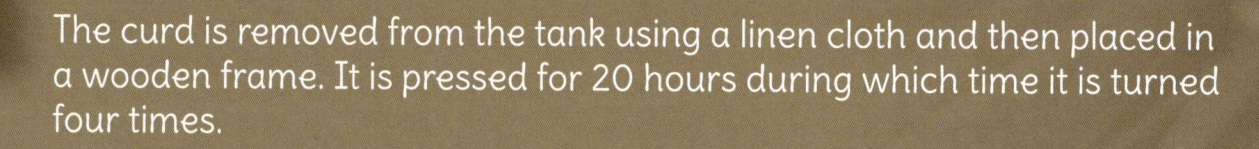

The curd is removed from the tank using a linen cloth and then placed in a wooden frame. It is pressed for 20 hours during which time it is turned four times.

It is allowed to rest in a cellar for 24 hours, then immersed in saturated brine for the first stage of salting.

Each round of cheese is weighed before going into the cellar for maturing. This takes from a minimum of 5 months until 18 months. It is left in a constant temperature of about 8°C and 96% humidity. Twice a week it is turned and brushed with brine.

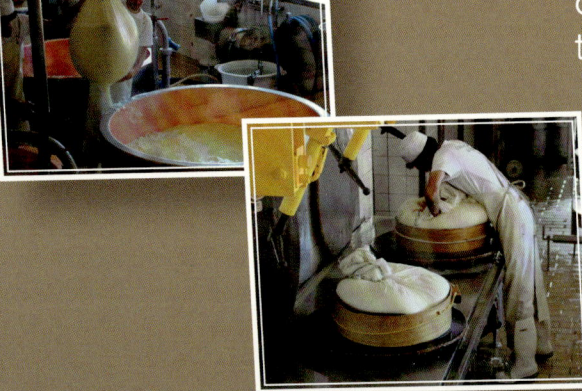

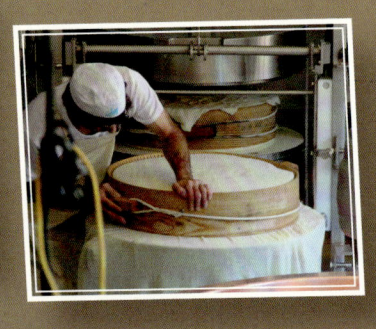

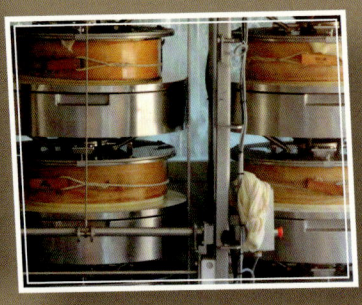

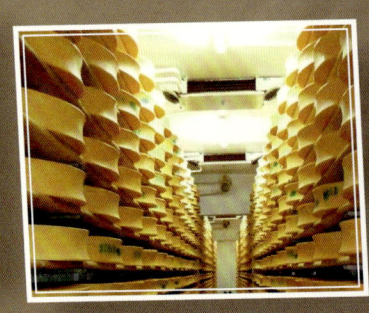

Maturing process of blue cheese Fourme de Montbrison

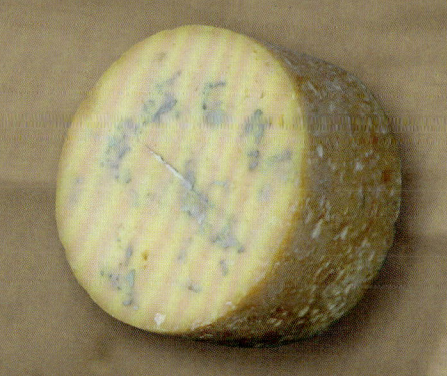

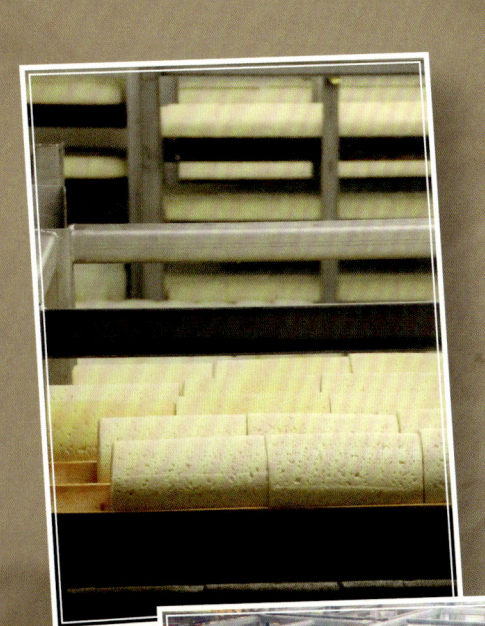

Cheeses are removed from their moulds and then placed on spruce channels.
It is during this time that the beautiful orange crust develops.

The cheeses are turned twice a day for 4 - 8 days, before being placed in a refining cellar.

After a few weeks, they are pricked with long needles.
Oxygen enables the blue to develop.

Cheeses remain in the cellar for about two and a half months before being sold.
The cellar is fed by a very cold stream and remains at a constant temperature of approximately 10°C.

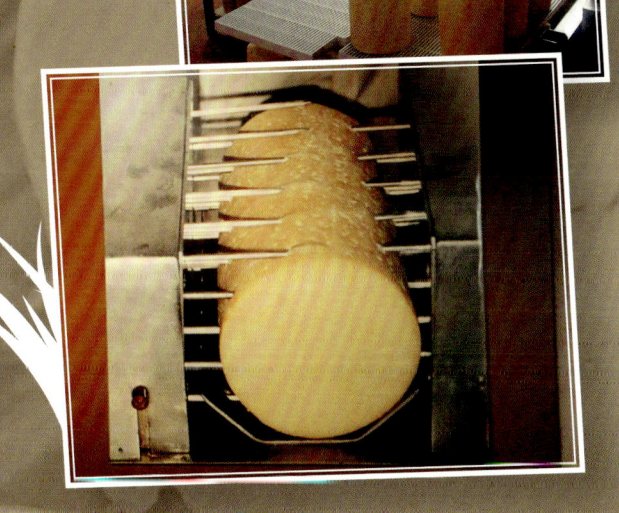

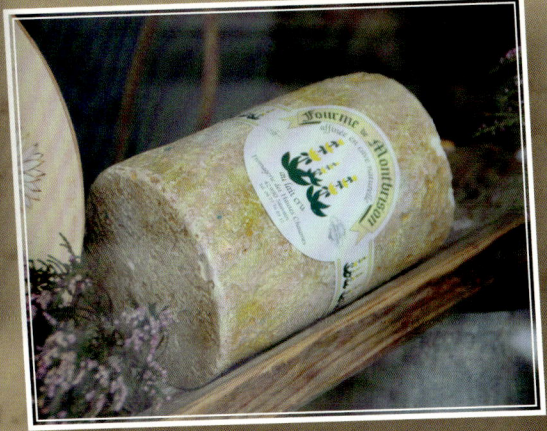

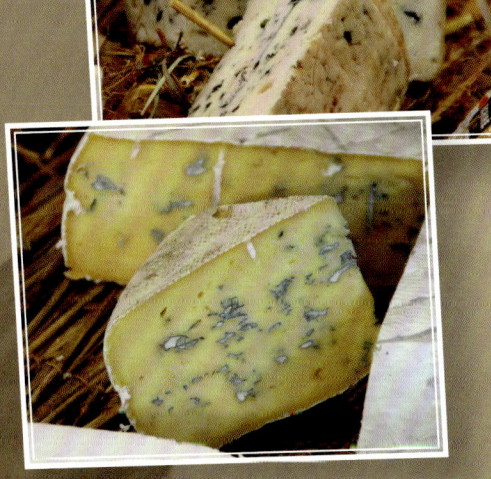

Cheese *Le fromage*

Other types of blue cheeses:

267

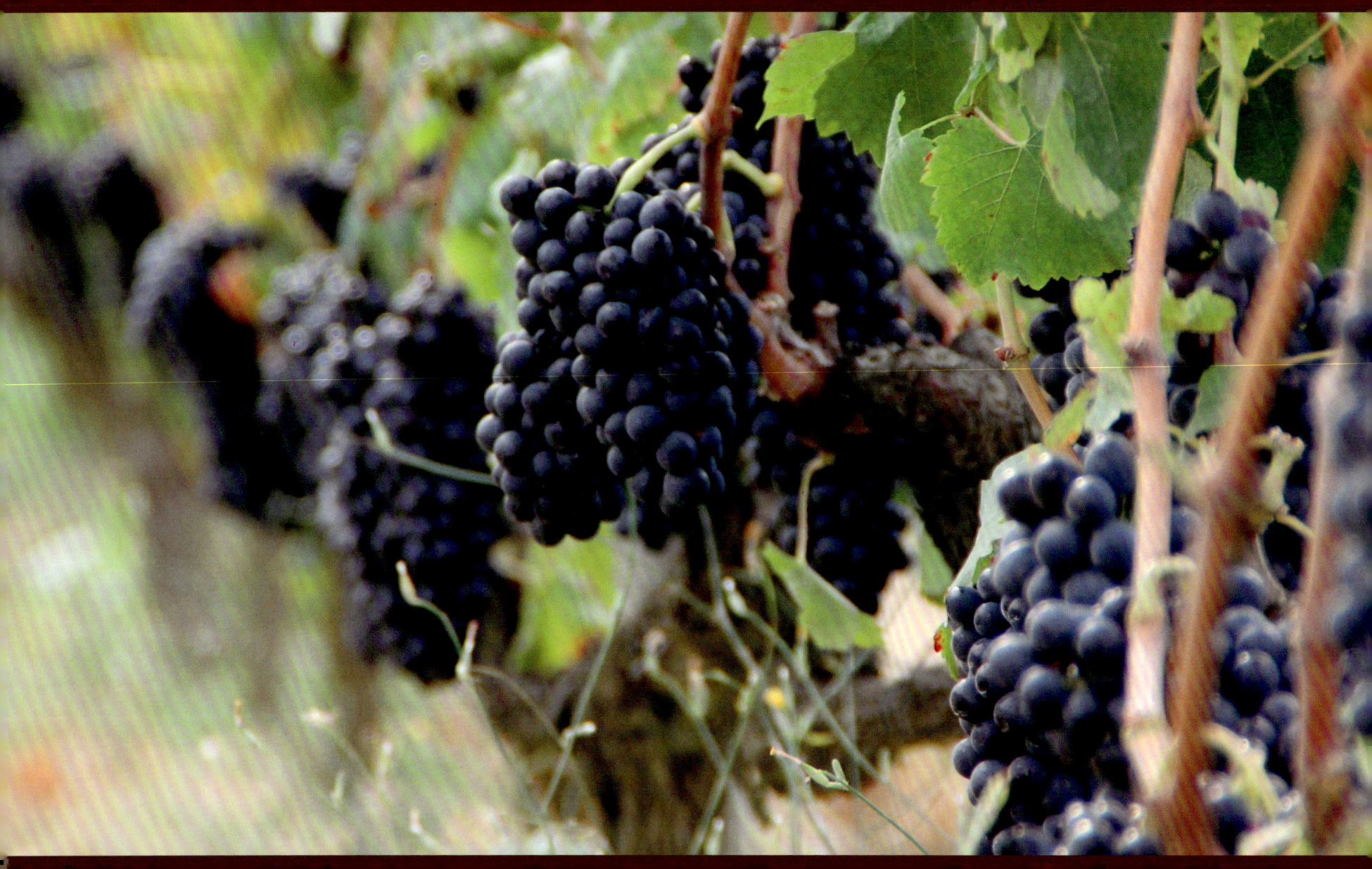

French Wines

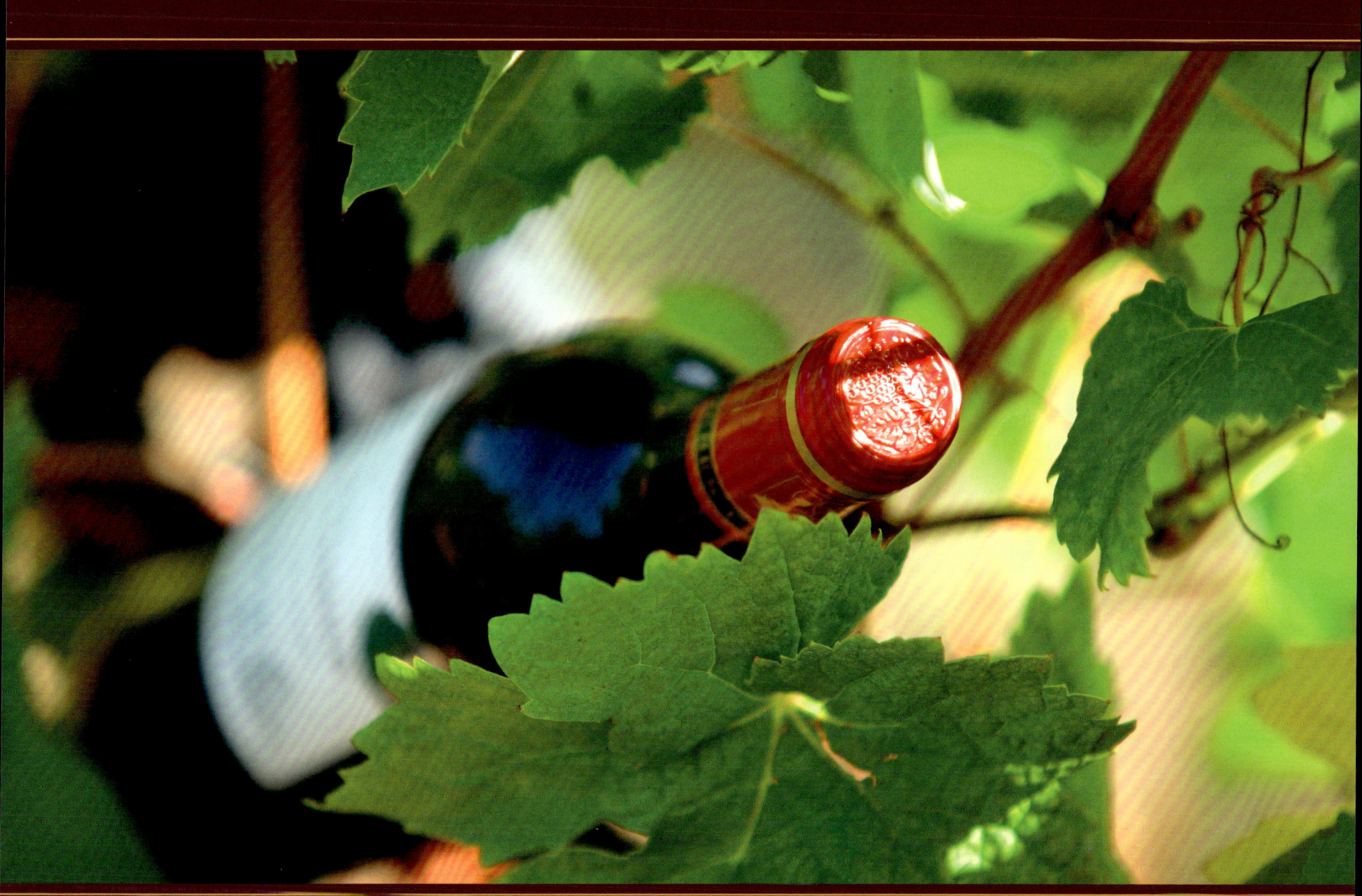

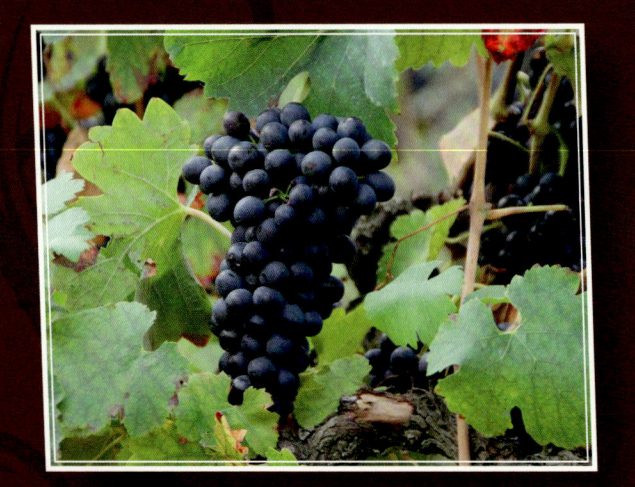

From the vineyard... to the bottle

Wine is not produced by itself, and the profession of a winegrower is perhaps one of the most difficult and delicate that there is. Firstly, harvesting is crucial. A conscientious winemaker will gather cluster samples three times a week during harvest time to analyse the grapes. Once they have reached their peak sweetness and acidity has sufficiently decreased, he will start harvesting without further delay, as long as the weather remains dry and clear. While gathering clusters, any damaged grapes are discarded.

The different stages during the development of a wine will differ depending on the type of wine: red, rosé or white.

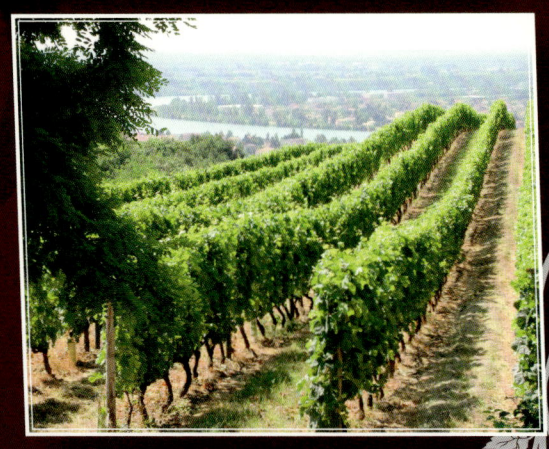

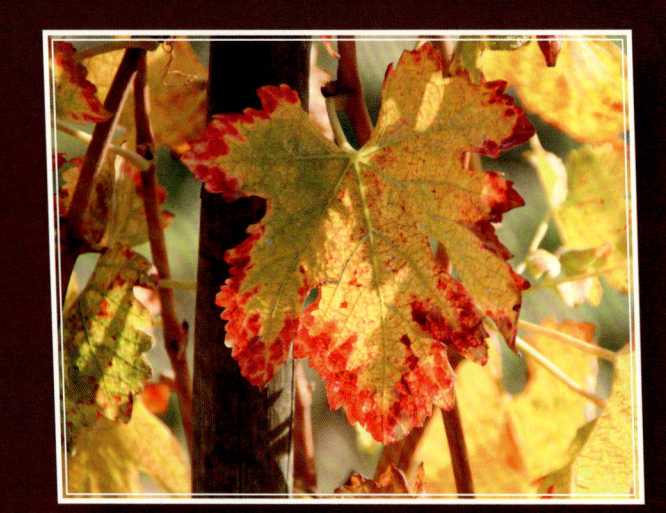

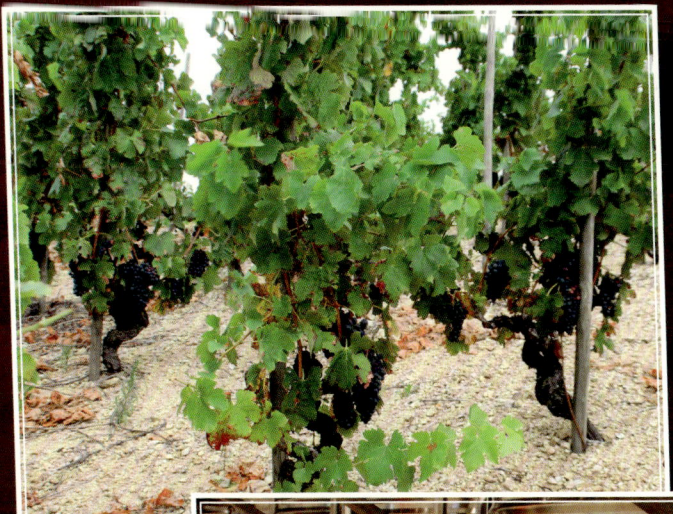

The quality of grapes varies from one year to another, according to the weather conditions which have a significant impact on the character of the wine. They are allowed to ferment without any addition of sugars, acids, water or enzymes. If there is a particularly good year, the quality of the wine is greatly improved, and many wine-enthusiasts would save bottles of a good vintage wine for future consumption; good-quality wine improves in flavour, if it is stored correctly.

The quality of each vintage year is described as either excellent (*excellente*), very good (*très bonne*), good (*bonne*), or average (*moyenne*). **Those with an *excellente* vintage date are the ones which improve with keeping!** The vintage date shown on the label of the wine bottle corresponds with the year the fruits were harvested and not the date when it was bottled.

The sweetness of wine is determined by the amount of residual sugar in the wine after fermentation as compared to the acidity in the wine.

Because of their composition, some wines should be drunk when they are still new, whereas others improve with age. A new wine is fruitier, sharper and fresher compared to an older wine, which is softer and its aroma and flavours are heavier and more complex.

Wine
Le vin

Storing wine

Some wines can improve with age, but they can also rapidly deteriorate if kept in inadequate conditions. **The three factors that have the most direct impact on wine are light, humidity and temperature.**

Ideally, the bottles must be stored on their sides—so that the cork is in contact with the wine—in a cellar, with a constant temperature of 12°C - 16°C and an airy atmosphere.

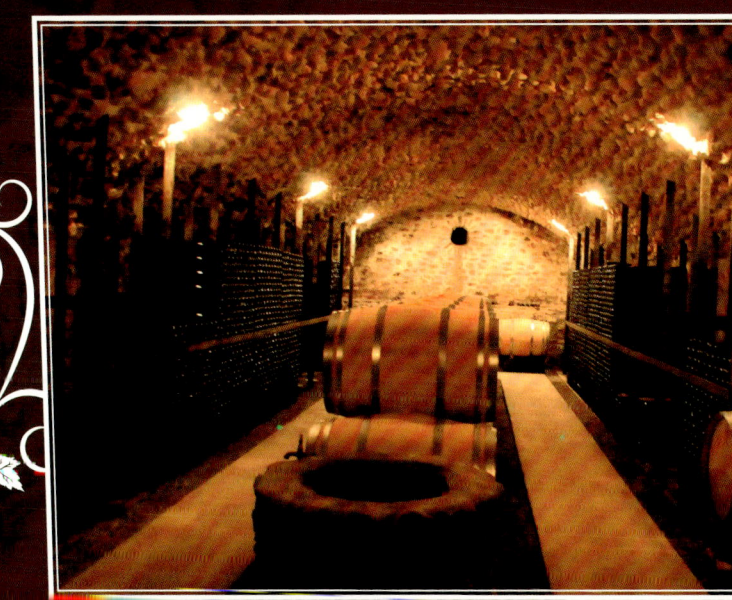

Serving wine

The art of choosing a wine from the vast selection available to accompany a given dish is a challenging one. The season and the occasion need to be taken into account.

In summer a white or rosé wine is preferred whereas in winter a stronger red is appreciated.

In general, the order of serving wine is as follows:

- If offering both red and white wine during a meal, the white would always be served before the red.
- Light wines precede those which are full bodied, and dry wines are drunk before sweet wines or liqueurs.
- New wines are served before older ones.
- Dry sparkling wine (e.g. champagne) should be served as an *apéritif* to open up the taste buds and not a sweet wine or liqueur that would overpower all the flavours of the meal to come.

WHITE WINE:

- Sharp, dry white wines are a good accompaniment to seafood, cold first courses and fried fish.
- Softer white wines go well with fish, certain white meats (especially poultry), shellfish in sauce, *foie gras* and soft blue cheeses.

RED WINE:

- Soft, fruity red wines are served with *charcuterie*, tarts, white meats, goat's cheese and other milder cheeses.
- Full-bodied red wine is reserved for red meats, game, duck and strong flavoured cheese.

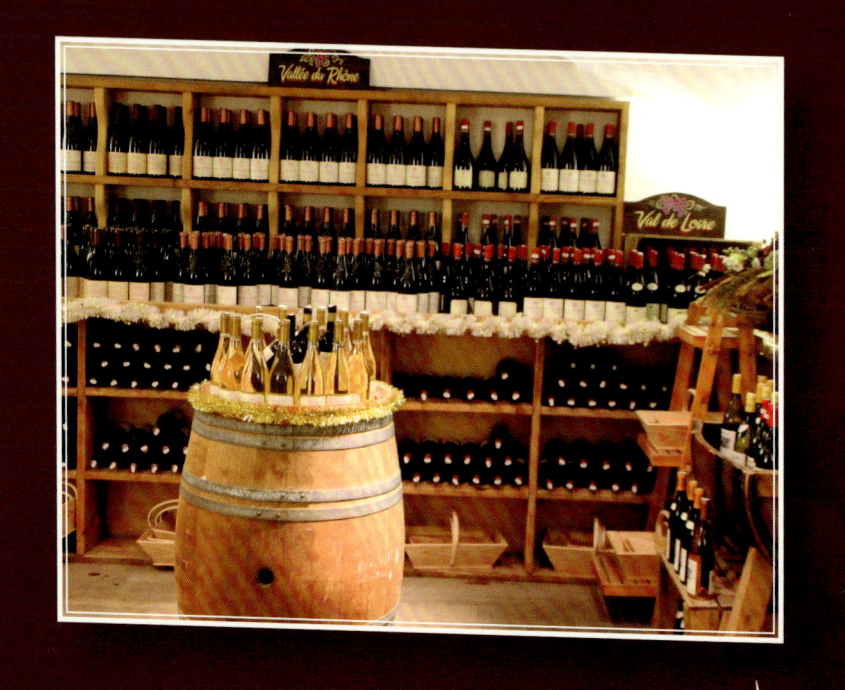

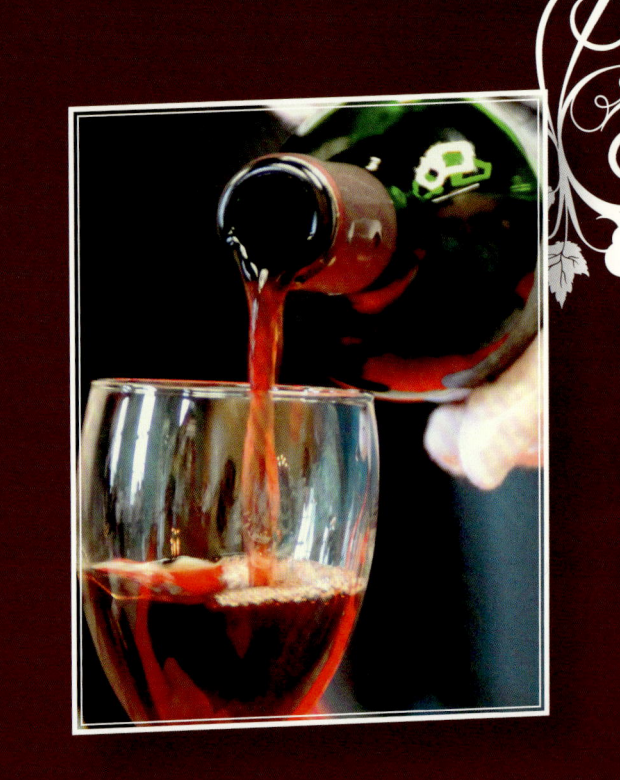

Opening a bottle of wine

When opening a bottle of wine take care not to shake it first, in case there is any sediment at the bottom.

Some wines should be opened for at least an hour before serving and allow them to 'breathe' whilst others are best served immediately after opening. Older red wines, and particularly *Bordeaux*, should be opened in advance, although in some cases the older wines can lose their flavour if allowed to aerate for too long. Sometimes younger wines 'relax' the flavour if allowed to be exposed to the air for a little while, making it smoother.

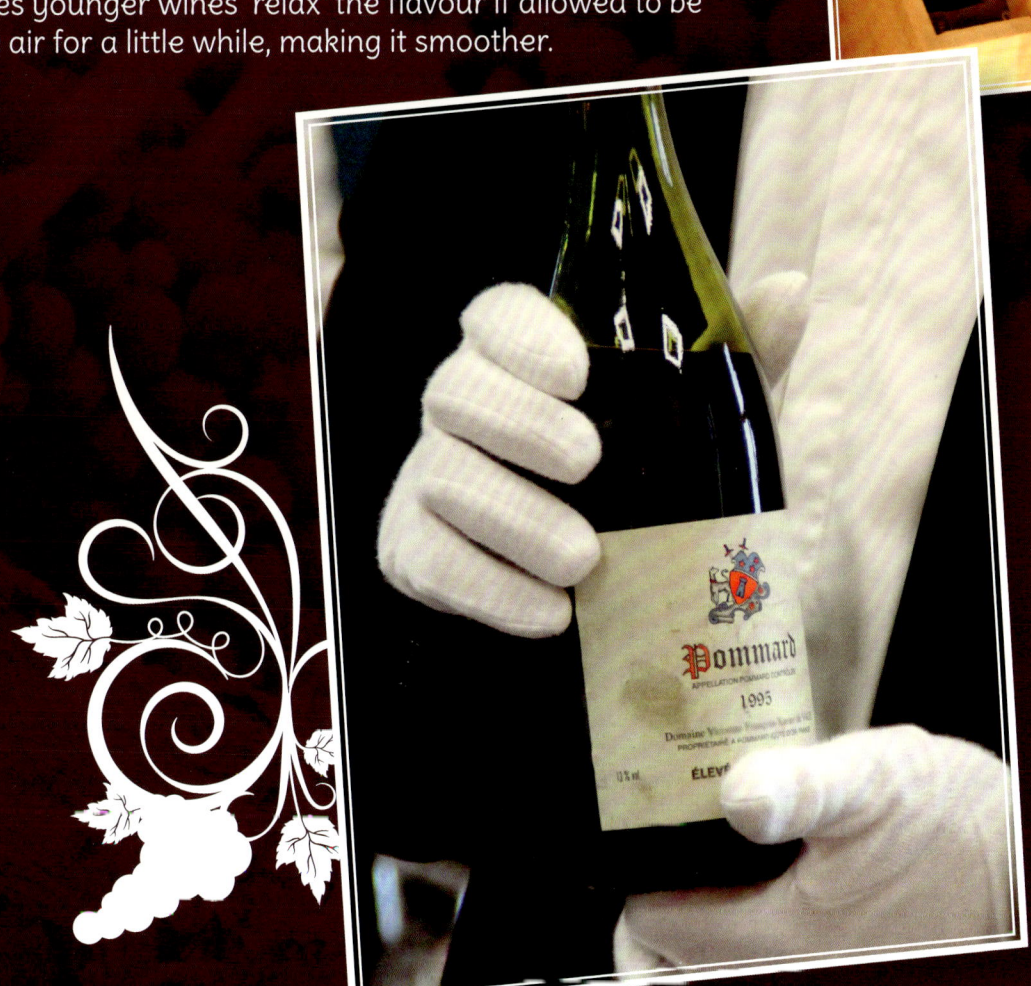

Wine
Le vin

A good temperature for serving wine

WHITE WINES (normally served at cellar temperature)

- Sweet or dry, light wines: 9°C – 10°C
- Dry and medium dry wines: 11°C – 12°C
- Good quality, dry wines: 13°C – 14°C

ROSÉ WINES

- Light wines: 9°C – 10°C
- Classic wines: 11°C – 12°C

RED WINES (normally served at room temperature)

- Light, fruity wines: 11°C -12°C
- *Beaujolais*, sweet red wines: 13°C – 14°C
- *Bourgogne, Rhône, Loire* and medium red wines: 15°C – 16°C
- *Pinot noir*: 16°C - 18°C
- *Bordeaux* and good quality red wines: 17°C – 18°C
- Red wines of exceptional quality: 18°C – 21°C

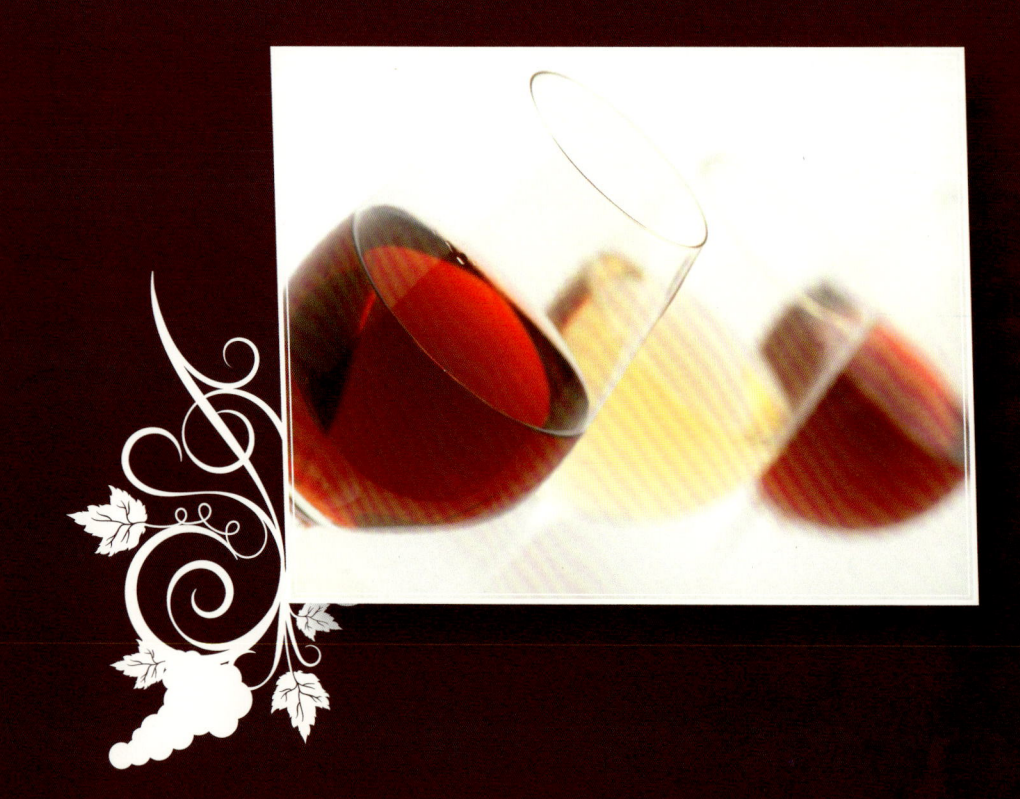

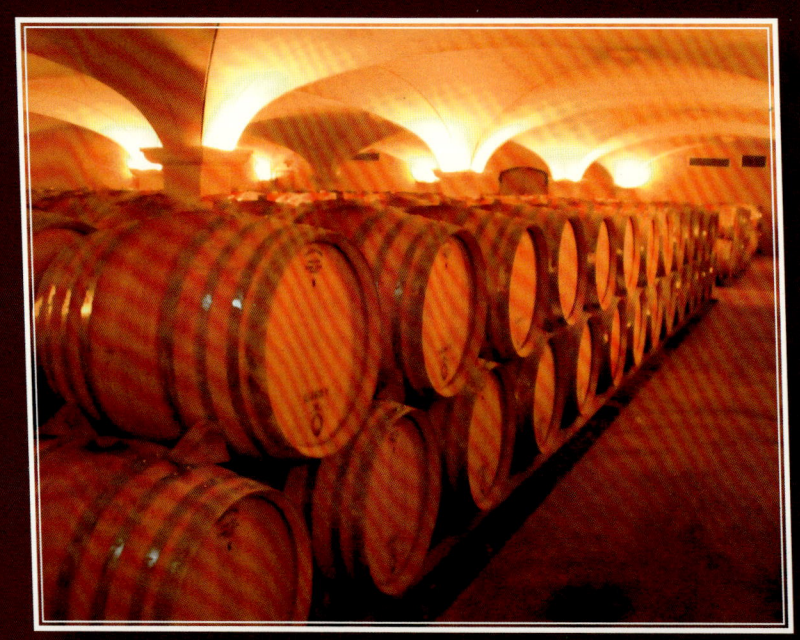

ENJOY RESPONSIBLY

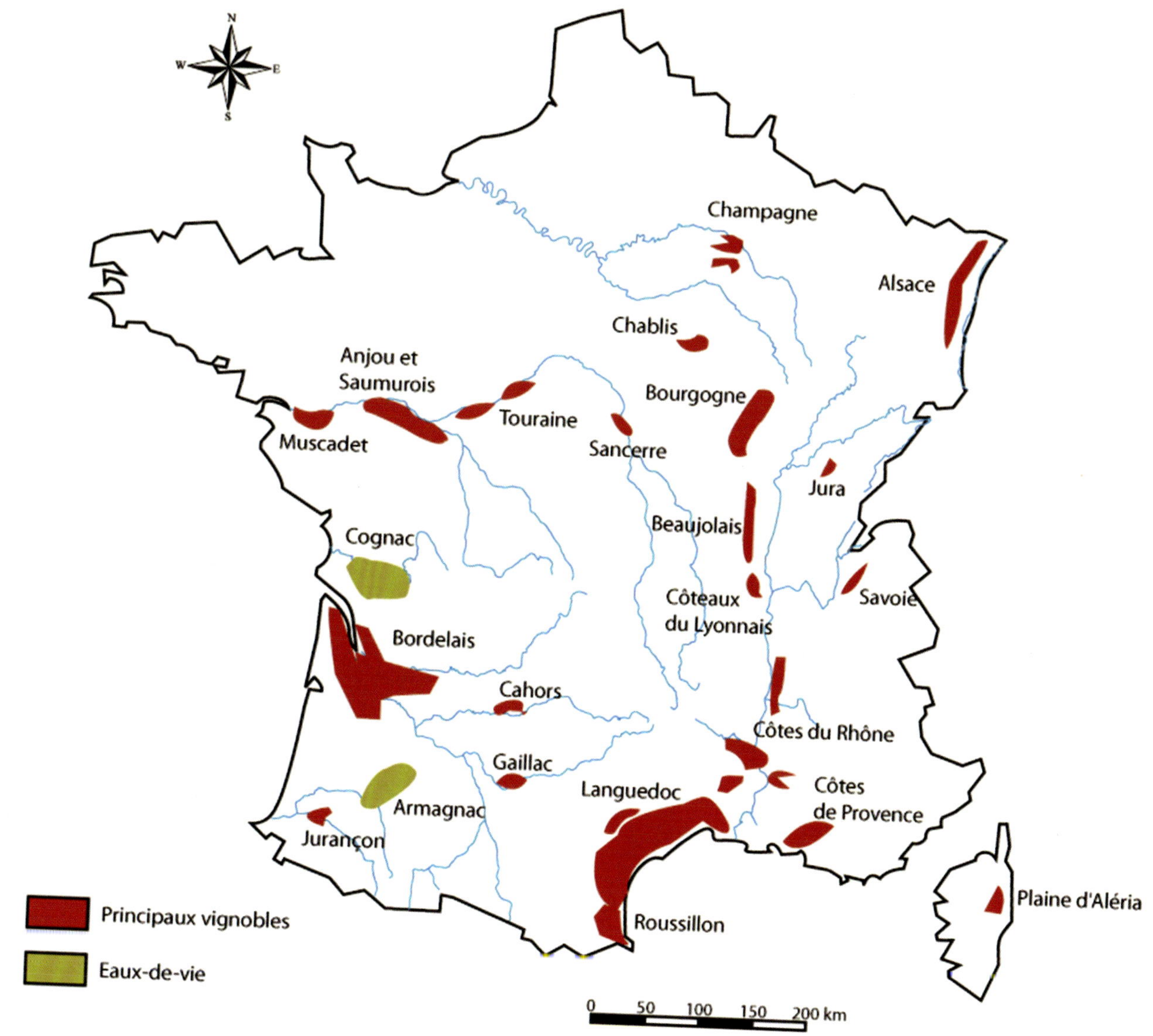
N
S
E
W
Champagne
Alsace
Chablis
Anjou et Saumurois
Bourgogne
Touraine
Muscadet
Sancerre
Jura
Beaujolais
Cognac
Côteaux du Lyonnais
Savoie
Bordelais
Cahors
Côtes du Rhône
Gaillac
Languedoc
Côtes de Provence
Armagnac
Jurançon
Plaine d'Aléria
Roussillon
Principaux vignobles
Eaux-de-vie
0 50 100 150 200 km

Champagne

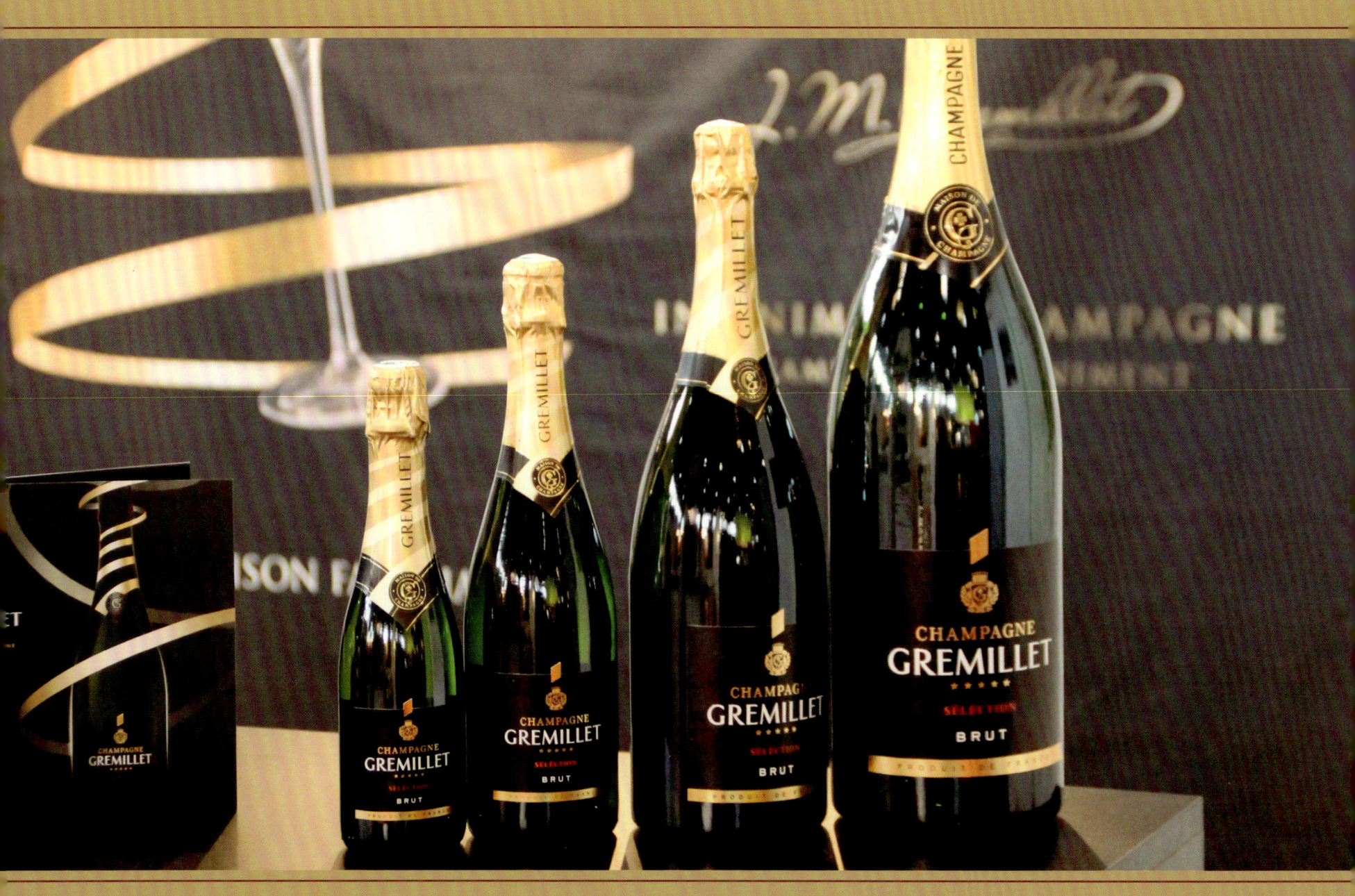

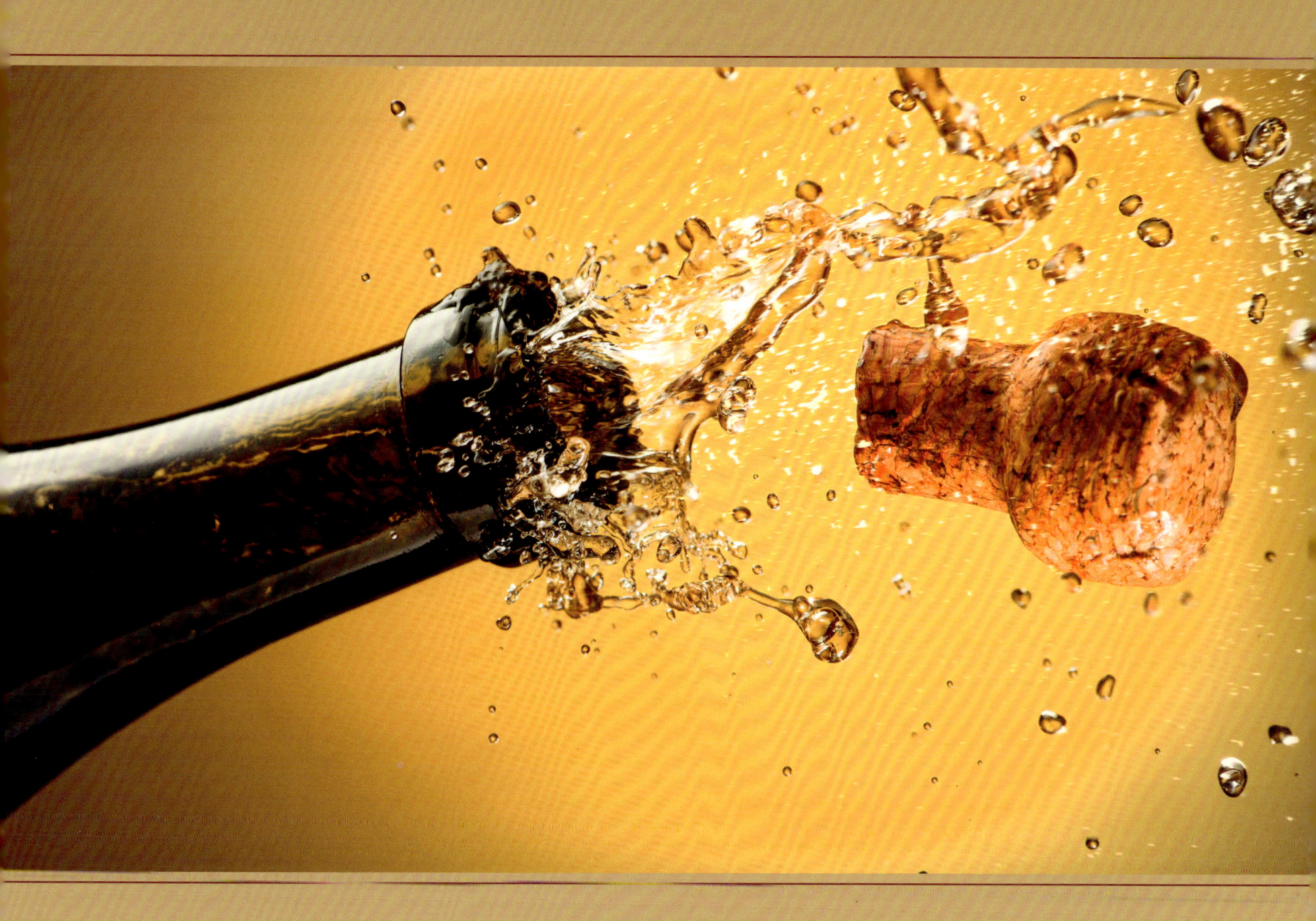

Champagne
Le champagne

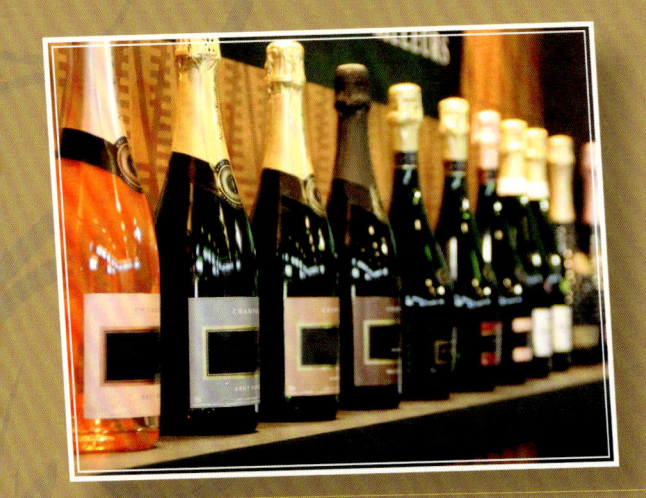

Champagne is a sparkling wine produced from grapes which are grown on chalky, sun-exposed hillsides in the Champagne region. Certain requirements of viticulture such as pruning, vineyard yield, degree of pressing and the length of time that the wine must stay on its lees before bottling, must be adhered to before a sparkling wine can be called 'champagne'.

The types of grapes used are *pinot noir*, *pinot meunier* and *chardonnay* although there are some other types allowed. The wine produced can be a blend of the types selected.

Production of champagne

The initial quality of the grapes is necessary for producing good champagne. The chalk, clay and limestone soil in the Champagne region is ideal for the vineyards: it reflects the sun, absorbs the heat and retains the necessary moisture to the roots. However, it requires many complex operations and skill of oenologists (wine experts).

Harvesting and pressing
In September the grapes are hand-picked when they are at optimum ripeness. They are sorted by vintages and varieties and are gently pressed to obtain the juice (known as the must) which is then decanted to clear any impurities.

Fermentation
The must is poured into vats for a first fermentation. A still wine is produced from this process.

Blending of wines
Originally champagne was produced from a single harvest but quality was inconsistent due to the variable weather conditions in Champagne, and therefore variation in quality of grapes. Blending together different harvests helps to promote regularity and consistency of style and quality.

This can be done by blending wines from different *crus* (growth)—as no two *crus* are the same—or by blending wines made from different but complementary types of grapes or adding wines from previous years. This stage is the masterpiece of champagne requiring experienced talent to balance and harmonise flavours and aromas.

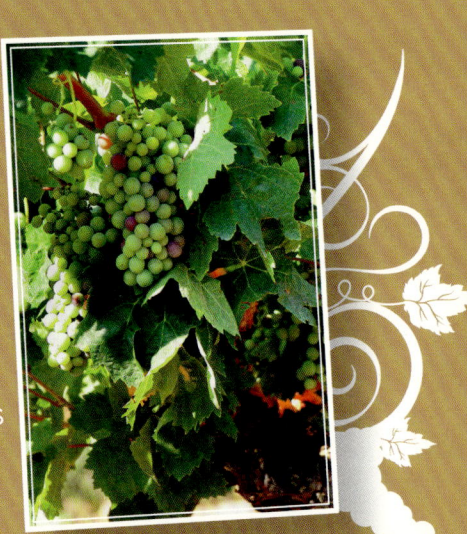

Secondary fermentation

Before bottling, a quantity of *liqueur de tirage* is added to the wine. This is a still champagne wine with sugar and yeast added. It is then bottled and sealed with a stopper then held in place by a wire cage or metal cap. The bottles are kept in a cellar (11°C - 12°C) and left on their sides. This second fermentation lasts for six to eight weeks and it is during this time that the still wine is transformed to sparkling wine (*prise de mousse*).

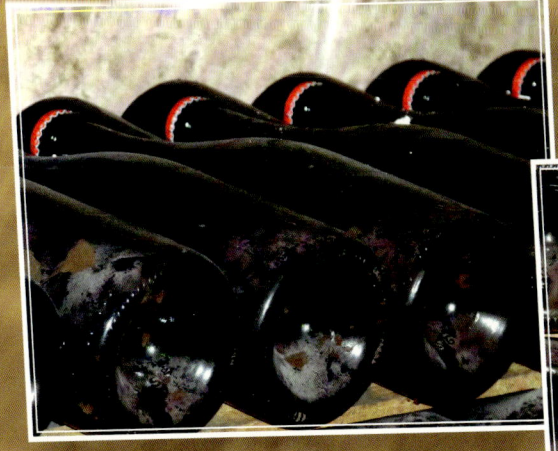

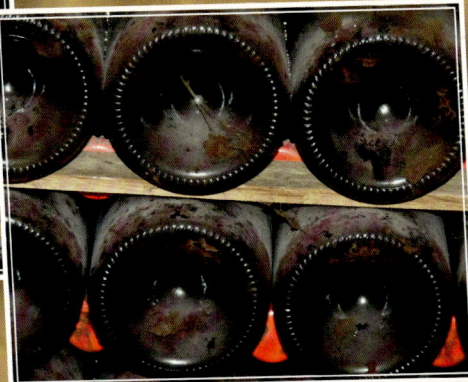

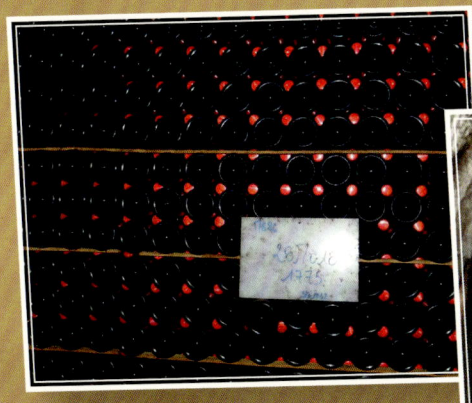

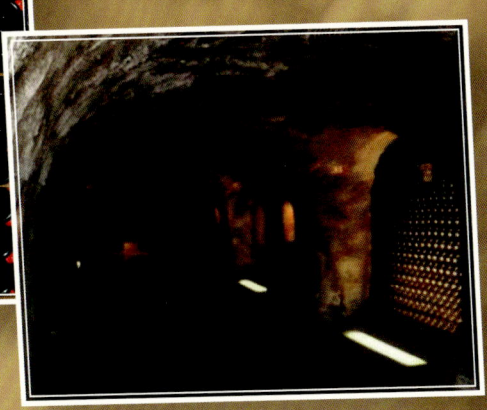

Ageing

The bottles remain deep inside the cellars at a constant temperature of 12°C for a long time—the greatest champagnes can spend several decades maturing in the cellar. The minimum ageing periods required by law for champagne are much longer than any other sparkling European wine. During this time the special stopper allows minute quantities of oxygen to enter the bottles and minute quantities of carbon dioxide to escape. The sugar is consumed and the yeast decomposes.

Champagne
Le champagne

Turning the bottles-riddling

Towards the end of their resting period, the bottles are rotated to loosen the sediment. To eliminate the build-up of these deposits, bottles are arranged on rotation stands or pallets with the neck down. They are rotated daily an eighth or a quarter turn for six to eight weeks. Finally, the deposit concentrates in the neck of the bottle.

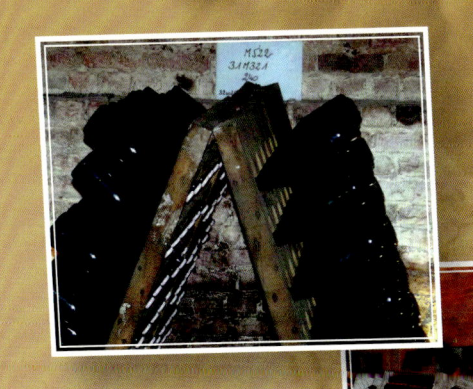

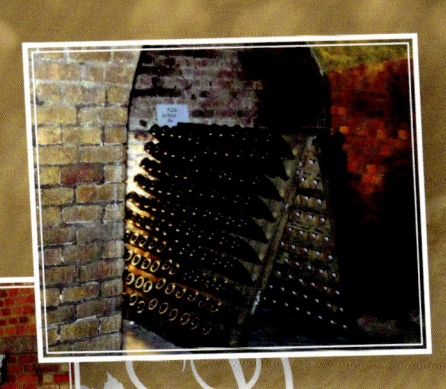

Disgorgement and dosage

This is the critical point after years of ageing. The neck of the bottle is plunged into a refrigerating solution (-27°C), freezing the collected sediment. When the bottle is opened, the sediment is ejected due to the pressure of the trapped carbon dioxide. A small quantity of *liqueur de dosage* is added to replenish the bottle. The dosage is varied in proportions of sugar to suit the style of wine.

Bottling

The bottles are immediately sealed with a cork covered with a protective metal cap. It is then shaken vigorously to allow the dosage to mix with the wine.

Below is a list of the different types of champagne with the residual sugar per litre:

Extra Brut	up to 6 g
Brut	6 g - 12 g
Extra sec	12 g - 17 g
Sec	17 g - 32 g
Demi-sec	32 g - 50 g
Doux	50 g and over

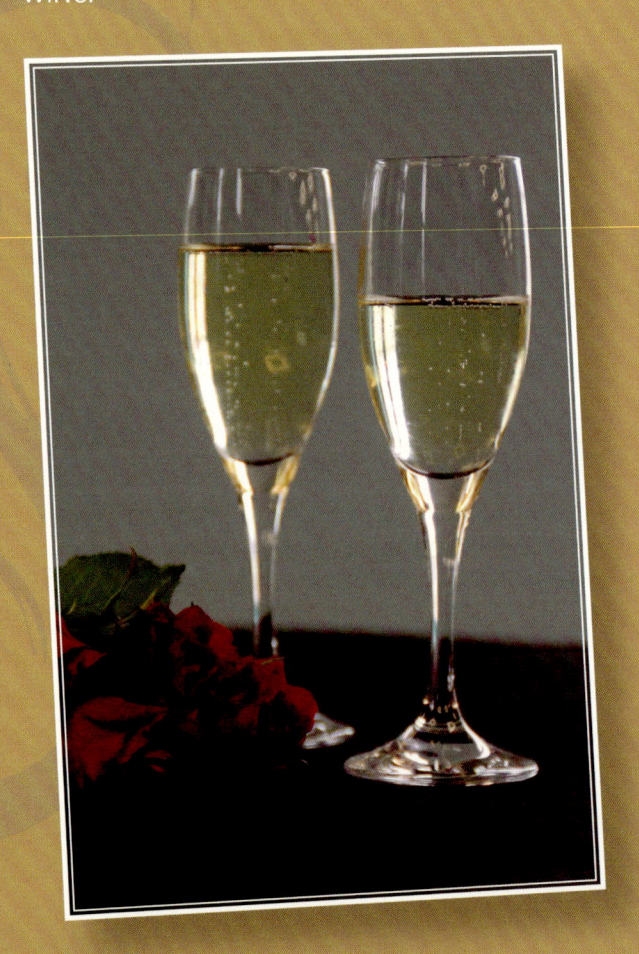

Champagne-a developing history

Champagne wine has a long history but since its first real steps in the 17th century it has experienced explosive growth.

Champagne was accidently discovered in France when wine was bottled before it had finished fermentation, causing the bottles to explode or their corks to be forced out. This was due to the pressure built up inside during fermentation. It seems that it was Dom Pérignon, a monk, who actually designed the process of this sparkling wine in the late 17th to early 18th century.

In 1728, King Louis XV authorised champagne to be transported in bottles rather than casks and this was the beginning of the champagne trade. It was about this time that the first champagne houses began.

During the 19th century, champagne really expanded internationally and many more champagne houses were created.

Thanks to production being modernised in the 20th century, the champagne market has become more efficient and has grown remarkably—to the delight and pleasure of the rest of the world!

A wine of distinction

Kings were traditionally crowned in Reims and according to history, champagne was used at the coronation banquets, it being recognised for its superior taste and finesse.

Back in the 17th, 18th and 19th centuries, champagne producers used innovative marketing, consistently promoting the image of royalty or aristocracy and presenting it as a luxurious drink but at a reasonable price. **Its fame and reputation spread rapidly beyond its national borders.**

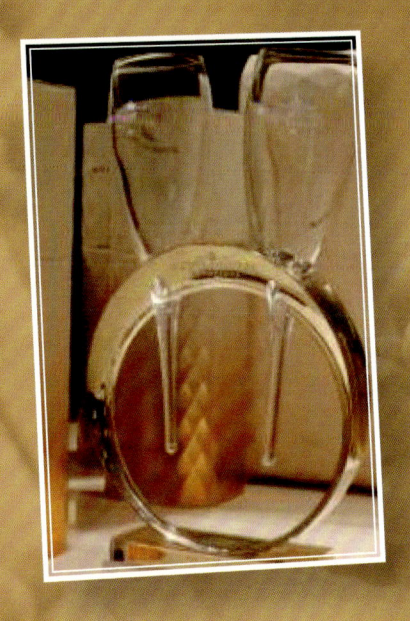

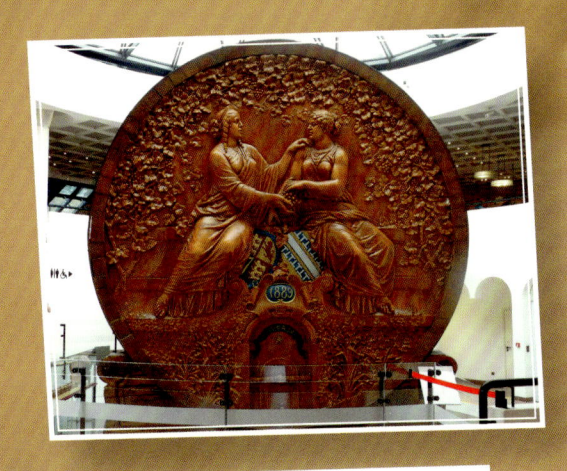

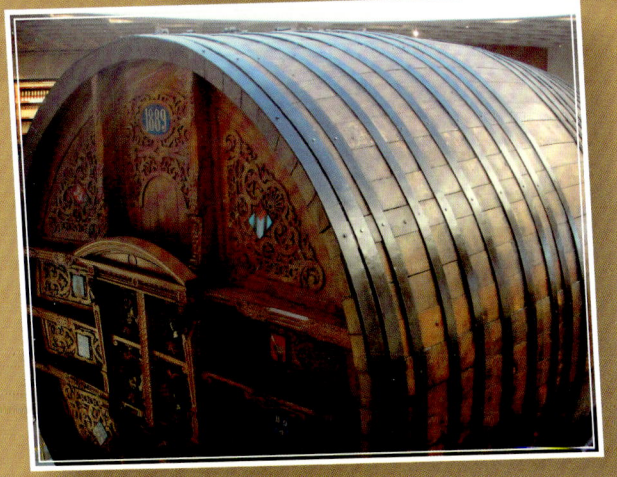

Eugène Mercier exhibited champagne at the Paris world exhibition in 1889 where it won second prize after the Eiffel Tower. He ordered a huge cask to be constructed holding 1600 hectolitres (213 000 bottles of 75 cl). With the help of 24 oxen and 10 men, the cask was taken to Paris where it was exhibited to the rest of the world! Today, it stands in the entrance hall of Mercier's champagne producing house in Epernay.

Champagne has become the favourite choice of wine at many famous and precious moments—whether it is at a christening, marriage, birthday or celebrating a victorious occasion. For example:
- Since the 19th century, champagne has appeared at royal weddings.
- Queen Victoria smashed a bottle of champagne against the hull of HMS Royal Arthur in 1891 as it was being launched, and since then it has become a custom at the inauguration of great ships.
- Champagne was drunk in celebration of Concorde's maiden voyage.
- As the French and English sections of the Channel tunnel met, it was celebrated with champagne.
- Sport victories are celebrated by spraying champagne on both the champions and the public.

Even Sir Winston Churchill (1874-1965) understood champagne's true value as he is quoted to have said, "Remember gentleman, it's not just France we are fighting for, it's Champagne".

Whatever the reason, without question, champagne is the aristocrat of wine and whatever celebration—it has to be champagne!

Champagne
Le champagne

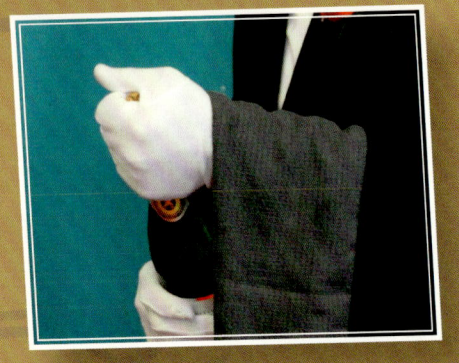

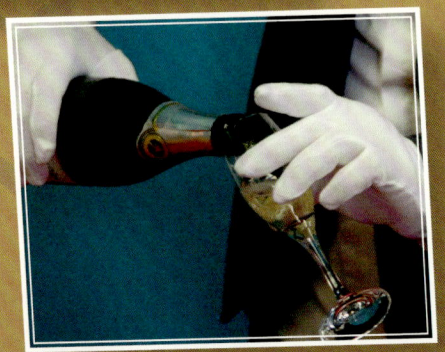

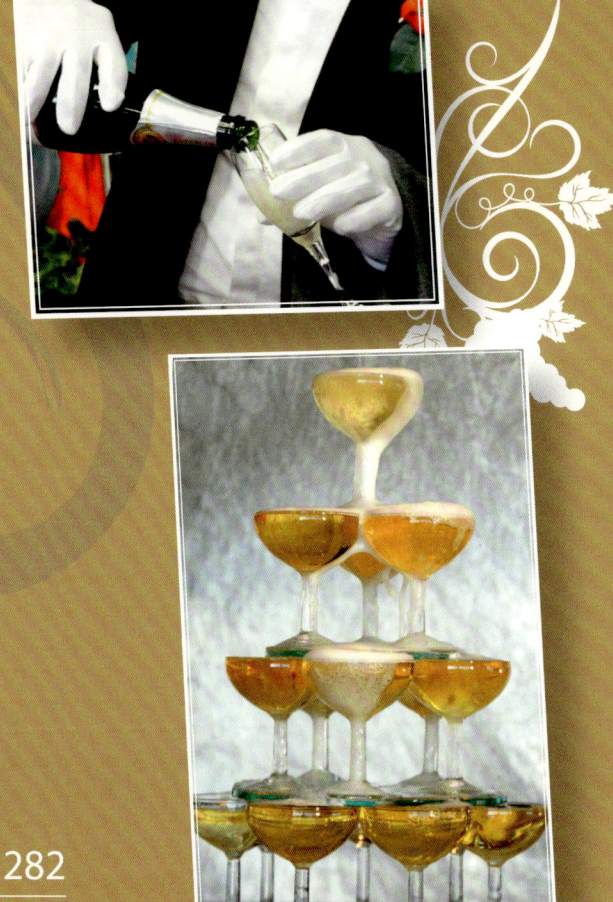

Serving Champagne

At what point in the meal should champagne be served

Champagne should be drunk primarily as an *apéritif*, but it can also be served at any time during a meal, if the menu is appropriate.

However, **it is an error to serve most champagne, especially dry champagne, with the dessert,** as the sugar in the dessert does not suit the slight acid flavour of the wine. An exception is rosé champagne, which can be served with fruit-based desserts.

Champagne should never be served with chocolate.

At what temperature should champagne be served

It is best to serve champagne at 8°C - 10°C. This temperature allows for better development of the flavour whilst maintaining the bubbles. Below this temperature it is too cold making aromas harder to detect, but above 10°C it appears heavy and less bright.

It is best to immerse a bottle for half an hour in an ice bucket filled halfway with cool water and ice. Remember, champagne is delicate. It should not be stored for a long time in the fridge. A bottle should only be left in the fridge for no more than 2-3 hours before serving.

After purchase, the storage conditions are very important. It should preferably be stored in a cellar at a constant temperature of between 7°C - 10°C.

How to open a bottle of champagne correctly

To open bottles correctly, untwist the wire which surrounds the cork and hold the bottle at a tilt. Slowly turn the cork and gradually it should come out without effort. If necessary, this can be speeded up by shaking the bottle slightly.

To prevent the foam from escaping, hold the bottle at 45° and pour slowly.

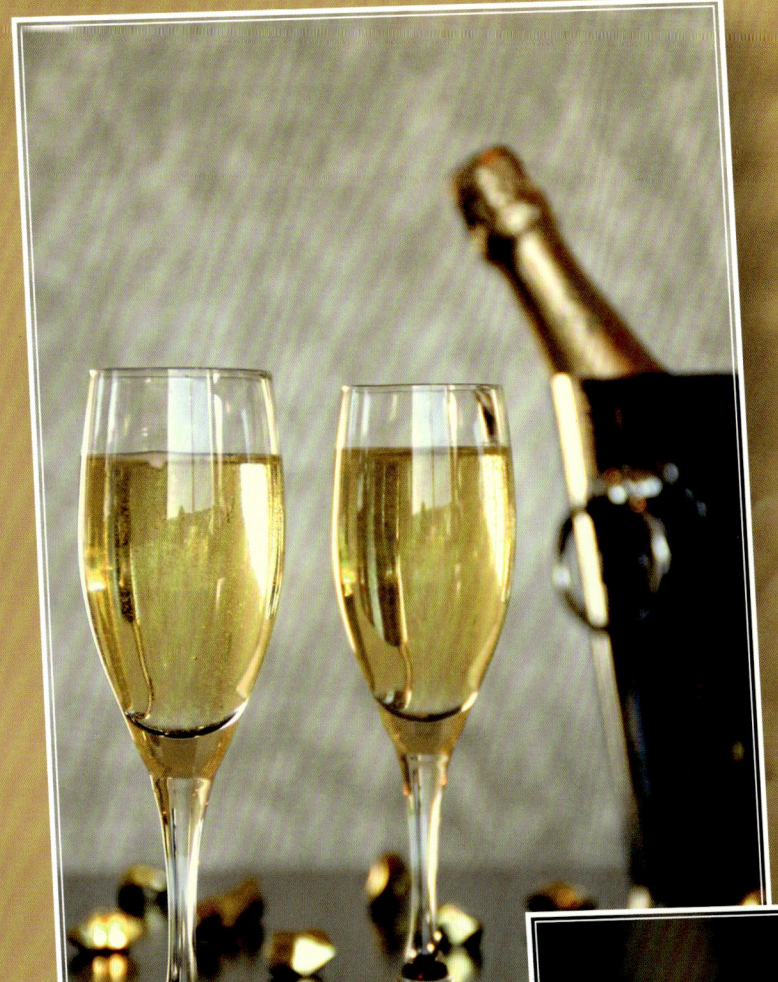

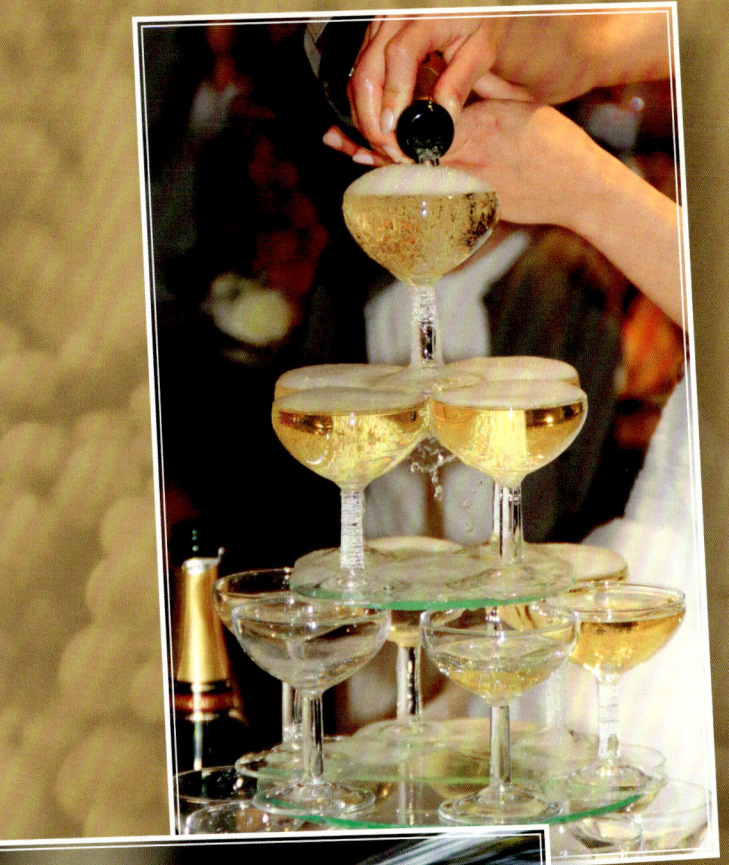

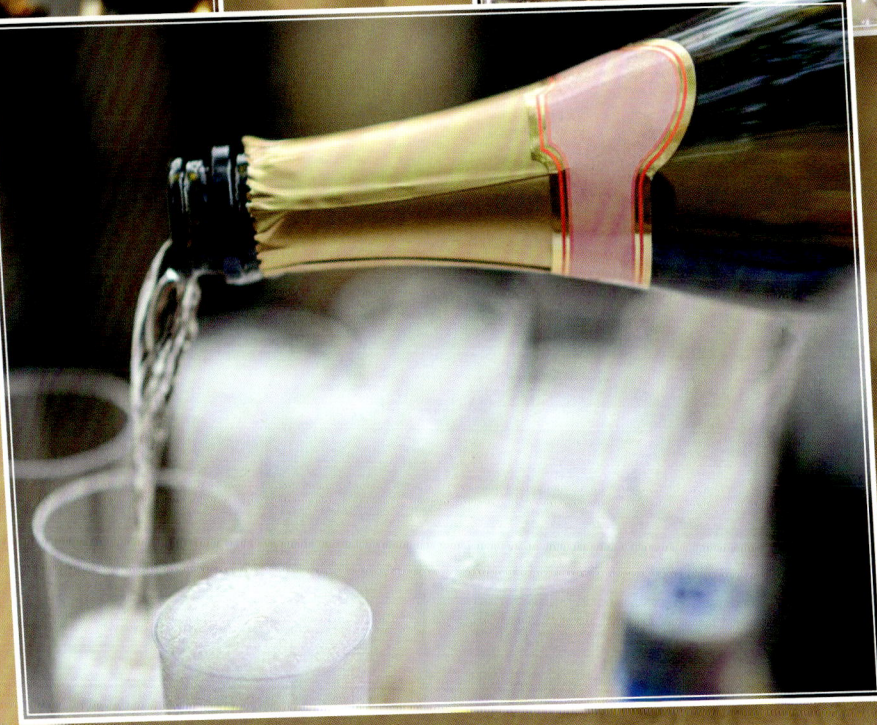

Champagne
Le champagne

283

Freezing recommendations

Whilst nothing can beat freshly baked food served straight from the oven, some foods freeze very well. It's always a satisfying feeling to cook in advance and fill the freezer with dishes ready to use at a moment's notice! What better way to impress those unexpected guests or satisfy a hungry family after a busy day!

The following table includes all the recipes found in the Art of French Cuisine and they have been actually tested to prove whether they do or do not freeze.

- **NEVER REFREEZE FOOD** once it has been defrosted.

- **ALWAYS LEAVE FOOD TO DEFROST COMPLETELY** before reheating unless otherwise stated.

- **FREEZER MUST BE KEPT AT A CONSTANT TEMPERATURE OF -18°C.**

- **ENSURE FOOD IS COVERED WELL AND LABELLED CLEARLY WITH THE CONTENTS AND THE DATE.**

- **DO NOT FREEZE OLD FOOD.** Freezing does not kill bacteria therefore it does not improve flavour or texture of food.

- **FOOD DOES NOT KEEP FOREVER IN THE FREEZER!**

LIST OF RECIPES	SUITABLE	NOT RECOMMENDED	NOTES
SOUPS / *SOUPES*			

Although soups are not complicated to make they require a bit of time for cooking, and often when the vegetables are at hand, soup is not required! Think in advance and avoid throwing those slightly overripe vegetables away—make soup!

If preferred, pour hot soup into warmed, glass bottles and close the lid tightly immediately—the soup can be stored in the fridge for several weeks. (Ensure the bottles are filled to the top.)

LIST OF RECIPES	SUITABLE	NOT RECOMMENDED	NOTES
VEGETABLE SOUP/ *Potage de légumes*	√		
FRENCH ONION SOUP/ *Soupe à l'oignon gratinée*	√		Freeze without the bread topping.
CARROT SOUP/ *Soupe à la carotte*	√		Freeze without the cream.
CREAM OF MUSHROOM SOUP/ *Velouté de champignons*	√		Freeze without the cream.
CREAM OF COURGETTE SOUP/ *Velouté de courgettes*	√		If lumps appear after reheating, blend slightly.
CREAM OF PUMPKIN SOUP/ *Velouté de potiron*	√		Freeze without the cream.

Freezing recommendations

LIST OF RECIPES	SUITABLE	NOT RECOMMENDED	NOTES
SALADS / *SALADES*			
All salads should be prepared fresh, although the *vinaigrette* can be prepared a few days in advance. Save time and make a big jar of *vinaigrette* ready to use at any time—you'll feel more like eating plenty of fresh salad!			
WALNUT SALAD / *Salade aux noix*		X	
CHICORY SALAD / *Salade d'endives*		X	
FRENCH BEAN SALAD / *Salade de haricots verts*		X	
LENTIL SALAD WITH BACON AND TOMATOES *Salade de lentilles aux lardons et tomates*		X	
LENTIL SALAD WITH BROCCOLI *Salade de lentilles au brocoli*		X	
DANDELION AND BACON SALAD *Salade de pissenlits aux lardons*		X	
LAMB'S LETTUCE WITH *RAVIOLES* AND WALNUTS *Salade de mâche aux ravioles et noix*		X	
NICOISE SALAD / *Salade niçoise*		X	

LIST OF RECIPES	SUITABLE	NOT RECOMMENDED	NOTES
STARTERS / *ENTREES*			
ASPARAGUS WITH *VINAIGRETTE* SAUCE *Asperges à la vinaigrette*		X	
ASPARAGUS WITH HOLLANDAISE SAUCE *Asperges avec sauce hollandaise*		X	
ARTICHOKES WITH *VINAIGRETTE* SAUCE *Artichauts à la vinaigrette*		X	
HAM AND MUSHROOM FILLED CREPES *Aumonières au jambon et champignons*	√		
ROLLED CREPES WITH HAM / *Crêpes roulées au jambon*	√		
CRAB-FILLED AVOCADOS / *Avocats garnis*		X	
HAM AND OLIVE CAKES / *Cakes au jambon et olives*	√		
COURGETTES AND GOAT'S CHEESE CAKES *Cakes aux courgettes et au fromage de chèvre*	√		
CREAMY PIZZA / *Crémière*	√		
ASSORTMENT OF CRUDITES / *Assortiment de crudités*		X	
GRATED CARROTS / *Carottes rapées*		X	
BAKED CAMEMBERT SERVED WITH CRUDITES *Camembert au four accompagné de crudités*		X	
LEEK PIE / *Flamiche aux poireaux*	√		

Freezing recommendations

LIST OF RECIPES	SUITABLE	NOT RECOMMENDED	NOTES
ENTREES / *STARTERS*			
FOUGASSE/ *Fougasse*	√		
BACON FOUGASSE/ *Fougasse aux lardons*	√		
GOUGERES/ *Gougères*	√		Cooked or uncooked.
MELON WITH CURED HAM/ *Melon au jambon cru*		X	
MELON WITH PORT/ *Melon au Porto*		X	
MIMOSA EGGS/ *Oeufs mimosa*		X	
PROVENCALE-STYLE PIZZA/ *Pissaladière*	√		
QUICHE LORRAINE/ *Quiche Lorraine*	√		Before freezing, place in a fridge overnight before removing from the tin. Freeze. Leave to defrost completely before reheating.
CHEESE SOUFFLE/ *Soufflé au fromage*		X	
ONION TART/ *Tarte à l'oignon*	√		Before freezing, place in a fridge overnight before removing from the tin. Freeze. Leave to defrost completely before reheating.
PROVENCALE-STYLE TART/ *Tarte à la provençale*	√		
CHEESE SOUFFLE TARTLETS *Tartelettes soufflées au fromage*	√		
FOIE GRAS WITH SPICED HONEY LOAF *Toasts au foie gras*		X	
RED ONION CHUTNEY/ *Confit d'oignons rouges*	√		Not necessary to freeze. Best to bottle while still hot.
AVOCADO-FILLED TOMATOES/ *Tomates garnies*		X	

LIST OF RECIPES	SUITABLE	NOT RECOMMENDED	NOTES
FISH AND SHELLFISH / *POISSONS ET FRUITS DE MER*			
CREAMED COD/ *Brandade de morue*	√		
CREAMED COD ON TOAST/ *Toasts à la brandade de morue*	√		Only freeze if serving hot.
CREAMED COD PIE/ *Brandade de morue parmentière*	√		
BOUCHEES A LA REINE WITH CREAMED COD / *Bouchées à la reine à la brandade de morue*		X	
SCALLOPS/ *Coquilles Saint-Jacques*	√		
PROVENCALE-STYLE BAKED SEA BREAM / *Dorade provençale au four*		X	
OYSTERS/ *Huitres*		X	
MUSSELS IN WHITE WINE/ *Moules marinières*		X	
SALMON PARCELS WITH HERB SAUCE / *Saumon en papillote et sauce aux herbes*	√		When defrosted, the sauce curdles. Reheat well, whisking continuously.
TROUT WITH ALMONDS/ *Truite aux amandes*		X	

Freezing recommendations

LIST OF RECIPES	SUITABLE	NOT RECOMMENDED	NOTES
MEATS / *VIANDES*			
VEAL BLANQUETTE/*Blanquette de veau*	✓		
BEEF STEW/*Boeuf bourguignon*	✓		
MEATBALLS WITH CABBAGE/*Caillettes au chou*	✓		
MEATBALLS WITH GREEN VEGETABLES *Caillettes au légumes verts*	✓		
DUCK WITH ORANGE/*Canard à l'orange*		X	
COQ AU VIN/*Coq au vin*	✓		
BEEF FONDUE/*Fondue bourguignonne*		X	
ACCOMPANIMENTS FOR A BEEF FONDUE *Accompagnements pour fondue bourguignonne*		X	
RABBIT IN MUSTARD SAUCE/*Lapin à la moutarde*	✓		
DUCK BREAST WITH HONEY AND PEARS *Magret de canard au miel et aux poires*		X	
DUCK BREAST WITH COCOA/*Magret de canard au cacao*		X	
HOT POT/*Pot au feu*		X	
PEPPERED STEAKS/*Steaks au poivre*		X	

290

LIST OF RECIPES	SUITABLE	NOT RECOMMENDED	NOTES
VEGETABLES AND STARCHES / *LEGUMES ET FECULENTS*			

Vegetables are always best eaten fresh as they can lose some of their valuable vitamins. However, some of these bakes can be prepared in advance and frozen. Defrost thoroughly before reheating.

LIST OF RECIPES	SUITABLE	NOT RECOMMENDED	NOTES
VICHY CARROTS / *Carottes Vichy*	√		Freezes better if cooked with butter than if cooked with olive oil.
RAW SAUERKRAUT / *Choucroute crue*		X	
SAUERKRAUT FROM ALSACE / *Choucroute d'Alsace*	√		
CARROT BAKE / *Fondant aux carottes*	√		
PROVENCALE-STYLE BAKE / *Gratin à la provençale*		X	
CHICORY BAKE WITH HAM / *Gratin d'endives au jambon*		X	
GRATIN DAUPHINOIS / *Gratin dauphinois*	√		Ensure that the potatoes are cooked before freezing or they will turn grey. Defrost slowly at room temperature then bake as indicated in the recipe.
SWISS CHARD BAKE / *Gratin de blettes*	√		Defrost slowly and bake as indicated.
SWISS CHARD IN TOMATO SAUCE / *Blettes en sauce tomate*		X	
CARDOON BAKE / *Gratin de cardon*	√		Defrost slowly and bake as indicated.
PUMPKIN BAKE / *Gratin de potiron*	√		Defrost slowly and bake as indicated.
POTATO AND LEEK BAKE *Gratin de pommes de terre aux poireaux*		X	
POTATO AND TOMATO BAKE *Gratin de pommes de terre aux tomates*		X	

Freezing recommendations

LIST OF RECIPES	SUITABLE	NOT RECOMMENDED	NOTES
VEGETABLES AND STARCHES / *LEGUMES ET FECULENTS*			
FRENCH BEANS WITH CHERRY TOMATOES / *Haricots verts aux tomates cerises*		X	
FRENCH BEANS WITH TOMATOES / *Haricots verts aux tomates*		X	
LENTILS WITH SAUSAGES / *Lentilles aux saucisses*	√		Turns slightly drier when frozen—still just as good.
SAUTEED POTATOES / *Pommes de terre sautées*		X	
DUCHESS POTATOES / *Pommes duchesses*	√		Freeze uncooked, laid out on a tray covered with greaseproof paper. Cook from frozen.
SEMOLINA QUENELLES / *Quenelles à la semoule*	√		Freeze uncooked without the *sauce financière*
FLOUR QUENELLES / *Quenelles à la farine*	√		Freeze uncooked without the *sauce financière*
GRATED POTATO CAKES / *Rapée de pommes de terre*		X	
RATATOUILLE / *Ratatouille*	√		
COURGETTE SOUFFLE / *Soufflé à la courgette*		X	
BROCCOLI SOUFFLE / *Soufflé au brocoli*		X	
SEMOLINA SOUFFLE / *Soufflé de semoule*	√		Freeze uncooked. Defrost slowly and bake as indicated.
PROVENCALE-STYLE TOMATOES / *Tomates à la provençale*		X	
STUFFED TOMATOES / *Tomates farcies*	√		Can be frozen once cooked.

LIST OF RECIPES	SUITABLE	NOT RECOMMENDED	NOTES
**CHEESE FAVOURITES	*AUTOUR DU FROMAGE***			
SAVOIE-STYLE FONDUE/*Fondue savoyarde*		X	
SAVOIE-STYLE POTATOES/*Pommes de terre savoyardes*		X	
SAVOIE-STYLE RACLETTE/*Raclette savoyarde*		X	Uncooked raclette cheese can be frozen.
TARTIFLETTE/*Tartiflette*		X	
**BASIC RECIPES	*RECETTES DE BASE***			
VINAIGRETTE SAUCE/*Vinaigrette*		X	Can be made a few days in advance and kept in a jar.
MAYONNAISE/*Mayonnaise*		X	
HOLLANDAISE SAUCE/*Sauce hollandaise*		X	
COCKTAIL SAUCE/*Sauce cocktail*		X	
TOMATO COULIS/*Coulis de tomates*	√		
TOMATO SAUCE/*Sauce tomate*	√		
BECHAMEL SAUCE/*Sauce béchamel*	√		
BECHAMEL SAUCE WITH CHEESE/*Sauce béchamel au fromage*	√		
FINANCIERE SAUCE/*Sauce financière*	√		
PIZZA DOUGH/*Pâte à pizza*	√		Cooked or uncooked.
SHORTCRUST PASTRY/*Pâte brisée*	√		Cooked or uncooked.

Gluten free

GLUTEN

What is gluten?

Gluten is what provides the elasticity of kneaded dough, and the delicious texture of breads and pastry products. It is a vegetable-based compound of proteins, fatty acids and sugar, combined with starch, and is found in the more common cereals such as wheat, oats, rye and barley.
Gluten is ubiquitous in the modern diet, because of its binding and consistency properties to foods.
It has, however, become one of the main triggers of food allergy.

Gluten hypersensitivity

This is a disorder affecting a great number of people which for some is a mild reaction but for others is a serious disease.
In the less severe form, it causes unpleasant symptoms that occur for several days, such as bloating, colitis, fatigue, disturbed sleep, migraine, skin disorders, etc.
The more serious form of gluten disorder causes an immunological reaction which can result in the destruction of the intestinal villi. This is what is called coeliac disease. To this, there is only one solution and that is to permanently avoid gluten.

Foods to avoid for a gluten-free diet

All gluten-containing cereals such as wheat, barley, rye, oats, spelt and kamut.
All traditional breads, pasta in any form, breakfast cereals, couscous, bulgur, wheat germ, wheat and oats, breadcrumbs and croutons, bechamel sauce, sweet and savoury baked goods (grissini, crackers, pizza, quiches, cookies, cakes, buns, etc.), breaded products (meat, poultry, fish and vegetables), any desserts made with flour.
Drinks such as whisky, beer, vodka made from wheat, soluble coffee containing barley malt.

Foods suitable for a gluten-free diet

Rice, buckwheat, quinoa, potatoes, chestnut, corn, millet, sesame, sorghum, tapioca, cassava.

All fruit and vegetables raw or cooked, homemade soups with vegetables, dried vegetables (lentils, split peas, chickpeas, nuts and other oilseeds).

Dairy products, butter, yogurts without wheat starch, natural cheese, meat, poultry, fish, eggs.

Vinegars, pure spices (certified gluten-free), all vegetable oils (except wheat germ oil), and traditional salad dressings (without soya sauce or *arome Maggi®*).

Sugar, maple syrup, honey and almond paste.

Desserts made from gluten-free flour (i.e. flour made from rice, maize, tapioca, and arrowroot).

Guar gum is a valuable food aid as it acts as an alternative to traditional gluten in baking and pastry preparations.

Note: Use rice flour when flouring greased baking tins.

Carefully read the labels on food packets to ensure they do not contain hidden gluten, such as in: ham, sausages, ice cream and chocolate, etc. (It is often recommended to buy a better quality brand of these foods as they are less likely to contain gluten.)

Gluten free

RECIPES	GLUTEN FREE	WITH GLUTEN	HOW TO ALTER A RECIPE INTO GLUTEN FREE
SOUPS / *SOUPES*			
VEGETABLE SOUP/ *Potage de légumes*	√		
FRENCH ONION SOUP/ *Soupe à l'oignon gratinée*		X	Use gluten-free bread and replace the flour with the same quantity of cornflour.
CARROT SOUP/ *Soupe à la carotte*	√		
CREAM OF MUSHROOM SOUP/ *Velouté de champignons*	√		
CREAM OF COURGETTE SOUP/ *Velouté à la courgette*	√		Use cornflour.
CREAM OF PUMPKIN SOUP/ *Velouté de potiron*	√		

RECIPES	GLUTEN FREE	WITH GLUTEN	HOW TO ALTER A RECIPE INTO GLUTEN FREE
SALADS / *SALADES*			
WALNUT SALAD/*Salade aux noix*		X	Make croutons using gluten-free bread.
CHICORY SALAD/*Salade d'endives*	√		
FRENCH BEAN SALAD/*Salade de haricots verts*	√		
LENTIL SALAD WITH BACON AND TOMATOES / *Salade de lentilles aux lardons et tomates*	√		
LENTIL SALAD WITH BROCCOLI / *Salade de lentilles au brocoli*	√		
DANDELION AND BACON SALAD / *Salade de pissenlits aux lardons*		X	Make croutons using gluten-free bread.
LAMB'S LETTUCE WITH *RAVIOLES* AND WALNUTS / *Salade de mâche aux ravioles et noix*		X	Do not use *ravioles*.
NICOISE SALAD/*Salade niçoise*	√		

Gluten free

RECIPES	GLUTEN FREE	WITH GLUTEN	HOW TO ALTER A RECIPE INTO GLUTEN FREE
STARTERS / *ENTREES*			
ASPARAGUS WITH VINAIGRETTE SAUCE *Asperges à la vinaigrette*	✓		
ASPARAGUS WITH HOLLANDAISE SAUCE *Asperges avec sauce hollandaise*	✓		
ARTICHOKES WITH VINAIGRETTE SAUCE *Artichauts à la vinaigrette*	✓		
HAM AND MUSHROOM FILLED CREPES *Aumonières au jambon et champignons*		X	Make the crèpes by replacing the flour with 100 g of rice flour, 100 g of potato starch, 50 g of buckwheat and 2 level teaspoons of bicarbonate of soda. Replace the *sauce béchamel* with a gluten-free *sauce béchamel* but using 40 g of cornflour instead of 20 g.
ROLLED CREPES WITH HAM / *Crêpes roulées au jambon*		X	Make the crèpes by replacing the flour with 100 g of rice flour, 100 g of potato starch, 50 g of buckwheat and 2 level teaspoons of bicarbonate of soda. Replace the *sauce béchamel* with a gluten-free *sauce béchamel* but using 40 g of cornflour instead of 20 g.
CRAB-FILLED AVOCADOS / *Avocats garnis*	✓		
HAM AND OLIVE CAKES / *Cakes au jambon et olives*		X	Replace the flour with 150 g of rice flour, 100 g of potato starch, 2 teaspoons of guar gum and replace the baking powder with bicarbonate of soda.

RECIPES	GLUTEN FREE	WITH GLUTEN	HOW TO ALTER A RECIPE INTO GLUTEN FREE
STARTERS / *ENTREES*			
COURGETTE AND GOAT'S CHEESE CAKES / *Cakes aux courgettes et au fromage de chèvre*		X	Replace the flour with 100 g of rice flour, 70 g of potato starch, 1 teaspoon of guar gum and replace the baking powder with bicarbonate of soda.
CREAMY PIZZA / *Crémière*		X	Replace the pizza base with a gluten-free *pâte à pizza*.
ASSORTMENT OF CRUDITES / *Assortiment de crudités*	✓		
GRATED CARROTS / *Carottes rapées*	✓		
BAKED CAMEMBERT SERVED WITH CRUDITES / *Camembert au four accompagné de crudités*	✓		
LEEK PIE / *Flamiche aux poireaux*		X	
FOUGASSE / *Fougasse*		X	
BACON FOUGASSE / *Fougasse aux lardons*		X	
GOUGERES / *Gougères*		X	
MELON WITH CURED HAM / *Melon au jambon cru*	✓		
MELON WITH PORT / *Melon au porto*	✓		

Gluten free

RECIPES	GLUTEN FREE	WITH GLUTEN	HOW TO ALTER A RECIPE INTO GLUTEN FREE
STARTERS / *ENTREES*			
MIMOSA EGGS / *Oeufs mimosa*	✓		
PROVENCALE-STYLE PIZZA / *Pissaladière*		X	Make a gluten-free *pâte à pizza*.
QUICHE LORRAINE / *Quiche Lorraine*		X	Make a gluten-free *pâte brisée*. Do not bake blind. Spread the mustard onto the pastry and cook for 5 minutes, then pour over the filling.
CHEESE SOUFFLE / *Soufflé au fromage*	✓		
ONION TART / *Tarte à l'oignon*		X	Make a gluten-free *pâte brisée*. Do not bake blind.
PROVENCALE-STYLE TART / *Tarte à la provençale*		X	Make a gluten-free *pâte brisée*. Do not bake blind. Fill the uncooked pastry case with the filling and cook for about 30 minutes.
CHEESE SOUFFLE TARTLETS *Tartelettes soufflées au fromage*		X	
FOIE GRAS WITH SPICED HONEY LOAF *Toasts au foie gras*		X	Follow the recipe for the less-sweetened *pain d'épices* but replace the flour with 170 g rice flour, 100 g potato starch and 2 tablespoons of guar gum.
RED ONION CHUTNEY / *Confit d'oignons rouges*	✓		
AVOCADO-FILLED TOMATOES / *Tomates garnies*	✓		

RECIPES	GLUTEN FREE	WITH GLUTEN	HOW TO ALTER A RECIPE INTO GLUTEN FREE
FISH AND SHELLFISH / *POISSONS ET FRUITS DE MER*			
CREAMED COD/*Brandade de morue*	√		
CREAMED COD ON TOAST/*Toasts à la brandade de morue*		X	Use gluten-free bread.
CREAMED COD PIE/*Brandade de morue parmentière*		X	Use gluten-free breadcrumbs.
BOUCHEES A LA REINE WITH CREAMED COD *Bouchées à la reine à la brandade de morue*		X	
SCALLOPS/*Coquilles Saint-Jacques*		X	Make a gluten-free sauce: Fry the 3 shallots in a little olive oil. Mix 20 g of cornflour with 100 ml of milk then add 300 ml of milk. Pour over the shallots and heat, stirring continuously until the mixture thickens and boils. Remove from the heat and stir in the grated cheese. Season with salt and pepper.
PROVENCALE-STYLE BAKED SEA BREAM *Dorade provençale au four*	√		
OYSTERS/*Huitres*	√		
MUSSELS IN WHITE WINE/*Moules marinières*	√		
SALMON PARCELS WITH HERB SAUCE *Saumon en papillote et sauce aux herbes*	√		
TROUT WITH ALMONDS/*Truite aux amandes*		X	

Gluten free

RECIPES	GLUTEN FREE	WITH GLUTEN	HOW TO ALTER A RECIPE INTO GLUTEN FREE
MEATS / *VIANDES*			
VEAL BLANQUETTE / *Blanquette de veau*		X	Replace the flour with the same quantity of cornflour.
BEEF STEW / *Boeuf bourguignon*		X	Replace the flour with the same quantity of rice flour.
MEATBALLS WITH CABBAGE / *Caillettes au chou*	√		
MEATBALLS WITH GREEN VEGETABLES *Caillettes aux légumes verts*	√		
DUCK WITH ORANGE / *Canard à l'orange*	√		
COQ AU VIN / *Coq au vin*		X	Replace the flour with cornflour: dissolve 15 g of cornflour in 50 ml of water and add to the liquid. Heat until boiling.
BEEF FONDUE / *Fondue bourguignonne*	√		
ACCOMPANIMENTS FOR A BEEF FONDUE *Accompagnements pour fondue bourguignonne*	√		
RABBIT IN MUSTARD SAUCE / *Lapin à la moutarde*	√		
DUCK BREAST WITH HONEY AND PEARS *Magret de canard au miel et aux poires*	√		
DUCK BREAST WITH COCOA / *Magret de canard au cacao*	√		
HOT POT / *Pot au feu*	√		
PEPPERED STEAKS / *Steaks au poivre*	√		

RECIPES	GLUTEN FREE	WITH GLUTEN	HOW TO ALTER A RECIPE INTO GLUTEN FREE
VEGETABLES AND STARCHES / *LEGUMES ET FECULENTS*			
VICHY CARROTS / *Carottes Vichy*	√		
RAW SAUEKRAUT / *Choucroute crue*	√		
SAUERKRAUT FROM ALSACE / *Choucroute d'Alsace*	√		
CARROT BAKE / *Fondant aux carottes*	√		
PROVENCALE-STYLE BAKE / *Gratin à la provençale*	√		
CHICORY BAKE WITH HAM / *Gratin d'endives au jambon*		X	Make a gluten-free *sauce béchamel*.
GRATIN DAUPHINOIS / *Gratin dauphinois*	√		
SWISS CHARD BAKE / *Gratin de blettes*		X	Make a gluten-free *sauce béchamel*.
SWISS CHARD IN TOMATO SAUCE / *Blettes en sauce tomate*	√		
CARDOON BAKE / *Gratin de cardons*		X	Make a gluten-free sauce : Fry the onion in a little olive oil. Mix 25 g of cornflour with 100 ml of water. Make a meat stock by dissolving 1 beef stock cube in 500 ml of water and pour over the onion, then add the cornflour mixture. Heat, stirring continuously until the mixture is boiling.

Gluten free

RECIPES	GLUTEN FREE	WITH GLUTEN	HOW TO ALTER A RECIPE INTO GLUTEN FREE
VEGETABLES AND STARCHES / *LEGUMES ET FECULENTS*			
PUMPKIN BAKE / *Gratin de potiron*		X	It is not possible to use a gluten-free *sauce béchamel* as it curdles with the eggs.
POTATO AND LEEK BAKE / *Gratin de pommes de terre aux poireaux*	✓		
POTATO AND TOMATO BAKE / *Gratin de pommes de terre aux tomates*	✓		
FRENCH BEANS WITH CHERRY TOMATOES / *Haricots verts aux tomates cerises*	✓		
FRENCH BEANS WITH TOMATOES / *Haricots verts aux tomates*	✓		
LENTILS WITH SAUSAGES / *Lentilles aux saucisses*		X	Make a gluten-free *sauce rousse*: Make the stock as indicated in the recipe. Fry the shallot in the olive oil. Mix 15 g of cornflour with 50 ml of the stock and pour in the rest of the stock. Pour this mixture into the saucepan with the shallot and heat, stirring continuously until the mixture is thick and boiling. Use gluten-free sausages.
SAUTEED POTATOES / *Pommes de terre sautées*	✓		
DUCHESS POTATOES / *Pommes duchesses*	✓		
SEMOLINA QUENELLES / *Quenelles à la semoule*		X	
FLOUR QUENELLES / *Quenelles à la farine*		X	
GRATED POTATO CAKES / *Rapée de pommes de terre*	✓		

RECIPES	GLUTEN FREE	WITH GLUTEN	HOW TO ALTER A RECIPE INTO GLUTEN FREE
VEGETABLES AND STARCHES / *LEGUMES ET FECULENTS*			
RATATOUILLE/ *Ratatouille*	√		
COURGETTE SOUFFLE/ *Soufflé à la courgette*		X	Make a gluten-free *sauce béchamel*: Liquidise the courgettes with 80 ml of milk. Mix together 40 ml of milk with 30 g of cornflour and add to the courgette purée. Heat until boiling stirring constantly and leave to simmer for 3 minutes, stirring continuously.
BROCCOLI SOUFFLE/ *Soufflé au brocoli*		X	Replace the courgette with the broccoli and continue as in the recipe for gluten-free *soufflé à la courgette*.
SEMOLINA SOUFFLE/ *Soufflé de semoule*		X	
PROVENCALE-STYLE TOMATOES/ *Tomates à la provençale*		X	Omit the breadcrumbs or replace with the same quantity of breadcrumbs made from gluten-free bread.
STUFFED TOMATOES/ *Tomates farcies*		X	Replace the breadcrumbs with the same quantity of breadcrumbs made from gluten-free bread.

Gluten free

RECIPES	GLUTEN FREE	WITH GLUTEN	HOW TO ALTER A RECIPE INTO GLUTEN FREE
**CHEESE FAVOURITES	*AUTOUR DU FROMAGE***			
SAVOIE-STYLE FONDUE/ *Fondue savoyarde*	√		Use gluten-free bread
SAVOIE-STYLE POTATOES/ *Pommes de terre savoyardes*	√		
SAVOIE-STYLE RACLETTE/ *Raclette savoyarde*	√		
TARTIFLETTE/ *Tartiflette*	√		

RECIPES	GLUTEN FREE	WITH GLUTEN	HOW TO ALTER A RECIPE INTO GLUTEN FREE
**BASIC RECIPES	*RECETTES DE BASE***			
VINAIGRETTE SAUCE/ *Vinaigrette*	√		Do not add soya sauce or *arome Maggi®*
MAYONNAISE/ *Mayonnaise*	√		
HOLLANDAISE SAUCE/ *Sauce hollandaise*	√		
COCKTAIL SAUCE/ *Sauce cocktail*	√		
TOMATO COULIS/ *Coulis de tomates*	√		

RECIPES	GLUTEN FREE	WITH GLUTEN	HOW TO ALTER A RECIPE INTO GLUTEN FREE
BASIC RECIPES/ *RECETTES DE BASE*			
TOMATO SAUCE/ *Sauce tomate*		X	
BECHAMEL SAUCE/ *Sauce béchamel*		X	Replace the flour with 20 g of cornflour. Dissolve it in 100 ml of milk. Add 400 ml of milk then heat until boiling, stirring constantly. Cook gently for an extra 2 minutes, stirring continuously. Season with salt, pepper and nutmeg.
FINANCIERE SAUCE/ *Sauce financière*		X	
PIZZA DOUGH/ *Pâte à pizza*		X	Replace the flour with 200 g of rice flour, 50 g of cornflour, 50 g of potato starch, 1 teaspoon guar gum and add an egg to the liquids. Once the dough has been kneaded, sprinkle lightly with rice flour and make into a ball. Lightly roll out, place into the dish and finish spreading it out from the inside.
SHORTCRUST PASTRY/ *Pâte brisée*		X	Mix together 150g of rice flour, 100g of potato starch, 1 teaspoon of guar gum and a generous pinch of salt. Add 80g of butter, cubed, and mix together until the mixture becomes like fine breadcrumbs. Make a well in the centre and add 1 egg with 50ml of cold water. Mix together with a wooden spoon. Gather the pieces together and shape into a ball. Place between 2 sheets of greaseproof paper and roll out. Place into a buttered and rice-floured dish.

Glossary

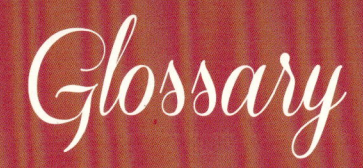

ANTIOXIDANTS
Antioxidants are natural compounds found in some foods. They prevent or reduce damage caused by free-radicals (chemicals containing oxygen) which attack other molecules. Well-known antioxidants include vitamins A, C and E.

APERITIF
A starter drink, generally alcoholic, taken before a meal which is meant to open the taste buds and stimulate the appetite for the forthcoming meal.

BAKE BLIND
A term used for lightly baking pastry by placing a sheet of greaseproof paper or foil on top of the pastry and placing heavy dried beans or baking beans on top to prevent the pastry from rising. Alternatively, have a container of old copper and silver coins handy—the metal reflects the heat and helps to cook the pastry!

BAIN-MAIRIE
This is a method of cooking or melting ingredients where they are put in a bowl which is placed in a shallow container of water and gently heated in the oven or on a hob.

BASTE
This is the term used to spoon or brush juice or fat over food during cooking. It helps to keep the food moist and seal in the flavour.

BLANQUETTE
A white stew of veal, chicken or lamb, bound with egg yolks and cream.

BLANCH
Blanching is done to vegetables, bacon and some meats, by boiling them very quickly in water then plunging them into cold water. This can help to destroy some damaging enzymes which are found in some vegetables before freezing them, preserve the colour and flavour or to loosen the skins.

BLEND
Liquidise to turn into a purée or liquid. This is normally done using an electric liquidiser or hand-held mixer.

BOUQUET GARNI
This is a tied bunch of herbs normally consisting of a bay leaf, parsley and thyme. It is placed in the cooking for flavouring and removed before serving.

BUCKWHEAT
Buckwheat is a gluten-free plant crop cultivated mainly for its grains. The dried grains can be ground with the outer bran and the resulting flour is a suitable substitute for people who are sensitive to wheat.

CALCIUM
Calcium is an essential chemical element found in many foods. Nearly all the calcium in our bodies is stored in the teeth and bones and is needed for the structure and maintenance of the skeleton.

CANAPÉ

Canapés are small finger foods traditionally made from thin slices of bread which are then decorated with savoury garnishes.

CARAMBAR® SWEETS

These are a type of toffees made in France, of varied flavours.

CARBOHYDRATE

A carbohydrate is a biological molecule consisting of carbon, hydrogen and oxygen atoms. In food science, the term carbohydrate generally refers to food that is rich in the complex carbohydrate starch (i.e. cereals, bread, pasta etc.) or simple carbohydrate such as sugar (i.e. sweets, jam, desserts, etc).

CARDIOVASCULAR DISEASE

CVD is a general term that describes a disease of the heart or blood vessels.

CASSAVA (MANIOC)

Also known as Brazilian arrowroot, cassava is a tropical plant with starchy roots from which tapioca is obtained.

CHLORINE

Chlorine is a chemical element and is a strong oxidizing agent. Common salt (sodium chloride) is the most common compound of chlorine.

CHOLESTEROL

Cholesterol is a waxy, fat-like substance made in the liver and is found in all cells of the body. It makes its way around the body in molecules called lipoproteins. Too much cholesterol in the blood is one of the risk factors in the development of coronary heart disease.

CLARIFY

This is a process to remove impurities from fat by heating. To clarify butter, slowly melt the butter to separate the milk solids, which sink to the bottom of the pan, skimming any foam off the top. The clarified butter can then be used for cooking at higher temperatures than normal butter without burning.

CORNFLOUR

(Known as cornstarch in some parts of the world.) This is a starch resembling a fine, powdery white flour and is often used as a thickening agent in sauces, soups and cakes.

CRUDITIES

Chopped, sliced or grated raw vegetables, served as a starter with *vinaigrette* or a dipping sauce.

CURDLE

When a mixture is curdled, it means that curds are formed by overheating or over mixing.

DEGLAZE

To remove the meat residue on the bottom of a saucepan etc. by adding water or wine.

Glossary

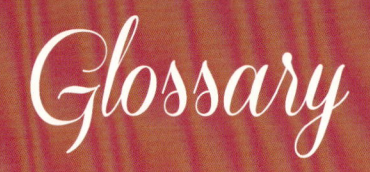

DEMERARA SUGAR
Brown raw cane sugar similar to *cassonade* in France.

DIGESTIF
A strong alcoholic drink served after a meal which is intended to aid the digestion.

EN PAPILLOTTE
This is a method of cooking food in a folded parcel of greaseproof paper to protect it from the high heat of the oven and help it retain moisture and flavour.

FIBRE
Also known as roughage, fibre is only found in foods that come from plants. There are two different types of fibre: soluble and insoluble. Soluble fibre can be digested and may help to reduce the cholesterol in the blood. Insoluble fibre cannot be digested and passes through the digestive system more easily, helping other foods also move through easier.

FLOUR
Plain flour is used in each of the recipes in this book. Consult the section on 'Mastering the art of bread making' for the differences in French flour.

FOIE GRAS
A special type of pâté made from the livers of ducks or geese which have been force-fed.

FOLD IN
This is the term used to combine a light ingredient such as a meringue with a heavier mixture. Use a spatula and cut through the mixture, turning one part over the other and making figures of 8.

FROMAGE BLANC
This is a white, sweet, slightly tart cheese which does not undergo lactic fermentation and has a texture similar to that of stirred yogurt. Can be eaten as a dessert and served with fruits or used in cooking for sweet or savoury dishes.

GANACHE
Hot cream and chocolate are mixed together until smooth then left to chill until stiff enough to spread as a covering or filling for cakes.

GELATINE
This is a setting agent derived from the protein of animal bones and is used to thicken sweet or savoury jellies.

GLAZE
Brush over the surface with a coating such as melted butter, lightly whisked egg, etc.

GUAR GUM

A powder which is used as a thickening agent and is especially useful for those who are allergic to gluten.

HERBES DE PROVENCE

A mixture of herbs from the South of France such as thyme, basil, oregano, parsley, marjoram, rosemary and tarragon.

HULL

To remove the cluster of leaves on a strawberry.

INFUSE

To immerse herbs or spices in a hot liquid then allow them to steep to flavour it.

KIRSCH

A cherry-flavoured liqueur.

KNEAD

This is the technique used to pull and stretch bread in order to develop the gluten in the flour so that the bread will keep its shape when it has risen. Use the dough hook for this process.

LAMB'S LETTUCE (CORN SALAD)

This is an edible, dark green leaf vegetable with a characteristic nutty flavour.

MACERATE

To make or become soft by steeping in a liquid.

MAGNESIUM

Magnesium is a mineral in the body and is naturally present in many foods. It is required, amongst other things for energy production and contributes to the structural development of the bones.

MARINIERE (A LA)

Literally meaning 'sailor's style'! This term is used when cooking seafood (such as mussels) in white wine and herbs.

MILLET

Millet is an ancient grain, cultivated in East Asia in early history. It is similar to wheat but is a non-gluten grain, making it an obvious substitute to wheat.

NOUGAT

A chewy sweet made of nuts, sugar or honey and egg whites.

OLEAGINOUS FRUITS

An oleaginous fruit is the part of a plant that is used to produce vegetable oil. It can be a fruit (e.g. olive), or a seed or nut (e.g. sesame or walnut).

ORANGE BLOSSOM WATER

A flavouring from the sweet-scented flowers of the orange tree.

PECTIN

This is a natural gelling agent which is extracted from ripe fruits and used in making jams and jellies.

Glossary

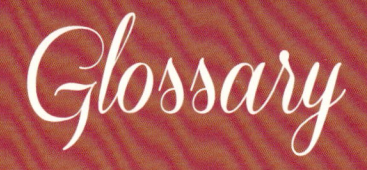

POACH
To cook delicate foods such as fish or eggs in a hot liquid, gently and just below boiling point.

POLYPHENOLS
Polyphenol is a generic term for several thousand plant-based molecules that have antioxidant properties.

POTASSIUM
Potassium is a mineral found in food and assists in a range of essential body functions, including blood pressure, normal water balance, muscle contractions, nerve impulses, digestion, heart rhythm and pH balance.

PURSLANE (VERDOLAGA OR PIGWEED)
Purslane is often considered a weed, but the stems, leaves and flower buds are all edible and contain high levels of omega 3 fatty acids, vitamins, and minerals such as magnesium, calcium, potassium and iron.

PRALINE
A sweet made by browning nuts (normally almonds or hazelnuts) then covered with a cooked sugar coating which is then coloured or flavoured.

PROTEIN
Proteins are large, complex molecules made up of amino acids which are required for the structure, functions and regulation of the body's tissues and organs.

PULSES (GRAIN LEGUMES)
Pulses are edible seeds that grow in pods such as beans, peas and lentils. They are a great source of protein, iron and fibre.

QUINOA
Quinoa is a seed, which can be prepared like whole grains such as rice or barley, or it can be ground into flour. It is gluten-free and is appreciated for its health benefits.

RENNET
This is found in the stomach lining membrane of young ruminant mammals and is used to curdle milk in cheese making.

SAUTE
Small pieces of food fried in butter or oil and moved around the frying pan to prevent it browning too rapidly.

SIMMER
Allow the food to cook gently just below boiling point. The bubbles will hardly break the surface. This method is often used where a food is first brought to the boil, then the heat is reduced and the food is allowed to simmer for a period of time.

SODIUM
Sodium is a chemical element and its most common form is table salt (sodium chloride). It is essential for helping maintain fluid balance and is a main nutrient used in nerve impulse transmissions and muscle contraction. Too much can lead to hypertension and kidney damage.

SORGHUM

Sorghum is a gluten-free cereal grain common in Africa and India. The wholegrain kernel is ground finely to make sorghum flour.

SPECULOOS BISCUITS

These are hard, spicy Belgian biscuits with a taste similar to gingerbread.

STARCH (AMYLUM)

Starch is a complex carbohydrate and is the chief storage form of carbohydrate in plants. It is obtained commercially especially from corn and potatoes.

STARTER CULTURE

This is a packet of dried lactic ferment available in most supermarkets and is used in helping yogurts to set.

STOCK

Liquid from meat or vegetables which is used as a basis for soup, stew, gravy or sauce.

TAPIOCA

Tapioca is the starch extracted from the cassava root and is used as a thickening agent in various foods.

VANILLA POD

These are sweet and fragrant dried pods which come from the vanilla orchid and are used to flavour many sweet dishes.

VITAMIN

Vitamins are organic compounds and are vital nutrients that the body requires in limited amounts.

Vitamins A, D, E and K are fat-soluble and stored in the fat tissues and the liver. They can be stored for days or even months.

Vitamin C and all the B vitamins are water-soluble and not stored for long as they get expelled through urine. These need to be replaced more often.

WHEAT GERM

Wheat germ is the embryo or germ of the wheat kernel which is separated in milling flour and used in food products as a source of vitamins.

WHISK

Whisking involves vigorously beating a light mixture such as egg whites or cream to incorporate as much air as possible. Always use a whisk attachment for this process.

ZEST

This is the outer layer of a citrus fruit. When removing the zest, leave the bitter white pith behind.

Conversion tables

Whilst these conversions are approximate only, any differences are only minimal and will not affect the cooking results.

OVEN TEMPERATURES

Celsius	Fahrenheit	Gas mark	Oven heat
110°	225°	¼	very cool
120°	250°	½	very cool
140°	275°	1	cool
150°	300°	2	cool
160°	325°	3	moderate
180°	350°	4	moderate
190°	375°	5	moderately hot
200°	400°	6	hot
210°	425°	7	hot
230°	450°	8	very hot
240°	475°	9	very hot

LIQUID MEASUREMENTS

Metric	Imperial	US Cups
60 ml	2 fl oz	¼ cup
100 ml	3½ fl oz	
125 ml	4 fl oz	½ cup
150 ml	5 fl oz	
185 ml	6 fl oz	¾ cup
200 ml	7 fl oz	
250 ml	8 fl oz	1 cup
300 ml	10 fl oz	
375 ml	12 fl oz	1½ cups
450 ml	16 fl oz	
500 ml	17 fl oz	2 cups
600 ml	20 fl oz (1 pint)	2½ cups
700 ml	1¼ pints	
750 ml	26 fl oz	3 cups
850 ml	30 fl oz (1½ pints)	
1 litre	35 fl oz (1¾ pints)	4 cups
1.5 litres	2¾ pints	
2.8 litres	5 pints	
3 litres	5¼ pints	

WEIGHT

Metric	Imperial
5 g	1/8 oz
10 g	1/4 oz
15 g	1/2 oz
25 g	1 oz
50 g	1¾ oz
75 g	2¾ oz
85 g	3 oz
100 g	3½ oz
150 g	5½ oz
225 g	8 oz
300 g	10½ oz
450 g	1 lb
500 g	1 lb 2 oz
1 kg	2 lb 4 oz
1.5 kg	3 lb 5 oz

LINEAR

Metric	Imperial
2 mm	1/16 inch
3 mm	1/8 inch
5 mm	1/4 inch
8 mm	3/8 inch
1 cm	1/2 inch
2 cm	3/4 inch
2.5 cm	1 inch
5 cm	2 inches
7.5 cm	3 inches
10 cm	4 inches
20 cm	8 inches
30 cm	12 inches / 1 foot
46 cm	18 inches / 1½ feet
50 cm	20 inches / 1⅔ feet

SPOON MEASUREMENTS

1 teaspoon of liquid = 5 ml
1 UK and US tablespoon of liquid = 15 ml
1 Australian tablespoon = 20 ml

Index - Recipes

164	Accompaniments for a beef fondue	190	Chicory bake with ham	251	*Financière* sauce
164	Andalusion sauce	64	Chicory salad	212	Flour *quenelles*
82	Artichokes with *vinaigrette* sauce	247	Cocktail sauce	126	*Foie gras* with spiced honey loaf
80	Asparagus with hollandaise sauce	168	Cooking the duck breast	102	Fougasse
80	Asparagus with *vinaigrette* sauce	160	*Coq au vin*	66	French bean salad
96	Assortment of crudités	92	Courgette and goat's cheese cakes	204	French beans with cherry tomatoes
128	Avocado-filled tomatoes	218	Courgette soufflé	204	French beans with tomatoes
104	Bacon fougasse	88	Crab-filled avocados	48	French onion soup
98	Baked camembert served with crudités	54	Cream of courgette soup	164	Garlic sauce
250	Bechamel sauce	52	Cream of mushroom soup	106	*Gougères*
250	Bechamel sauce with cheese	56	Cream of pumpkin soup	98	Grated carrots
162	Beef fondue	134	Creamed cod	214	Grated potato cakes
154	Beef stew	134	Creamed cod on toast	192	*Gratin Dauphinois*
134	*Bouchées-à-la-reine* with creamed cod	134	Creamed cod pie	84	Ham and mushroom filled crêpes
218	Broccoli soufflé	94	Creamy pizza	90	Ham and olive cakes
196	Cardoon bake	70	Dandelion and bacon salad	246	Hollandaise sauce
186	Carrot bake	208	Duchess potatoes	172	Hot pot
50	Carrot soup	170	Duck breast with cocoa	72	Lamb's lettuce with *ravioles* and walnuts
118	Cheese soufflé	170	Duck breast with honey and pears	100	Leek pie
124	Cheese soufflé tartlets	158	Duck with orange	68	Lentil salad with bacon and tomatoes

316

Index - Recipes

68	Lentil salad with broccoli	138	Provençale-style baked sea bream	164	Shallot sauce
206	Lentils with sausages	114	Provençale-style pizza	253	Shortcrust pastry
245	Mayonnaise	122	Provençale-style tart	224	Stuffed tomatoes
156	Meatballs with cabbage	222	Provençale-style tomatoes	194	Swiss chard bake
156	Meatballs with green vegetables	198	Pumpkin bake	194	Swiss chard in tomato sauce
108	Melon with cured ham	116	Quiche Lorraine	164	Tartare sauce
110	Melon with port	166	Rabbit in mustard sauce	240	*Tartiflette*
112	Mimosa eggs	216	*Ratatouille*	236	The origin of raclette
164	Moussed sauce	182	Raw sauerkraut	232	Tips for a successful cheese fondue
142	Mussels in white wine	126	Red onion chutney	248	Tomato coulis
74	Niçoise salad	86	Rolled crêpes with ham	249	Tomato sauce
120	Onion tart	144	Salmon parcels with herb sauce	146	Trout with almonds
120	Onion tart with bacon	184	Sauerkraut from Alsace	152	Veal blanquette
140	Oysters	208	Sautéed potatoes	46	Vegetable soup
164	Paprika sauce	230	*Savoie*-style fondue	180	Vichy carrots
174	Peppered steaks	234	*Savoie*-style potatoes	244	*Vinaigrette* sauce
252	Pizza dough	238	*Savoie*-style *raclette*	62	Walnut salad
200	Potato and leek bake	136	Scallops		
202	Potato and tomato bake	210	Semolina *quenelles*		
188	Provençale-style bake	220	Semolina soufflé		

Index - Recettes

164	Accompagnements pour fondue Bourguignonne	98	Carottes rapées	192	Gratin Dauphinois
82	Artichauts à la vinaigrette	180	Carottes Vichy	194	Gratin de blettes
80	Asperges à la vinaigrette	182	Choucroute crue	196	Gratin de cardons
80	Asperges avec sauce Hollandaise	184	Choucroute d'Alsace	200	Gratin de pommes de terre aux poireaux
96	Assortiment de crudités	126	Confit d'oignons rouges	202	Gratin de pommes de terre aux tomates
232	Astuces pour une bonne fondue	160	Coq au vin	198	Gratin de potiron
84	Aumônières au jambon et champignons	136	Coquilles Saint-Jacques	190	Gratin d'endives au jambon
88	Avocats garnis	248	Coulis de tomates	204	Haricots verts aux tomates
152	Blanquette de veau	94	Crémière	204	Haricots verts aux tomates cerises
194	Blettes en sauce tomate	168	Cuisson du magret de canard	140	Huîtres
154	Bœuf bourguignon	86	Crêpes roulées au jambon	166	Lapin à la moutarde
134	Bouchées à la reine à la brandade de morue	138	Dorade provençale au four	206	Lentilles aux saucisses
134	Brandade de morue	100	Flamiche aux poireaux	236	L'origine de la raclette
134	Brandade de morue parmentière	186	Fondant aux carottes	170	Magret de canard au cacao
156	Caillettes au chou	162	Fondue bourguignonne	170	Magret de canard au miel et aux poires
156	Caillettes aux légumes verts	230	Fondue savoyarde	245	Mayonnaise
90	Cakes au jambon et olives	102	Fougasse	108	Melon au jambon cru
92	Cakes aux courgettes et au fromage de chèvre	104	Fougasse aux lardons	110	Melon au porto
98	Camembert au four accompagné de crudités	106	Gougères	142	Moules marinières
158	Canard à l'orange	188	Gratin à la provençale	112	Œufs mimosa

Index - Recettes

252	Pâte à pizza	64	Salade d'endives	48	Soupe à l'oignon gratinée
253	Pâte brisée	74	Salade niçoise	174	Steaks au poivre
114	Pissaladière	164	Sauce à l'ail	122	Tarte à la provençale
208	Pommes de terre sautées	164	Sauce à l'échalote	120	Tarte à l'oignon
234	Pommes de terre savoyardes	164	Sauce Andalouse	120	Tarte à l'oignon aux lardons
208	Pommes duchesses	164	Sauce au paprika	124	Tartelettes soufflées au fromage
172	Pot au feu	250	Sauce béchamel	240	Tartiflette
46	Potage de légumes	250	Sauce béchamel au fromage	134	Toasts à la brandade de morue
212	Quenelles à la farine	247	Sauce cocktail	126	Toasts au foie gras
210	Quenelles à la semoule	251	Sauce financière	222	Tomates à la provençale
116	Quiche Lorraine	246	Sauce hollandaise	224	Tomates farcies
238	Raclette savoyarde	164	Sauce mousseuse	128	Tomates garnies
214	Râpée de pommes de terre	164	Sauce tartare	146	Truite aux amandes
216	Ratatouille	249	Sauce tomate	52	Velouté de champignons
62	Salade aux noix	144	Saumon en papillote et sauce aux herbes	54	Velouté de courgettes
66	Salade de haricots verts	218	Soufflé à la courgette	56	Velouté de potiron
68	Salade de lentilles au brocoli	218	Soufflé au brocoli	244	Vinaigrette
68	Salade de lentilles aux lardons et tomates	118	Soufflé au fromage		
72	Salade de mâche aux ravioles et noix	220	Soufflé de semoule		
70	Salade de pissenlits aux lardons	50	Soupe à la carotte		

319

Limit of Liability and Disclaimer of Warranty: We have used our best efforts in preparing the Art of French Cuisine Book, and the information is provided "as is." We make no representation or warranties with respect to the accuracy or completeness of the contents of the cookbook and we specifically disclaim any implied warranties of merchantability or fitness for any particular purpose.

All material in the Recipe Book is provided for your information only and may not be construed as medical advice or instruction. No action or inaction should be taken based solely on the contents of this information; instead, readers should consult appropriate health professionals on any matter relating to their health and well-being.

IMPORTANT: Any person who may be at risk of any form of adverse reaction to foodstuffs of any kind, including raw foods, should exercise due care with regard to recipes and foods included in this book. We accept no responsibility related to the consumption of foods included in this publication.

WE DO NOT CLAIM TO BE DOCTORS, NUTRITIONISTS OR DIETITIANS.
THE INFORMATION IN THIS RECIPE BOOK IS MERELY OUR OPINION AND DOES NOT REPLACE PROFESSIONAL MEDICAL OR NUTRITIONAL ADVICE.

ACKNOWLEDGEMENTS

Gratitude is expressed to Régis Marcon for writing the preface and allowing us to use his photography and video for marketing purposes.
Also to the following companies who kindly allowed us to disclose their brand name in various photographs:
Château du Tariquet, Moulin Dozol, Léon Bel (La vache qui rit, Apéricube) Maïzena,
Edmond Fallot, Fourme de Montbrison, Champagne Gremillet

Photography by K. Déaux except those listed below:
Régis Marcon: page 5; Antigone: page 21, 168, 266 (top right), 269, 274 (top); Fotolia: page 27, 28 (below left), 32, 33 (below), 34 (above), 277, 283 (below);
C. Malécot: page 29 (first left); C. Blanc: page 30 (top); L. Reiner: page 149; R. Ellett: page 266 (last on the right);
K. Malécot: page 278 (top 2 photos, middle left, 3 below), 281 (middle); W. Teissonnière: page 281 (below).

Published by:
UBT (Eu) Ltd, Exchange Place, Poseidon Way, Warwick CV 35 6BY
Copyright© Copyright Holders: K. L. Déaux, J. A. Reiner
Design: Antigone, 9, av du 8 mai 1945, 69500 Bron (France)
Printed and bound in China by: C & C Offset Printing Co.

ISBN: 978-0-9934810-0-0